Acne Scars

Classification and Treatment

Second Edition

Series in Dermatological Treatment

About the Series

Published in association with the *Journal of Dermatological Treatment*, the series in *Dermatological Treatment* keeps readers up to date with the latest clinical therapies to improve problems with the skin, hair, and nails. Each volume in the series is prepared separately and typically focuses on a topical theme. Volumes are published on an occasional basis, depending on the emergence of new developments.

Facial Skin Disorders
Ronald Marks

Textbook of Atopic Dermatitis
Sakari Reitamo, Thomas A. Unger and Martin Steinhoff

Acne Scares: Classification and Treatment, First Edition
Antonella Tosti, Maria Pia De Padova and Kenneth R. Beer

Abdominal Stomas and Their Skin Disorders, Second Edition
Callum C. Lyon and Amanda Smith

Nail Surgery
Bertrand Richert, Nilson Di Chiacchio and Eckart Haneke

Dermatoscopy in Clinical Practice, Second Edition: Beyond Pigmented Lesions
Giuseppe Micali and Francesco Lacarrubba

Phototherapy Treatment Protocols, Third Edition
Steven R. Feldman and Michael D. Zanolli

For more information about this series, please visit: https://www.crcpress.com/Series-in-Dermatological-Treatment/book-series/CRCSERDERTRE

Acne Scars
Classification and Treatment
Second Edition

Edited by

Antonella Tosti, MD
Dermatology and Cutaneous Surgery, University of Miami Health System, Miami, Florida, USA

Maria Pia De Padova, MD
Department of Dermatology, Ospedale Privato Nigrisoli, Bologna, Italy

Gabriella Fabbrocini, MD
Department of Dermatology, University of Naples Federico II, Naples, Italy

Kenneth R. Beer, MD
Beer Dermatology Associates, West Palm Beach and Jupiter, Florida, USA

CRC Press
Taylor & Francis Group
Boca Raton London New York

CRC Press is an imprint of the
Taylor & Francis Group, an **informa** business

CRC Press
Taylor & Francis Group
6000 Broken Sound Parkway NW, Suite 300
Boca Raton, FL 33487-2742

Printed in Canada on acid-free paper

International Standard Book Number-13: 978-1-138-89422-8 (Hardback)

Library of Congress Cataloging-in-Publication Data

Names: Tosti, A. (Antonella), editor. | De Padova, Maria Pia, editor. | Fabbrocini, Gabriella, editor. | Beer, Kenneth, editor.
Title: Acne scars : classification and treatment / edited by Antonella Tosti, Maria Pia De Padova, Gabriella Fabbrocini and Kenneth R. Beer.
Other titles: Series in dermatological treatment.
Description: Second edition. | Boca Raton, FL : CRC Press, [2019] | Series: Series in dermatological treatment | Includes bibliographical references and index.
Identifiers: LCCN 2018025044| ISBN 9781138894228 (hardback : alk. paper) | ISBN 9781315179889 (ebook : alk. paper)
Subjects: | MESH: Acne Vulgaris--complications | Cicatrix--therapy | Cicatrix--physiopathology
Classification: LCC RL131 | NLM WR 430 | DDC 616.5/3--dc23
LC record available at https://lccn.loc.gov/2018025044

Visit the Taylor & Francis Web site at
http://www.taylorandfrancis.com

and the CRC Press Web site at
http://www.crcpress.com

Contents

Contributors

Murad Alam, MD, MSCI, MBA
Departments of Dermatology, Otolaryngology, and Surgery
Feinberg School of Medicine Northwestern University
Chicago, Illinois

Gillian Beer
Beer Dermatology Associates
West Palm Beach, Florida

Kenneth R. Beer, MD
Beer Dermatology Associates
West Palm Beach and Jupiter, Florida

Enzo Berardesca, MD
San Gallicano Dermatological Institute
IRCCS
Rome, Italy

Katherine O. Brag, MD
Department of Dermatology
Tulane University School of Medicine
New Orleans, Louisiana

Norma Cameli, MD, PhD
San Gallicano Dermatological Institute
IRCCS
Rome, Italy

Jessica Cervantes, BS
University of Miami
Miller School of Medicine
Miami, Florida

Annie Chiu, MD
Private Practice
Redondo Beach, California

Maria Pia De Padova, MD
Department of Dermatology
Ospedale Privato Nigrisoli
Bologna, Italy

Marianna Donnarumma, MD
Section of Dermatology
University of Naples Federico II
Naples, Italy

Karin Eshagh, MD
Department of Dermatology
Icahn School of Medicine at Mount Sinai
New York City, New York

Gabriella Fabbrocini, MD
Department of Dermatology
University of Naples Federico II
Naples, Italy

Sabrina Fabi, MD, FAAD, FAACS
Cosmetic Laser Dermatology
La Jolla, California

and

University of California
San Diego Medical Center
San Diego, California

Aldo D. Galvez, MD
Department of Dermatology
Cayetano Heredia University
Lima, Peru

Giorgia Giuffrida
Department of Clinical and Experimental Medicine, Dermatology Unit
University Hospital "G. Martino"
Messina, Italy

and

Dermatology Clinic
University of Catania
Catania, Italy

Chee Leok Goh, MD, MBBS, MRCP
Senior Consultant Dermatologist
National Skin Centre
Singapore

Adrianna Gonzalez, MD
Beer Dermatology Associates
West Palm Beach, Florida

Evangeline B. Handog, MD, FPDS
Department of Dermatology
Asian Hospital and Medical Center
Muntinlupa, Philippines

and

YLL School of Medicine
National University of Singapore
Singapore

Deirdre Hooper, MD
Department of Dermatology
Tulane University
New Orleans, Louisiana

Daniele Innocenzi, MD (Deceased)
University of Bologna
Bologna, Italy

Rohit Kakar, MD
Skin Care and Laser Physicians of Beverly Hills
Los Angeles, California

Jonette Keri, MD, PhD
Department of Dermatology and Cutaneous Surgery
University of Miami
Miller School of Medicine
and
Miami VA Healthcare System
Dermatology Service
Miami, Florida

Francesco Lacarrubba, MD
Dermatology Clinic
University of Catania
Catania, Italy

Marina Landau, MD
Department of Dermatology
Wolfson Medical Center
Holon, Israel

Maria Juliet E. Macarayo, MD
Dermatology Department
Angeles University Foundation Medical Center
Angeles City, Pampanga, Philippines

and

University of Bologna
Bologna, Italy

Maria Mariano, MD
San Gallicano Dermatological Institute
IRCCS
Rome, Italy

Amy J. McMichael, MD
Department of Dermatology
Wake Forest School of Medicine
Winston-Salem, North Carolina

Giuseppe Micali, MD
Dermatology Clinic
University of Catania
Catania, Italy

Vic A. Narurkar, MD
Bay Area Laser Institute
and
Department of Dermatology
California Pacific Medical Center
San Francisco, California

and

Associate Clinical Professor of Dermatology
University of California Davis School of Medicine
Sacramento, California

Megan Pirigyi, MD
Department of Dermatology
Feinberg School of Medicine Northwestern University
Chicago, Illinois

Concetta Potenza, MD
Dermatology Unit "Daniele Innocenzi"
Department of Medical-Surgical Sciences and Biotechnologies
Sapienza University of Rome
Rome, Italy

Ilaria Proietti, MD, PhD
Dermatology Unit "Daniele Innocenzi"
Department of Medical-Surgical Sciences and Biotechnologies
Sapienza University of Rome
Rome, Italy

Farhaad Riyaz, MD
Department of Dermatology
Feinberg School of Medicine Northwestern University
Chicago, Illinois

Aurora Tedeschi, MD, PhD
Dermatology Clinic
University of Catania
Catania, Italy

Antonella Tosti, MD
University of Miami
Miller School of Medicine
Miami, Florida

and

University of Bologna
Bologna, Italy

Maria Vastarella
Section of Dermatology
University of Naples Federico II
Naples, Italy

Patrick M. Zito, DO
Beer Dermatology Associates
West Palm Beach, Florida

and

Department of Dermatology
Larkin Community Hospital-Palm Springs
Hialeah, Florida

1

Classification of Acne Scars: Clinical and Instrumental Evaluation

Giuseppe Micali, Francesco Lacarrubba, and Aurora Tedeschi

KEY FEATURES

- Several classifications of acne scars have been proposed but a consensus is still lacking.
- A standard method for evaluation of scar depth represents an unmet need and is essential for therapeutic and prognostic purposes.
- Non-invasive instrumental techniques such as high-frequency ultrasound and three-dimensional digital photography may help for a more accurate and reproducible evaluation and classification of acne scars.

Introduction

Scar is defined as "the fibrous tissue that replaces normal tissue destroyed by injury or disease" [1]. Causes of acne scar formation can be broadly categorized as the result of increased tissue formation or, more commonly, loss or damage of local tissue [2]. Clinical manifestations of acne scars and severity of scarring are generally related to the degree of inflammatory reaction, to tissue damage, and to time lapsed since the onset of tissue inflammation [3,4].

Clinical Classifications of Acne Scars

There have been several attempts to classify acne scars in order to standardize severity assessments and treatment modalities [3,4]. However, consensus concerning acne scar nomenclature and classification is still lacking, even among acne experts [3,5].

In 1987, Ellis and Mitchell proposed an acne scar classification system and first utilized the descriptive terms ice pick, crater, undulation, tunnel, shallow-type, and hypertrophic scars [6]. Langdon, in 1999, distinguished three types of acne scars: type 1—shallow scars that are small in diameter; type 2—ice pick scars; type 3—distensible scars [7]. Lately, in 2000, Goodman proposed that atrophic acne scars may be divided into superficial macular, deeper dermal, perifollicular scarring, and fat atrophy based on pathophysiologic features [8].

According to the grading system proposed by Jacob et al., acne scars may be clinically classified as atrophic or hypertrophic [9]. Atrophic scars are subclassified into three basic types depending on width, depth, and three-dimensional architecture:

- *Ice pick scars*: Narrow (diameter <2 mm), deep, sharply marginated, and depressed tracks that extend vertically to the deep dermis or subcutaneous tissue.
- *Boxcar scars*: Round to oval depressions with sharply demarcated vertical edges. They are wider at the surface than ice pick scars and do not taper to a point at the base. These scars may be shallow (0.1–0.5 mm) or deep (≥0.5 mm) and the diameter may vary from 1.5 to 4.0 mm.

- *Rolling scars*: Occur from dermal tethering of otherwise relatively normal-appearing skin and are usually wider than 4–5 mm in diameter. An abnormal fibrous anchoring of the dermis to the subcutis leads to superficial shadowing and to a rolling or undulating appearance of the overlying skin.

Other clinical entities included in this classification are *hypertrophic scars, keloidal scars,* and *sinus tracts* [9]. Both hypertrophic and keloidal scars result from an abnormal excessive tissue repair: clinically, hypertrophic scars are raised within the limits of primary lesion, whereas keloidal scars transgress this boundary and may show prolonged and continuous growth [10]. Sinus tracts may appear as grouped open comedones histologically showing a number of interconnecting keratinized channels [8].

Another classification is that proposed by Kadunc and de Almeida in 2003 [3]. Acne scars in this system are classified as elevated, dystrophic, or depressed. Other parameters include shape, consistency, color, and distensibility. This classification system may also serve to assess the efficacy of various therapeutic options based on acne scar types [3]. Kadunc's classification is summarized in Table 1.1.

In 2006, Goodman and Baron proposed a qualitative grading system that differentiates four grades according to scar severity (Table 1.2): grade I corresponds to macular involvement (including erythematous, hyperpigmented or hypopigmented scars), while grades II, III, and IV correspond, respectively, to mild, moderate, and severe atrophic, and hypertrophic lesions [11]. Interestingly, the authors consider lesion severity also according to visibility at a social distance ($\geq$50 cm). Moreover, since patients may present various types of acne scars at numerous anatomic sites (i.e., one cheek, the neck, the chest, etc; these single areas are defined by the authors as "cosmetic units"), scars are further subdivided into four grades of severity by anatomic sites involved: localized disease (up to three involved areas) is classified as A (focal, one cosmetic unit involvement) or B (discrete, two to three cosmetic units), whereas the involvement of more cosmetic units is classified as generalized disease, previously described in Table 1.2. The same authors also suggested a quantitative numeric grading system based on lesion counting (1–10, 11–20, >20), scar type (atrophic, macular, boxcar, hypertrophic, keloidal), and severity (mild, moderate, severe). Final scoring depended on the addition of points assigned to each respective category and reflected disease severity, ranging from a minimum of 0 to a maximum of 84 (Table 1.3) [12].

TABLE 1.1

Kadunc and de Almeida's Morphologic Classification of Acne Scars

Scars Types	Clinical Description
1. Elevated	
1a. Hypertrophic	Hypertrophic lesions raised above the skin surface and limited to the original injured area
1b. Keloidal	Usually found in patients with genetic predisposition; their dimensions exceed the initial injured tissue
1c. Papular	Soft elevations, like anetodermas, frequently observed on the trunk and chin area
1d. Bridges	Fibrous strings over healthy skin
2. Dystrophic	Irregular or star-like scar shapes with a white and atrophic floor
3. Depressed	
3a.1. Distensible retractions	Scars attached only by their central area after skin distension
3a.2. Distensible undulations (valleys)	Lesion that does not completely disappear after skin distension
3b.1. Nondistensible superficial	Shallow, dish-like defects
3b.2. Nondistensible medium	Crater-like, with a scar base that is relatively smooth, has normal color and texture, and has a wide diameter
3b.3. Nondistensible deep	Narrow and fibrotic scars, ice pick or pitted scars with sharp shoulders perpendicular to the skin surface that may appear as epithelial invaginations sometimes reaching the subcutaneous layer
3b.4. Tunnels	Two or more ice pick scars connected by epithelialized tracts

Source: Data from Kadunc BV and Trindade de Almeida AD. *Dermatol Surg.* 2003;29:1200–9.

TABLE 1.2

Goodman and Baron's Qualitative Global Scarring Grading System

Grade	Level of Disease	Clinical Features	Examples of Scars
1	Macular	• Erythematous, hyper- or hypopigmented flat marks • Visible to patient or observer irrespective of distance	• Erythematous flat marks • Hyperpigmented flat marks • Hypopigmented flat marks
2	Mild	• Mild atrophy or hypertrophy • May not be obvious at social distances of 50 cm or greater • May be covered adequately by make-up; the normal shadow of shaved beard hair in males, or normal body hair if extrafacial	• Rolling • Small soft papular
3	Moderate	• Moderate atrophy or hypertrophy • Obvious at social distances of 50 cm or greater • Not covered easily by make-up, the normal shadow of shaved beard hair in males, or body hair if extrafacial • Able to be flattened by manual stretching of the skin	• More significant rolling • Shallow boxcar • Mild-to-moderate hypertrophic or papular scars
4	Severe	• Severe atrophic or hypertrophic scarring • Obvious at social distances of 50 cm or greater • Not covered easily by make-up, the normal shadow of shaved beard hair in males, or body hair if extrafacial • Not able to be flattened by manual stretching of the skin	• Punched out atrophic (deep boxcar) • Ice-pick • Bridges and tunnels • Gross atrophy • Dystrophic scars • Significant hypertrophy • Keloid

Source: From Goodman GJ and Baron JA. *Dermatol Surg*. 2006;32:1458–66, with permission.

TABLE 1.3

Goodman and Baron's Quantitative Global Acne Scarring Grading System

Grade/Type	Grade 1 (1–10 lesions)	Grade 2 (11–20 lesions)	Grade 3 (>20 lesions)
A) Milder scarring (1 point each)	1 point	2 points	3 points
Macular erythematous or pigmented			
Mildly atrophic dish-like			
B) Moderate scarring (2 points each)	2 points	4 points	6 points
Moderately atrophic dish-like			
Punched out with shallow bases, small scars (<5 mm)			
Shallow but broad atrophic areas			
C) Severe scarring (3 points each)	3 points	6 points	9 points
Punched out with deep but normal bases, small scars (<5 mm)			
Punched out with deep abnormal bases, small scars (<5 mm)			
Linear or troughed dermal scarring			
Deep, broad atrophic areas			
D) Hyperplastic			
Papular scars	2 points	4 points	6 points
Keloidal/hypertrophic scars	Area <5 cm^2 6 points	Area 5–20 cm^2 12 points	Area >20 cm^2 18 points

Source: From Goodman GJ and Baron JA. *J Cosmet Dermatol*. 2006;5:48–52, with permission.

TABLE 1.4

Acne Scar Severity Score (SCAR-S), to be Independently Applied to the Face, Chest, and Back; the Overall Scar Score is the Sum of Scores from Each of these Three Sites

Category	Score	Description
Clear	0	No visible scars from acne
Almost clear	1	Hardly visible scars from 2.5 m away
Mild	2	Easily recognizable; less than half the affected area (e.g., face, back, or chest) is involved
Moderate	3	More than half the affected area (e.g., face, back, or chest) is involved
Severe	4	Entire area is involved
Very severe	5	Entire area with prominent atrophic or hypertrophic scars

Source: From Tan JK et al. *J Cutan Med Surg*. 2010;14:156–60, with permission.

According to the ECCA (échelle d'évaluation clinique des cicatrices d'acné) grading scale of Dreno et al. in 2007, morphological aspects of lesions define the type of scars as follows: atrophic scars (V-shaped, U-shaped, and M-shaped), superficial elastolysis, hypertrophic inflammatory scars (<2 years since onset), and keloid and hypertrophic scars (>2 years since onset). Each scar type is associated with a quantitative score (0, 1, 2, or 3 depending on the number of lesions) multiplied by a weighting factor that varies according to severity, evolution, and morphological aspect. The final global score is directly correlated with clinical severity and ranges from 0 to 540, depending on the type and number of acne scars [4].

In 2010, another acne scar severity score (SCAR-S) was proposed (Table 1.4). It was based on a six-point scale: 0 = clear (no visible scars from acne); 1 = almost clear (hardly visible scars from 2.5 m away); 2 = mild (easily recognizable, less than half the affected area [e.g., face, back, or chest] is involved); 3 = moderate (more than half the affected area [e.g., face, back, or chest] is involved); 4 = severe (entire area involved); 5 = very severe (entire area with prominent atrophic or hypertrophic scars) [13]. This scale was independently applied to the face, chest, and back, and finally a composite scar score (overall SCAR-S) was computed for each patient by summation of the three regional scar scores (range 0–15). Similar to previous scales, it is inclusive of both atrophic and hypertrophic scar, but it does not involve acne scar counting [13].

A recent study evaluating classification of atrophic acne scars by shape, size, and location that aimed to establish reliability in assessments by different dermatologists, has shown that shape-based evaluations of acne scars are subjective and do not readily yield strong agreement [14]. For this reason, the authors suggested a new, simpler classification system of atrophic acne scars based only on their size: <2, 2–4, and >4 mm, affecting diagnostic and therapeutic choices [14].

Finally, some authors have proposed adding an additional type of acne scar to the existing classification schemes: the papular scar [15,16]. They are 2–4-mm wide soft, skin-colored papules affecting most commonly the chin and nose, which can be misdiagnosed as closed comedones, inflammatory acne, and granulomas, thus leading to a delay in the appropriate treatment [15,16].

Instrumental Evaluation of Acne Scars

An accurate evaluation and classification of acne scars is crucial for the selection of the optimal therapeutic approach. Histopathologic examination, which may most precisely depict scar morphology, is not feasible in routine clinical practice, and non-invasive instrumental techniques could be useful for this purpose.

High-frequency ultrasound (≥20 MHz) represents a technique long used in clinical and experimental dermatology [17]. In a study aimed at assessing and correlating clinical and ultrasound morphologic features of acne scars, 81 lesions (atrophic and/or hypertrophic scars, according to the classification of Jacob et al. [9]) from 41 patients were evaluated [18]. Digital clinical images of each patient's face (full front, left, and right views) were obtained by VISIA-CR Complexion Analysis System (Canfield Imaging Systems, Fairfield, NJ, USA). Cross-sectional B-mode scans were obtained using a 22-MHz ultrasound system (maximal axial resolution: 72 μm, depth of penetration: 8 mm, scan width: 12.8 mm linear).

At the end of the study, scarring lesions were clinically classified as boxcar (n = 32), rolling (n = 24), ice pick (n = 16), keloidal (n = 6), and hypertrophic (n = 3).

Ultrasound examination allowed a more precise evaluation of scar morphology. In particular:

- *Atrophic scars*: Appeared as invaginations of the skin in which all skin layers were normally represented:
  a. *Ice pick scars*: Uniformly had a sharp, demarcated, V-shaped appearance; they were characterized by a narrow diameter at the surface (usually <2 mm) and a vertical extension that reached a depth corresponding to the deep dermis (Figure 1.1).
  b. *Boxcar scars*: Uniformly presented with a sharp, demarcated, U-shaped aspect; they were characterized by a superficial diameter usually ranging from 2 to 4 mm and a vertical extension that reached a depth corresponding to the superficial or deep dermis (Figure 1.2).
  c. *Rolling scars*: Appeared as poorly demarcated depressions of the skin or "waves" of the epidermal layer that were difficult to evaluate due to the ultrasound probe-induced spread compression, which hampers sample size measurement. (Figure 1.3).
- *Hypertrophic and keloidal scars*: Uniformly appeared as dome-shaped areas of increased skin thickness (Figures 1.4 and 1.5); the dermis usually was less echogenic than normal skin. In most cases, with the 22-MHz probe, keloidal scars were not entirely visualized with the probe due to their large size.

In general, ultrasound results correlated well with clinical features, as expected. However, half of clinically designated ice pick lesions (eight out of 16) were more precisely categorized as boxcar lesions upon ultrasound examination. Moreover, this technique allowed precise width and depth measurements that were useful for therapeutic purposes [18].

Another promising non-invasive technique that could be used for the objective evaluation of acne scars is represented by the three-dimensional digital photography (Figure 1.6). In a recent study, the results obtained with a facial modelling device allowing quantitative computer-generated volumetric measurements (Clarity 3D Research Ti System, BrighTex Bio-Photonics, San Jose, CA, USA) [19] have

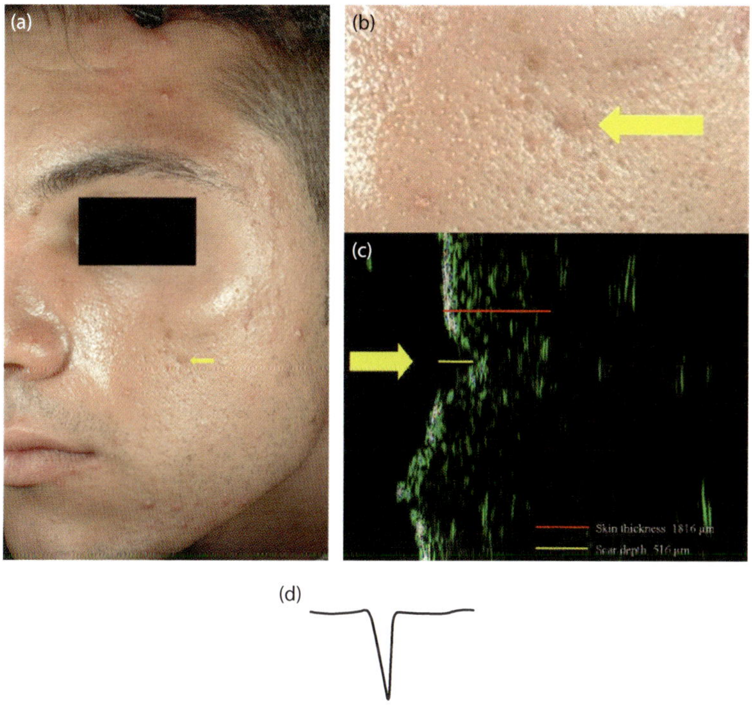

FIGURE 1.1 Ice pick scar: (a,b) clinical and (c) ultrasound appearance; (d) cross-sectional profile.

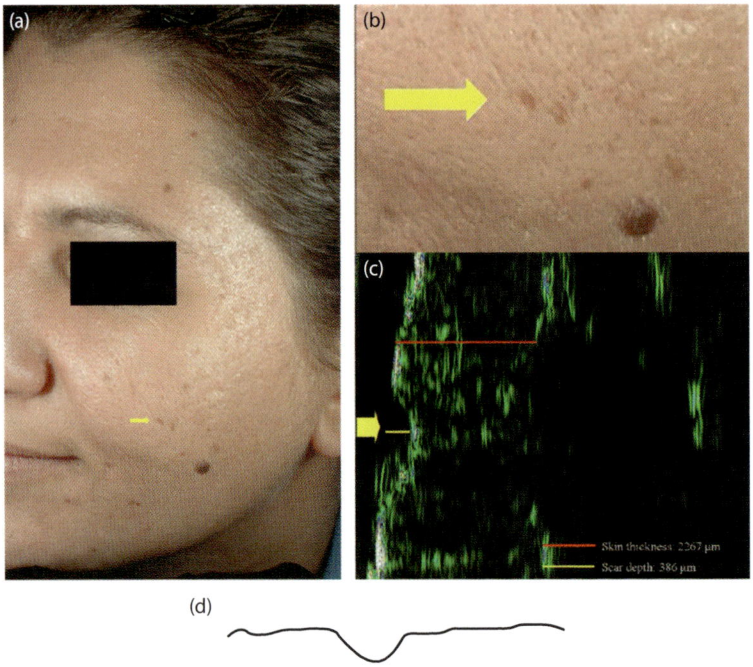

FIGURE 1.2 Boxcar scar: (a,b) clinical and (c) ultrasound appearance; (d) cross-sectional profile.

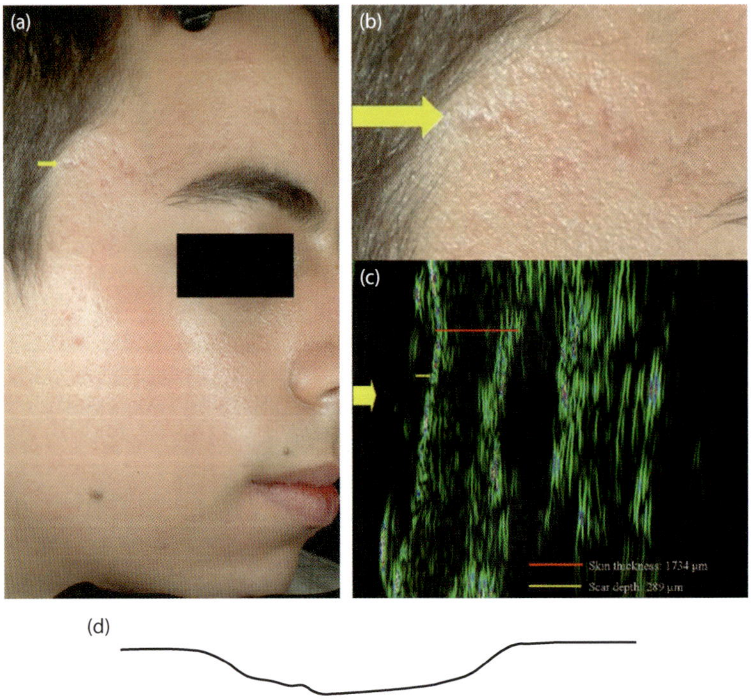

FIGURE 1.3 Rolling scar: (a,b) clinical and (c) ultrasound appearance; (d) cross-sectional profile.

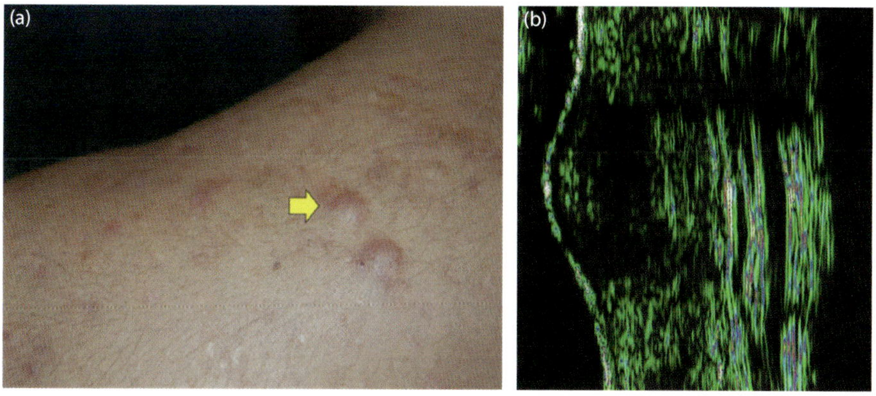

FIGURE 1.4 Hypertrophic scar: (a) clinical and (b) ultrasound appearance.

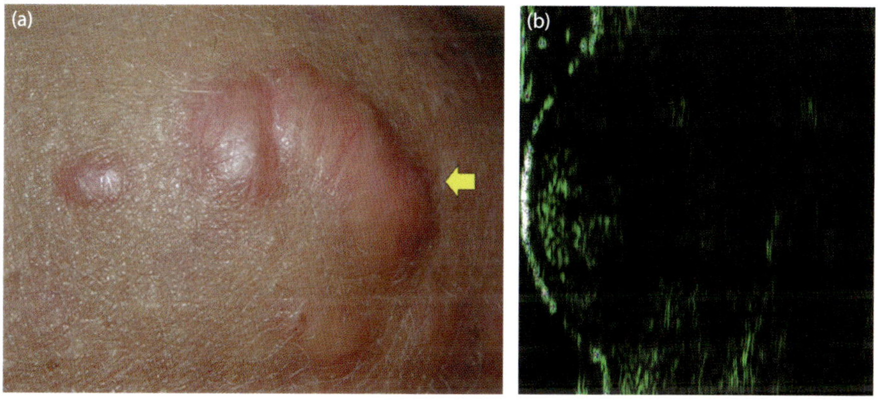

FIGURE 1.5 Keloidal scar: (a) clinical and (b) ultrasound appearance.

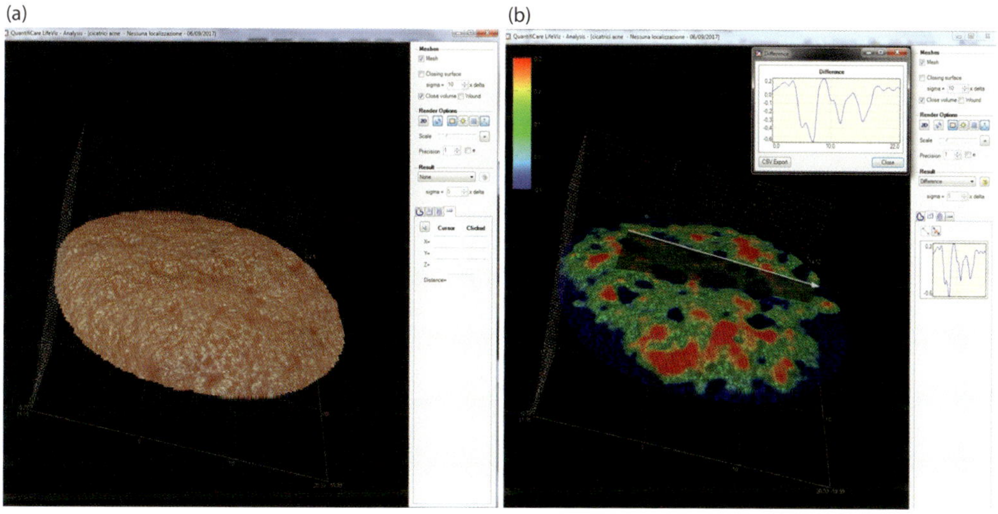

FIGURE 1.6 (a) Three-dimensional capture of an area of the face presenting with several atrophic scars. (b) The same area after digital processing showing colored zones corresponding to different scars depth from red (superficial) to blue (deep).

been compared with direct evaluation of Goodman and Baron scores by board-certified dermatologists, resulting in a statistically significant linear correlation, suggesting that facial imaging may help quantify post-acne scarring [19]. However, these preliminary results should be further confirmed by other studies.

Conclusions

There is still a lack of consensus in the literature regarding acne scar nomenclature and classification. A major problem is represented by the pleomorphic appearance of these lesions that may cause variable interpretation at clinical examination. A standard method for evaluation of scar depth represents an unmet need and is essential for therapeutic and prognostic purposes. The use of new technologies for objective and reproducible analysis of acne scars, such as ultrasound and digital photography, may help for a more accurate evaluation and classification and for high-quality research.

REFERENCES

1. "Scar." The American Heritage® Stedman's Medical Dictionary. Houghton Mifflin Company. February 10, 2009. Available from: http://dictionary.reference.com/browse/scar.
2. Rivera AE. Acne scarring: A review and current treatment modalities. *J Am Acad Dermatol.* 2008;59:659–76.
3. Kadunc BV, Trindade de Almeida AD. Surgical treatment of facial acne scars based on morphologic classification: A Brazilian experience. *Dermatol Surg.* 2003;29:1200–9.
4. Dreno B, Khammari A, Orain N, Noray C, Mérial-Kieny C, Méry S. ECCA grading scale: An original validated acne scar grading scale for clinical practice in dermatology. *Dermatology.* 2007;214:46–51.
5. Finlay AY, Torres V, Kang S, Bettoli V, Dreno B, Goh CL, Gollnick H. Global alliance. Classification of acne scars is difficult even for acne experts. *J Eur Acad Dermatol Venereol.* 2013;27(3):391–3.
6. Ellis DA, Michell MJ. Surgical treatment of acne scarring: Non-linear scar revision. *J Otolaryngol.* 1987;16:2116–9.
7. Langdon RC. Regarding dermabrasion for acne scars [letter]. *Dermatol Surg.* 1999;25:919–20.
8. Goodman GJ. Postacne scarring: A review of its pathophysiology and treatment. *Dermatol Surg.* 2000;26:857–71.
9. Jacob CI, Dover JS, Kaminer MS. Acne scarring: A classification system and review of treatment options. *J Am Acad Dermatol.* 2001;45:109–17.
10. Jemec GB, Jemec B. Acne: Treatment of scars. *Clin Dermatol.* 2004;22:434–8.
11. Goodman GJ, Baron JA. Postacne scarring: A qualitative global scarring grading system. *Dermatol Surg.* 2006;32:1458–66.
12. Goodman GJ, Baron JA. Postacne scarring—A quantitative global scarring grading system. *J Cosmet Dermatol.* 2006;5:48–52.
13. Tan JK, Tang J, Fung K, Gupta AK, Richard Thomas D, Sapra S, Lynde C, Poulin Y, Gulliver W, Sebaldt RJ. Development and validation of a scale for acne scar severity (SCAR-S) of the face and trunk. *J Cutan Med Surg.* 2010;14:156–60.
14. Kang S, Lozada VT, Bettoli V, Tan J, Rueda MJ, Layton A, Petit L, Dréno B. New atrophic acne scar classification: Reliability of assessments based on size, shape, and number. *J Drugs Dermatol.* 2016;15(6):693–702.
15. Gan SD, Graber EM. Papular scars: An addition to the acne scar classification scheme. *J Clin Aesthet Dermatol.* 2015;8(1):19–20.
16. Ali FR, Kirk M, Madan V. Papular Acne Scars of the nose and chin: An under-recognised variant of acne scarring. *J Cutan Aesthet Surg.* 2016;9(4):241–43.
17. Lacarrubba F, Patania L, Perrotta R, Stracuzzi G, Nasca MR, Micali G. An open-label pilot study to evaluate the efficacy and tolerability of a silicone gel in the treatment of hypertrophic scars using clinical and ultrasound assessments. *J Dermatol Treat.* 2008;19:50–3.
18. Lacarrubba F, Verzì AE, Tedeschi A, Catalfo P, Nasca MR, Micali G. Clinical and ultrasonographic correlation of acne scars. *Dermatol Surg.* 2013;39(11):1683–8.
19. Petukhova TA, Foolad N, Prakash N, Shi VY, Sharon VR, O'Brecht L, Ali IA, Feldstein S, Halls J, Wang Q, Li CS, Sivamani RK. Objective volumetric grading of postacne scarring. *J Am Acad Dermatol.* 2016;75(1):229–31.

2

Pathophysiology of Acne Scars

Enzo Berardesca, Maria Mariano, and Norma Cameli

KEY FEATURES

- Acne
- Inflammation
- Scar
- Ice pick
- Boxcar

Introduction

Acne is a very common skin disease affecting 90% of 16–17-year-old boys and 80% of 16–17-year-old girls. Acne recovers in the majority of cases after 25 years of age but in approximately 1% of males and 5% of females it persists until the age of 40 [1–4]. Acne is neither a primary disease of the sebaceous gland or a bacterial infection. It is instead best viewed as an abnormal hyperkeratinization of the follicular epithelium [5,6] with secondary effects on the sebaceous glands due to the effects of *Propionibacterium acnes* and the cellular immunity of the host.

Scarring occurs early in acne and may affect some 95% of patients with this disease. It relates to both its severity and delay before treatment. All types of acne, from papulopustular through to nodulocystic disease may scar and adequate treatment must be started early.

The Role of Inflammation

Scarring indeed occurs as a consequence of deep inflammation. Inflammation in acne is a two-stage process, with lymphocytes and neutrophils affecting the attenuated follicular wall of the closed comedone and, if this wall is breached, the extravasation of irritating follicular contents into the dermis leads to a variety of lesions [7]. The search for the cause of the breach of the follicular wall has been a long one. Initially it was blamed on the free fatty acids from hydrolysis of sebaceous gland triglycerides courtesy of the lipases liberated by *P. acnes*. These irritating substances are hypothesized to allow penetration of the follicular wall. It is, however, doubtful that physiologically there is enough production of free fatty acids to exert this inflammatory effect [8,9]. Moreover, *P. acnes* is important in generating inflammation, with the ability to chemoattract polymorphonuclear leukocytes by the liberation of a low molecular weight chemotactic substance [10] that can diffuse through intact follicular walls and be responsible for the intrafollicular location of leucocytes. The neutrophils neutralize the *P. acnes* with the release of intracellular hydrolytic enzymes, but do not appear to kill the bacteria [11]. There have also been antibodies found to *P. acnes* in microcomedones and interaction with these antibodies may liberate hydrolytic proteases that weaken the follicular wall and allow extrusion of irritating intrafollicular contents into the dermis [7].

Hairs, lipids, keratin, and bacteria induce a foreign body inflammation as they enter the dermis from the disrupted follicle. Degradation of bacteria and other structures occur but with incomplete intracellular digestion and destruction. As a consequence, neutrophils release enzymes and pro-inflammatory factors into the extracellular dermal environment. The released substances activate both classic and alternative complement pathways, including when C5a neutrophil chemotactic factor recruits more neutrophils to amplify the inflammatory response [13]. The severity of inflammation in acne has been correlated to the level of *P. acnes* antibodies [14]. Those unfortunate patients with severe inflammatory acne appear to have elevated indices of lymphocyte transformation to *P. acnes* antigens, abnormal neutrophil chemotaxis and phagocytosis, and excess activation of macrophages. There is considerable evidence against *P. acnes* causing actual dermal infection, as they tend to perish rapidly in human tissue. It also seems to be unimportant whether the organisms are alive or dead in terms of their ability to incite an inflammatory response. Thus, the role of *P. acnes* is to incite the breach in the follicular wall and to be part of the chemotactic and pro-inflammatory cascade that follows [7].

Innate Immunity and Inflammation

Innate immunity seems to play a role in acne scars. In a recent study [15], two different profiles of innate immunity of the epidermis between acne patients prone to scars or not have been identified. The absence of the development of scars is associated (both in normal and inflammatory skin) with a low expression in epidermis/superficial dermis of pro-inflammatory markers (toll-like receptor 4 [TLR4], IL-2), remodeling markers (TIMP-2, cJUN), and the immunosuppressive cytokine (IL-10). The expression of IL-2 (a pro-inflammatory cytokine), two remodeling factors (TIMP-2, cJUN), and IL-10 was higher in the acne inflammatory lesions evolving towards atrophic scars than in acne inflammatory lesions not developing scars. Identification of these different levels of expression of inflammatory markers implicated in the early phase of development of healing in patients prone to scars confirms the data that shows that excessive inflammation in healing tissue of the dermis leads to scarring [16].

The activation of keratinocytes is also an early event in the cascade of inflammation that precedes dermal inflammation. The keratinocytes in acne are activated as soon as the microbiome is modified by *P. acnes* [17]. In particular, toll-like receptors trigger the production of inflammatory cytokines such as IL-8, TNF-α, and IL-12 that diffuse from the epidermis to follicles in the dermis, increasing local inflammation in the deep dermis with a rupture of follicle [18].

In addition, expression of the inflammatory cytokine IL-2, which characterizes a Th1 (CD4) immune response, is significantly overexpressed in both the epidermis/superficial dermis of apparently normal skin and in acne papules of patients prone to scars compared with patients not prone to scars [15]. Furthermore, IL-2 expression is significantly higher both in clinically normal skin and in the inflammatory skin of patients developing scars. This cytokine helps persistent chronic activation of innate immunity by maintaining the activation and proliferation of CD4+ T lymphocytes around the follicle and in the epidermis [19]. CD4 T-cell infiltration is greater around the follicle in acne patients with scars than without scars [16]. High IL-10 levels in the apparently normal skin of acne patients prone to scars compared with patients not prone to scars have also been reported [15]. A high expression of IL-10 could encourage the development of chronic inflammation maintained by the presence of *P. acnes*, specifically resistant *P. acnes* strains [20].

Concerning the remodeling markers, cJUN and AP-1 expression is weaker both in clinically normal skin and in papules of patients not prone to scars as confirmed in different studies [15,21]. These results confirm that, even in the epidermis, AP-1 activation is higher in prone to scars (PS) patients.

Metalloproteinases (MMPs) and their inhibitors (TIMPs) determine the architecture of the extracellular matrix. Modulation of the TIMP/MMP ratio is strictly important in healing by controlling collagen production and metabolism. MMP-9 has been reported to be increased in papules compared with apparently normal skin in patients prone to scars [15]. In conclusion, clinically normal epidermis of acne patients prone to scars is associated with a profile of activation of innate immunity that is different from patients not prone to scars. This profile is characterized by an increase in TLR2, IL-2, cJUN, TIMP-2, MMP-9, and IL-10 expressions. Interestingly, this protein profile affected two crucial ratios involved in scar development: one was control of inflammation duration (IL-10/IL-2) and the other one was healing remodeling (MMP-9/TIMP-2).

Other factors such as platelets may play an important role. Platelets have primary importance in wound healing and activated platelets can also interact with microbes and immune cells. Human platelets express a range of bacterial recognition receptors such as TLR4. Activation of TLR4 on a platelet's surface leads to the production of cytokines and chemokines, recruitment of neutrophils, bacterial degradation as well as adaptive immunity activation and stimulation of immune-mediated inflammatory reaction [22,23]. *P. acnes* infection may lead to the activation of platelets. The activated platelets recruit MMPs to the site of acne lesion initiation and lead to wound healing accompanied with scarring. Increased level of platelet activation marker PF4 in patients with severe acne suggests the importance of platelets in abnormal healing and scar formation [24].

Scar Formation

Collagen and other tissue damage from the inflammation of acne leads to permanent skin texture changes and fibrosis. The type of immune response of patients predisposed to scar may be different from those who do not scar [15,16]. It has been reported that in inflamed lesions of known duration the number of CD4+ T cells present in lesions from scarrers was approximately half those found in lesions of non-scarrers [24]. However, a high percentage of these cells were skin homing memory/effector cells, suggesting that patients who scar were sensitive to the causative antigen(s). In lesions of >6 hours to 48 hours the numbers of macrophages, blood vessels, and vascular adhesion molecules were high and comparable in scarrers and non-scarrers, while the numbers of Langerhans cells and the level of cellular activation was low in lesions from scarrers, indicative of an ineffective response to the causal antigen(s). However, in resolving lesions from scarrers there was an upregulation of the response with greater cellular activation and a further influx of macrophages and skin homing memory/effector cells [25].

Scars normally proceed through the specific phases of the wound-healing cascade: inflammation, granulation, and remodeling. Dermal damage results in either an increase or decrease of tissue and often worsens in appearance with age as a result of normal skin changes. In contrast, damage limited to the epidermis or papillary dermis can heal without scar formation.

From an histopathological point of view, scars demonstrate thicker, abundant collagen that is stretched and aligned in the same plane as the epidermis. More specifically, hypertrophic scars have islands of dermal collagen fibers, small vasculature, and fibroblasts throughout [26]. Scars have an incidence 5–15 times

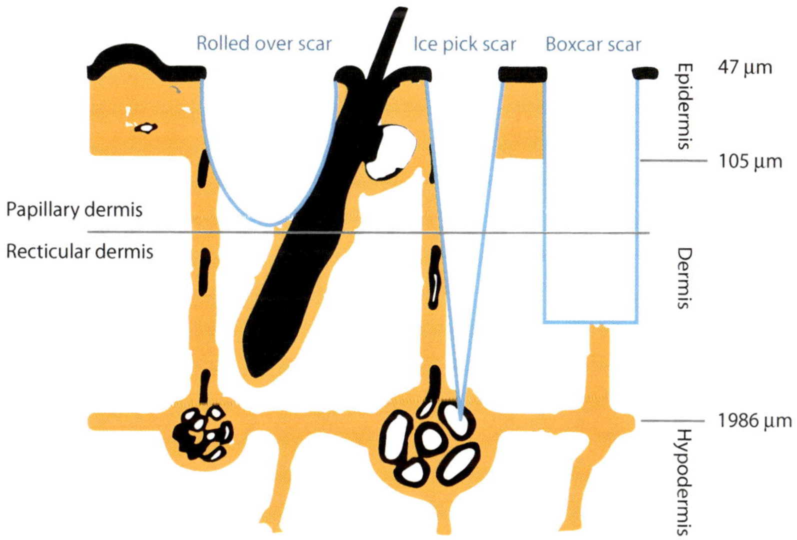

FIGURE 2.1 Appearance of acne scars. (From Sánchez Viera M. *Br J Dermatol.* 2015;172:47–51, with permission [12].)

higher in African Americans and 3–5 times higher in Asians compared with Caucasians. It is estimated that they affect between 4.5% and 16% of both the African American and Hispanic populations [27].

Acne scars can be classified as: ice pick, rolling, and boxcar [12,28]. The ice pick scars are usually smaller in diameter (<2 mm) and deep, with the possibility of tracts to the dermis or subcutaneous tissue. Although the orifice is smaller and steep-sided, there may be a wide base that could evolve into a depressed, boxcar scar. Commonly these are seen on the cheeks. Depressed or boxcar scars are described as shallow (<0.5 mm) or deep (>0.5 mm) and are often 1.5–4 mm in diameter. They have sharply defined edges with steep, almost vertical walls. Soft rolling scars can be circular or linear, are often greater than 4 mm in diameter, and have gently sloped edges that merge with normal-appearing skin (Figure 2.1).

REFERENCES

1. Burton JL, Cunliffe WJ, Stafford I, Shuster S. The prevalence of acne vulgaris in adolescence. *Br J Dermatol.* 1971;85:119–26.
2. Munro-Ashman D. Acne vulgaris in a public school. *Trans St John's Hosp Dermatol Soc.* 1963;49:144–8.
3. Rademaker M, Garioch JJ, Simpson NB. Acne in schoolchildren: No longer a concern for dermatologists. *BMJ.* 1989;298:1217–19.
4. Bloch B. Metabolism, endocrine glands and skin disease, with special reference to acne vulgaris and xanthoma. *Br J Dermatol.* 1931;43:61–87.
5. Knaggs HE, Holland DB, Morris C, Wood EJ, Cunliffe WJ. Quantification of cellular proliferation in acne using monoclonal antibody Ki-67. *J Invest Dermatol.* 1994;102:89–92.
6. Holmes RL, Williams M, Cunliffe WJ. Pilosebaceous duct obstruction and acne. *Br J Dermatol.* 1972;87:327–32.
7. Downing DT, Stewart ME, Wertz PW, Strauss JS. Essential fatty acids and acne. *J Am Acad Dermatol.* 1986;14:221–5.
8. Strauss JS, Pochi PE. Intracutaneous injection of sebum and comedones: Histological observations. *Arch Dermatol.* 1965;92:443–56.
9. Puhvel SM, Sakamoto M. An *in vivo* evaluation of the inflammatory effect of purified comedonal components in human skin. *J Invest Dermatol.* 1977;69:401–6.
10. Webster GF, Leyden JJ. Characterization of serum independent polymorphonuclear leukocyte chemotactic factors produced by *Propionebacterium acnes. Inflammation.* 1980;4:261–9.
11. Webster GF, Leyden JJ, Tsai CC, Baehni P, McArthur WP. Polymorphonuclear leukocyte lysosomal release in response to *Propionebacterium acnes in vitro* and its enhancement by sera from inflammatory acne patients. *J Invest Dermatol.* 1980;74:398–401.
12. Sánchez Viera M. Management of acne scars: Fulfilling our duty of care for patients. *Br J Dermatol.* 2015;172:47–51.
13. Webster GF, Leyden JJ, Nilsson UR. Complement activation in acne vulgaris: Consumption of complement by comedones. *Infect Immun.* 1979;26:183–6.
14. Puhvel SM, Hoffman LK, Sternberg TH. Presence of complement fixing antibodies to *Corynebacterium acnes* in the sera of acne patients with acne vulgaris. *Arch Dermatol.* 1966;93:364–6.
15. Saint-Jean M, Khammari A, Jasson F, Nguyen J-M, Dréno B. Different cutaneous innate immunity profiles in acne patients with and without atrophic scars. *Eur J Dermatol.* 2016;26(1):68–74.
16. Holland DB, Jeremy AH, Roberts SG et al. Inflammation in acne scarring: A comparison of the responses in lesions from patients prone and not prone to scar. *Br J Dermatol.* 2004;150:72–81.
17. Beylot C, Auffret N, Poli F et al. *Propionibacterium acnes*: An update on its role in the pathogenesis of acne. *J Eur Acad Dermatol Venereol.* 2014;28:271–8.
18. Kim J. Review of the innate immune response in acne vulgaris: Activation of Toll-like receptor 2 in acne triggers inflammatory cytokine responses. *Dermatology.* 2005;211:193–8.
19. Malek TR. The biology of interleukin-2. *Annu Rev Immunol.* 2008;26:453–79.
20. Weiss E, Mamelak AJ, La Morgia S et al. The role of interleukin 10 in the pathogenesis and potential treatment of skin diseases. *J Am Acad Dermatol.* 2004;50:657–75.
21. Kang S, Cho S, Chung JH et al. Inflammation and extracellular matrix degradation mediated by activated transcription factors nuclear factor-kappaB and activator protein-1 in inflammatory acne lesions *in vivo. Am J Pathol.* 2005;166:1691–9.

22. Younis S, Rana F, Blumenberg M, Javed Q. Role of activated platelets in severe acne scarring and adaptive immunity activation. *Clin Chem Lab Med (CCLM)*. 2017;55(7):e152–3.
23. Semple JW, Italiano JE Jr, Freedman J. Platelets and the immune continuum. *Nat Rev Immunol*. 2011;11:264–74.
24. Kaplan KL, Owen J. Plasma levels of beta-thromboglobulin and platelet factor 4 as indices of platelet activation *in vivo*. *Blood*. 1981;57:199–202.
25. Holland DB, Jeremy AHT. The role of inflammation in the pathogenesis of acne and acne scarring. *Sem Cutan Med Surg*. 2005;24(2):79–83.
26. Tuan TL, Nichter LS. The molecular basis of keloid and hypertrophic scar formation. *Mol Med Today*. 1998;4:19–24.
27. Ketchum LD, Cohen IK, Masters FW. Hypertrophic scars and keloids. *Plast Reconstr Surg*. 1974;53:140–54.
28. Jacob CI, Dover JS, Kaminer MS. Acne scarring: A classification system and review of treatment options. *J Am Acad Dermatol*. 2001;45:109–17.

3

Topical Drugs for Prevention and Treatment of Acne Scars

Jonette Keri

KEY FEATURES

- Discuss the mechanism of action of topical agents which have been found to be helpful for acne scarring.
- Review clinical studies showing positive results with topical treatments showing improvement in acne scarring.

Introduction

Acne scarring is a major concern of most acne patients. Patients come to the dermatologist looking for a topical medication to help with the acne scarring. Although there are many topical treatments for acne, there is little information about how these medications can prevent and treat acne scars, and scarring occurs in patients with acne about 95% of the time [1]. Atrophic acne scars represent the majority of acne scarring with hypertrophic and keloidal scars being much less. Evidence supports the topical use of retinoids, glycolic acid, and benzoyl peroxide when combined with adapalene for the treatment of acne scarring. Surprisingly, there are very few published reports on the use of topical agents for acne scarring.

In this chapter we will review the data that is available to date so that practitioners are aware of what is available.

Scar Formation and Mechanism of Action of Topical Agents

The scar starts with inflammation, followed by granulation tissue formation, and then matrix remodeling [2]. The matrix remodeling stage is characterized by the interplay between various mediators. An imbalance between the ratio of matrix metalloproteinases (MMPs) to tissue inhibitors of matrix metalloproteinases (TIMPs), can lead to either atrophic or hypertrophic scarring [2]. Gene array analysis of acne lesions shows a number of upregulated genes that are involved in inflammation and matrix remodeling including matrix MMPs 1 and 3, IL-8, human beta-defensin 4, and granzyme B [3]. Interest in topical treatments that target points along the above pathways represent possible therapeutic options. For example, it is known that topical retinoids can stimulate the production of procollagen by fibroblasts as well as decrease the amount of matrix MMP 1 [4,5]. Glycolic acid is known to be keratolytic [6] and benzoyl peroxide is known to decrease inflammation and thus decrease scar formation.

Prevention of Acne Scars

The best bet for prevention of acne scarring is to quickly and effectively treat early inflammatory lesions. Topical agents are a mainstay in the treatment of inflammatory lesions. Surprisingly, there are only a few references where prevention of scarring by the use of topical agents was discussed. These will be noted.

Topical Treatments for Acne Scarring

An early review of the uses of topical vitamin A suggested that keloidal or hypertrophic scars could be treated with some success with topical vitamin A acid [7]. However, it was years later when the first reported case of atrophic acne scarring was treated successfully with topical tretinoin cream. In this case report, a 25-year-old female was given tretinoin 0.05% cream to use nightly and after 4 months had significant improvement in her acne scarring [8]. Glycolic acid cream at 15% was compared with glycolic acid peeling and was found not to be as effective as the peeling but did give some patients a statistically significant partial response compared with placebo [9]. After this time, there were few papers concerning the use of topicals to treat acne scarring. There was some use of iontophoresis with tretinoin. In this setting, the tretinoin is applied and then an iontophoresis mask is placed on the face to facilitate the tretinoin going deeper into the skin. This procedure was done in physicians' offices [10,11]. More recent literature uses retinoids in combination with other agents. These remaining studies will be reviewed in the following sections.

Retinaldehyde and Glycolic Acid

The first report is a double-blind, vehicle-controlled trial of 145 patients treated with 0.1% retinaldehyde/6% glycolic acid cream for patients with moderate acne from three European nations: France, Italy, and Greece [12]. The patients were treated for 3 months and were assessed for a number of factors including a global acne scarring score. Although there was improvement in both the vehicle group and the active ingredient group, there was a trend towards a greater improvement with the retinaldehyde/glycolic acid treatment group. The authors concluded that by treating the inflammatory lesions this helped to prevent scarring. The scars which already existed were treated through effects of retinaldehyde on keratinocytes by affecting differentiation and proliferation. The scars were also treated by the keratolytic effect of the glycolic acid. Specifically, the patients did better with respect to the erythema and hyperpigmentation of their scars.

Retinoic Acid and Glycolic Acid Combination

A study involving 35 patients using topical retinoic acid 0.025% and glycolic acid 12%, evaluated for the presence of acne scarring after 12 weeks of use [13]. The patients gradually increased use from a half hour to a few hours to overnight over the 12-week period. The patients were not on any other treatment. The patients were evaluated by two methods: one for atrophic acne scarring and the other for what was labeled as macular erythematous pigmented lesions. This was used to help determine the difference between the atrophic scars and the pigmented macular lesions. For the patients evaluated for scarring the Goodman and Baron quantitative global scarring grading system was used before and at the end of the 12-week period. Numerical scoring was defined by the appearance and number of scars. The numerical values were then tallied and divided into no improvement, mild, moderate, good, and very good improvement. Three out of 35 showed no improvement, 16 showed mild improvement, 13 had moderate improvement, two had good improvement, and one had very good improvement.

For the pigmentary change, of the macular lesions, improvement was categorized as no improvement, or mild, moderate, or good improvement. The results of this section of the study showed five out of 35 having no improvement, two having mild improvement, eight having moderate improvement, and 20 having good improvement.

TABLE 3.1 Topical Agents Shown to Help Acne Scars

Retinaldehyde and glycolic acid
Retinoic acid and glycolic acid
Adapalene/benzoyl peroxide

Note: Theoretically, short course of potent topical steroids in acne fulminans patients.

The study makes a valid observation that many (mainly patients) perceive scars as pigmentary changes, thus complimentary evaluation of this physical finding was prudent by the authors.

Adapalene/Benzoyl Peroxide

The most recent assessment of acne scars with a topical medication is a split-face randomized controlled trial using adapalene 0.1%/benzoyl peroxide 2.5% gel in adult patients with moderate acne who were followed for 6 months [14]. Very importantly, this study addressed the development of new scars. Fewer new atrophic scars were noted in the treated group, with an average of two fewer atrophic scars over 6 months. In addition, assessment of scarring showed the percentage of patients that were almost clear improved from 9.7% to 45.2% after treatment, where as in the vehicle group that percentage remained stable (9.7%–6.5%). The authors suggest a dual effect of adapalene/benzoyl peroxide by improving the overall severity of the atrophic acne scars and reducing the occurrence of new scars, thus prevention of acne scarring.

Acne Fulminans, Special Case

Potent topical steroids applied on all ulcerated nodules may have some beneficial effect to decrease inflammation in the first 7–10 days [15]. Theoretically, the decrease in inflammation may help with scarring.

Conclusion

There is evidence that retinoids, glycolic acid, and benzoyl peroxide in combination with adapalene can treat acne scarring (Table 3.1). There isn't evidence to support scar prevention except for limited data from the aforementioned three topicals. In preparation for this review, other topical acne treatments and their effect on acne scarring was searched in the medical literature and there were no published reports to support the use of topical azelaic acid, sulfur, sulfacetamide, and dapsone. Finally, there are anecdotal reports of potent topical steroids helping with acne fulminans lesions.

REFERENCES

1. Layton AM, Henderson CA, Cunliffe WJ. A clinical evaluation of acne scarring and its incidence. *Clin Exp Dermatol.* July 1994;19(4):303–8.
2. Fabbrocini G, Annunziata MC, D'Arco V et al. Acne scars: Pathogenesis, classification and treatment. *Dermatol Res Pract.* 2010;2010:893080. P 1–13.
3. Trivedi NR, Gilliland KL, Zhao W et al. Gene array expression profiling in acne lesions reveals marked upregulation of genes involved in inflammation and matrix remodeling. *Invest Dermatol.* May 2006;126(5):1071–9.
4. Fisher GJ, Datta S, Wang Z et al. c-Jun-dependent inhibition of cutaneous procollagen transcription following ultraviolet irradiation is reversed by all-trans retinoic acid. *J Clin Invest.* September 2000;106(5):663–70.
5. Quan T, Qin Z, Shao Y et al. Retinoids suppress cysteine-rich protein 61 (CCN1), a negative regulator of collagen homeostasis, in skin equivalent cultures and aged human skin *in vivo*. *Exp Dermatol.* July 2011;20(7):572–6.

6. Lewis AD, Radoszycki H. Alpha hydroxyl acids. In: *Comprehensive Dermatologic Drug Therapy*. 2nd ed. Wolverton SE, ed. Philadelphia, USA: Saunders Elsevier, 2007, 731–43.
7. Thomas JR 3rd, Doyle JA. The therapeutic uses of topical vitamin A acid. *J Am Acad Dermatol*. May 1981;4(5):505–13.
8. Harris DW, Buckley CC, Ostlere LS et al. Topical retinoic acid in the treatment of fine acne scarring. *Br J Dermatol*. July 1991;125(1):81–2.
9. Erbağci Z, Akçali C. Biweekly serial glycolic acid peels vs. long-term daily use of topical low-strength glycolic acid in the treatment of atrophic acne scars. *Int J Dermatol*. October 2000;39(10):789–94.
10. Schmidt JB, Donath P, Hannes J et al. Tretinoin-iontophoresis in atrophic acne scars. *Int J Dermatol*. February 1999;38(2):149–53.
11. Knor T. Flattening of atrophic acne scars by using tretinoin by iontophoresis. *Acta Dermatovenerol Croat*. 2004;12(2):84–91.
12. Dreno B, Katsambas A, Pelfini C et al. Combined 0.1% retinaldehyde/6% glycolic acid cream in prophylaxis and treatment of acne scarring. *Dermatology*. 2007;214(3):260–7.
13. Chandrashekar BS, Ashwini KR, Vasanth V et al. Retinoic acid and glycolic acid combination in the treatment of acne scars. *Indian Dermatol Online J*. March–April 2015;6(2):84–8.
14. Dreno B, Tan J, Rivier M et al. Adapalene 0.1%/benzoyl peroxide 2.5% gel reduces the risk of atrophic scar formation in moderate inflammatory acne: A split-face randomized controlled trial. *J Eur Acad Dermatol Venereol*. April 2017;31(4):737–42.
15. Zaba R, Schwartz R, Jarmuda S et al. Acne fulminans: Explosive systemic form of acne. *J Eur Acad Dermatol Venereol*. May 2011;25(5):501–7.

4

Superficial Peeling

Jessica Cervantes, Maria Pia De Padova, and Antonella Tosti

KEY FEATURES

- Very useful for treating pigmented macular scars.
- Useful for improving boxcar scars.
- Improve active acne lesions.
- Can be utilized in dark skin.

Introduction

Superficial chemical peeling (SCP) is the process of applying a chemical agent to the skin with the intention of destroying the outermost damaged skin layers and ultimately accelerating the restoration process for regeneration of epidermal and dermal tissues [1,2]. Specifically, the utilization of chemical peels induces damage in the epidermis and papillary dermis, leading to epidermal regeneration and post-inflammatory collagen neoformation [3]. For a chemical peel to be classified as superficial, it must exfoliate the epidermal layers without penetrating beyond the basal layer [4]. This treatment modality has many applications in dermatology including facial rejuvenation, photoaging, dyschromias, melasma, mild acne, acne scars (Figure 4.1), oily skin with enlarged pores, and rosacea [3]. For acne scars, the choice of chemical agent depends on the skin type and type of scar, among other factors [5,6] (Figure 4.2). Trichloroacetic acid (TCA) is the most utilized agent for mild acne scars, whereas active acne lesions are more commonly treated with pyruvic acid (PA) or TCA in combination with salicylic acid (SA).

The level of expected improvement is extremely variable and depends on the patient, type of scar, and potency of treatment. As superficial chemical peels are typically of mild potency, repeated treatments are necessary to obtain desired results. Among the different classifications of acne scars, macular and boxcar scars have been documented to be most responsive to chemical treatment [1]. The best treatment results are achieved in macular scars [1].

Superficial chemical peels are widely utilized worldwide in both men and women of all Fitzpatrick skin types and is relatively safe in light and dark phototypes [3,7]. Individuals of all ages can benefit from the improved appearance and quality of the epidermis after undergoing repeated peels [7].

History

As early as 1550 BC, caustic preparations for peeling procedures were described in Egyptian medicine [4]. In the nineteenth century, dermatologists began to show interest in peeling procedures. In 1882, Unna described the keratolytic properties of SA, resorcinol, TCA, and phenol [25]. At that time, treatment of acne scars had been approached only with medium-deep or deep peelings. More recently, acne scars have been treated with repeated sessions of superficial peels [4,7].

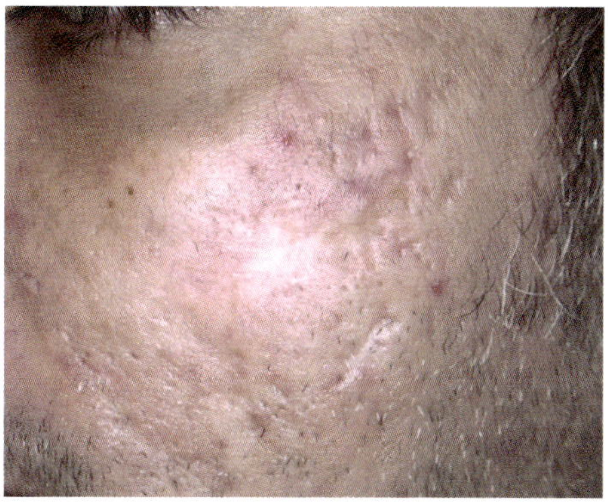

FIGURE 4.1 Patient with multiple types of scars: retracting, ice pick, and boxcar scars.

Advantages and Disadvantages

Advantages

SCP can be universally used on all Fitzpatrick skin types without any major risks. During the procedure, there is minimal discomfort that generally persists for no more than 30 minutes and is well tolerated by most patients. Sedation is not needed for the procedure. The post-peel recovering period is short, lasting only a few days. The desquamation that takes place is well accepted and can be avoided by using glycolic acid invisible peeling of the skin. Nonetheless, some patients prefer Jessner's exfoliation or the thin brown sheets of post-TCA peeling. Complications are rare and when present are of mild severity [3].

Disadvantages

Although clinically proven to work, not all patients achieve desirable results with SCP. The level of improvement is extremely variable and depends on factors such as skin type, type of scar, and intrinsic patient characteristics [1,5]. Every patient's expectation is different, and it is important to state that multiple peels may be necessary [3,5]. Specific drawbacks of each peeling agent are described under the respective section of "Peeling Agents."

Contraindications

Although generally limited, contraindications to superficial peelings exist. These include [3,4]:

- Connective tissue disorders
- Dermatitis
- Infection
- Immunosuppression
- Keloidal tendency or delayed/abnormal wound healing
- Isotretinoin or any systemic retinoid use within 6 months of treatment
- Oral anticoagulants, oral contraceptives, or tetracycline use
- Pregnant or nursing patients
- Active skin disorders or inflammation on the treatment site
- Active herpes simplex virus
- Glycolate hypersensitivity (glycolic acid contraindicated)

Peeling Agents

Trichloroacetic Acid

For many decades, TCA has been the gold standard in chemical peeling. With proper application, TCA is considered to be one of the most satisfying procedures for acne scars. Treatment regimens with 10%–20% TCA, mixed with 100 mL of distilled water, is generally recommended for superficial peels as it produces controlled coagulation and denaturation of skin proteins (keratocagulation) above the stratum granulosum [1,3]. The resultant effect is the visible white frost, which varies depending on the concentration and depth of penetration of the solution [8]. Following this induced damage, epidermal and dermal rejuvenation take place with new collagen deposition and normalization of elastic tissue [3]. It is not usually necessary to neutralize TCA, but neutralization with cold water can be done.

If TCA concentrations between 25% and 35% are used, the solution penetrates below the stratum granulosum to diffuse throughout the full thickness of the epidermis and provide a medium-depth peel. TCA (25%–30%) is indicated for boxcar scars without active lesions, rolling scars, and scars of different depths (Figure 4.2a,b). Concentrations beyond 35% are not recommended for general superficial peels as they can lead to undesirable scarring. However, TCA (35%) is the preferred strength for the treatment of isolated ice pick scars [1]. At 40%–50%, injury to the papillary dermis results, and at concentrations greater than 50%, injury extends into the reticular dermis [1]. Chemical reconstruction of skin scars (CROSS), a newer treatment technique, relies on the localized application of pressure to atrophic acne scars via manually pressing on the depressed areas with a TCA-containing wooden applicator. This method results in focal application of higher TCA concentrations of 65%–100% without significant complications as it avoids damage to adjacent skin [9].

Advantages of TCA include low cost, ease of treatment monitoring (via visualization of frost color), and homogeneity of application (Figures 4.2b and 4.3a). A stinging and burning sensation during application and the potential for hypo/hyper pigmentation are notable disadvantages [8]. Other expected skin changes include mild edema, erythema, and transient hyperpigmentation. No allergic reactions or systemic toxicity is expected [7]. In general, high concentrations of TCA are not indicated for dark skin (Fitzpatrick V-VI) due to the high risk of hyperpigmentation.

Glycolic Acid

α-hydroxy acids (AHAs) is a family of carboxylic acids consisting of glycolic, lactic, malic, oxalic, tartaric, and citric acid. Glycolic acid is the most popular AHA that is used as a peeling agent [8]. Superficial glycolic acid peels provide an overall improvement in the appearance of the skin with minimal post-peel recovery. The chemical effect of topical AHAs is to diminish corneocyte cohesion above the granular layer and diminish the quantity of desmosomes and tonofilament aggregates. This results in detachment

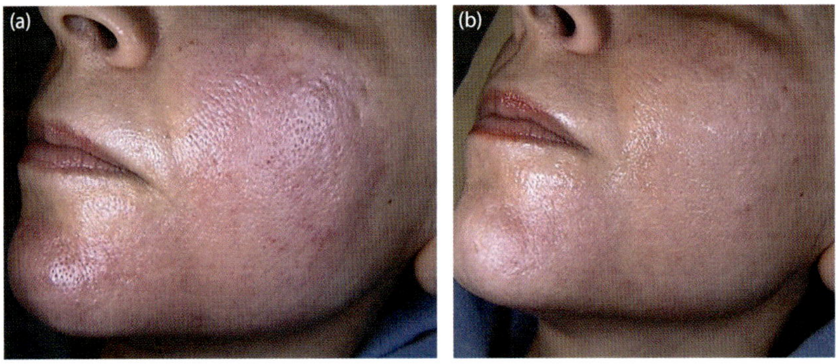

FIGURE 4.2 Boxcar scars (a) at first session and (b) after third session with 25% trichloroacetic acid peeling.

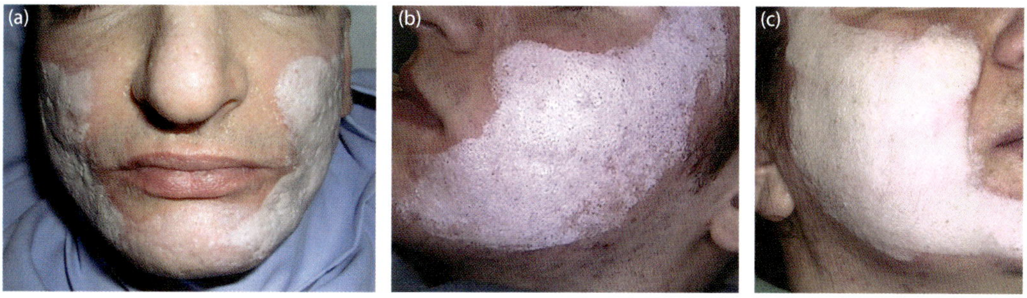

FIGURE 4.3 White frost after application of (a,b) 25% and (c) 30% trichloroacetic acid peel.

of the stratum corneum with subsequent desquamation within 24 hours post-treatment [3]. In summary, AHAs such as glycolic acid result in thinning of the stratum corneum, promotion of epidermolysis, and dispersion of basal layer melanin [8]. Furthermore, increased secretion of interleukin-6 causes increases in dermal hyaluronic acid and collagen gene expression [1].

Erythema, blanching, stinging, and spotted-like frosting are signs of intended epidermolysis. Glycolic acids are generally nontoxic and systematically safe. Hyperpigmentation, especially in dark skin, and allergic reactions have been reported as possible side effects [2,3]. Other undesirable reactions include erythema, desquamation, and a sensation of the facial skin being pulled [2]. Residual macular or atrophic scars may also result due to glycolic acid's fast and heterogeneous penetration.

Glycolic acid (30%–70%) is indicated for macular scars, especially in patients without active acne lesions. For best results, five sequential sessions applied for a variable time (2–20 minutes) every 2 weeks with 70% glycolic acid should be administered [1,8,10]. Neutralization with 8%–15% sodium bicarbonate solution is administered after the peel. Of special interest, glycolic acid has been documented to be efficacious in Asian skin, with minimal side effects [11].

Pyruvic Acid

PA is an alpha-ketoacid that physiologically coverts to lactic acid. With its keratolytic, antimicrobial, and sebostatic properties, PA is a very potent peeling agent that can be used in all skin types [8]. Additionally, PA may stimulate new collagen production and elastic fiber formation [1,8]. Neutralization is achieved with 10% sodium bicarbonate solution. After 5–7 days, healing is complete [3]. PA (40%–70%) is mostly indicated for patients with active acne, moderate macular scars, and very superficial boxcar scars [12] (Figure 4.4a–c). This regimen results in very rapid effects and provides a very homogenous peel with vast improvement in skin texture [12]. Advantages of PA peels include minimal desquamation, homogenous penetration, and short recovery periods.

Due to its high risk of scarring and respiratory side effects, PA peels are typically not the first choice. The stinging and irritating vapors released by PA have been reported to injure the upper respiratory

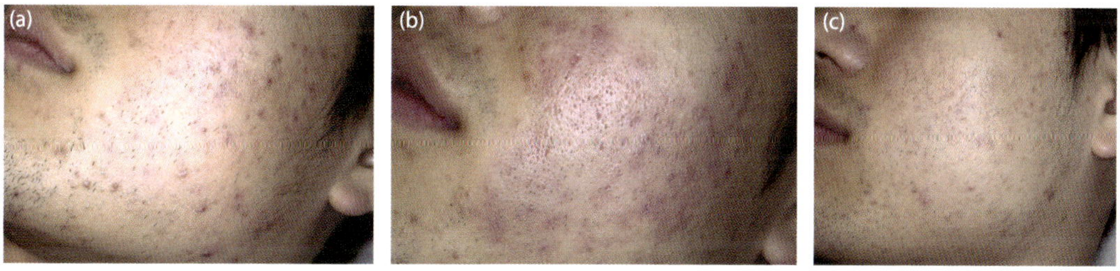

FIGURE 4.4 Active acne with boxcar and ice pick scars (a) before and (b) after two sessions with 60% pyruvic acid peeling, and (c) after two sessions with 25% trichloroacetic acid peeling.

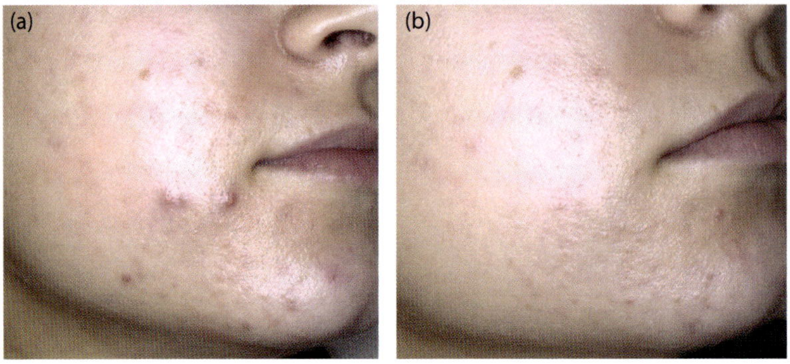

FIGURE 4.5 Active acne (a) before and (b) after four sessions with 25% salicilyc acid peeling.

mucosa. For this reason, adequate ventilation during the procedure is advised [1]. Furthermore, PA peels are commonly associated with intense pain and erythema.

Salicylic Acid

SA is a lipophilic, β-hydroxy acid that results in the activation of basal cells and fibroblasts and desquamation of the upper layers of the stratum corneum by removing intercellular lipids covalently linked to the surrounding envelope of keratinized cells [1,8].

For superficial peeling purposes, a hydroethanolic or polyethanol glycol vehicle is used with a 20%–30% SA concentration. For best results, a 25% SA concentrate should be applied three to five times, every 3–4 weeks [1,8] (Figure 4.5a,b). Upon administration, a progressively increasing stinging or burning sensation may be experienced. This rapidly decreases as SA's superficial anesthesia takes effect. Other side effects include erythema and dryness. A white precipitate, which correlates to evaporation of the vehicle, may be seen on the skin surface. Neutralization is generally not needed. Desquamation lasts for up to 7 days, usually appearing in the first 2–3 days, and results in a very homogenous peel.

Application can be repeated every 4 weeks if needed [3]. SA (25%) is safe for dark skin as it rarely causes post-inflammatory hyperpigmentation or scarring [1]. It is also indicated for active acne and macular scars, producing very rapid effects. SA (25%–30%) followed by TCA (30%) is indicated for patients with active acne, especially comedonic acne, and boxcar scars. SA (25%) followed by TCA (25%) is a less aggressive regimen indicated for active acne, superficial boxcar scars and macular scars. This combination leads to a shorter post-peeling healing phase [13]. Although rare, if SA toxicity should occur, adverse effects such as rapid breathing, tinnitus, hearing loss, dizziness, abdominal cramps, and central nervous system symptoms can appear. Overall, SA is considered one of the best peeling agents [1].

Resorcinol

Resorcinol is a potent reducing agent that is used in paste formulations of 10%–50% concentration. It is applied daily for three consecutive days, at which time water and topical creams should be avoided for at least 4–7 days to allow for potent desiccation. Each treatment should be applied for ~25 minutes and then wiped off. This peeling modality is time consuming and accounts of thyroid side effects have been reported [3].

Jessner's Solution

Jessner's solution (JS) is a peeling agent composed of resorcinol (14 g), lactic acid (85%, 14 g) and SA (14 g) in an alcohol base (ethanol 95%, 100 mL) [8]. The chemical effect is disruption of weak hydrogen bonds in keratin and separation of the stratum corneum, with intercellular and epidermal intraepithelial edema [1,3]. JS can be applied alone for light peels, or it can be applied in preparation for a TCA peel [8]. JS followed by TCA (25%–30%) is indicated for active acne and boxcar scars. In general, an intense burning sensation may occur during application. After application, mild erythema and powdery whitening of the skin is frequently seen. The whitening of the skin is due to precipitation of the chemical onto the skin. Peelings can be repeated monthly if needed.

Multiple coats of solution can be applied depending on the depth of peel desired. Level 1 peel is created with one to three coats of JS and results in mild flaking of the skin after 1–2 days. Level 2 is created with four to ten coats of JS and presents with erythema and pinpoints of white frosting. Mild red-brown discoloration and skin tightening occur 1–3 days after, followed by exfoliation and moderate flaking 2–4 days later. Additional coats of JS create a level 3 peel, resulting in moderate stinging and noticeable erythema and frosting.

Peel Procedure

Treatment Regimen

Regardless of the peeling agent used, treatment of acne scars requires an average of four to seven sessions at an interval of 30–40 days. The choice of superficial peeling agent depends on the type of scar, skin type, and skin thickness. These factors are influenced by previous topical treatments and environmental factors, such as cold weather, which enhances the penetration of chemical agents.

Medical History

It is critical to take a complete history prior to the SCP procedure to uncover any factors that may interfere with optimal results. Important features to look for include past issues with wound healing and propensity for scar formation. Rosacea, seborrheic or atopic dermatitis, and psoriasis are among the dermatological conditions that may increase the risk for post-operative complications. One should also inquire about previous resurfacing procedures or surgeries [14].

Priming/Pre-Treatment

Two to three weeks before the SCP procedure, several pre-peeling preparation tasks must take place. These steps are essential to obtain uniform penetration of the peeling agent, reduce healing time, prevent post-inflammatory hyperpigmentation (PIH), and determine personal skin tolerance to chemicals. Commonly used priming agents include retinoic acid (tretinoin 0.05%), SA (1%–2%), PA (2%–3%), glycolic acid (8%–12%), hydroquinone (2%), kojic acid with glycolic acid (5%–10%), and modified Kligman's formula [3]. Most topical products should be applied three times a week for 1 month, and should be interrupted 4 days before the SCP procedure to avoid excessive penetration of the peeling agent [3,4]. In patients of dark phototype, supplementary treatment with a hydroquinone-based preparation may be used to decrease the risk of PIH [4,14]. In patients with a history of recurrent herpes simplex infections, treatment with oral antivirals (e.g. Acyclovir) should be administered starting 2 days before the SCP and lasting 7–10 days after the SCP as exacerbations have been documented to occur [3,14].

Consent

Before the procedure, a detailed informed consent should be given to the patient to offer him/her the opportunity to understand the procedure and appreciate potential consequences. This also provides the patient a moment in time to ask possible questions and express any concerns. It is important to always provide written information about the procedure (Table 4.1). To avoid disappointments or flawed expectations, it is important to clearly explain to the patient that superficial peels can improve but not completely resolve acne scars [5].

TABLE 4.1

Patient Information about Chemical Peeling

- Superficial peeling is a cosmetic procedure that exfoliates the skin through application of chemicals that induce skin irritation and ultimately improve skin texture and appearance.
- Expect severe burning during the procedure. This will usually last for 3–4 minutes.
- Expect skin redness for 2–3 days.
- Two to 3 days after the peeling, the skin will turn reddish brown and start to peel. Rarely, blisters and crusts may appear.
- The procedure can cause pigmented or white spots that are usually temporary and resolve in 1–3 months. In some skin types, these pigmentary changes may persist and require specific treatments.
- For the first week after the procedure, apply a moisturizer three to four times a day.
- Don't scratch or remove the scales as it may result in scarring.
- Avoid sun exposure as it can lead to development of pigmentary spots. Wear a high protection sunscreen at all times for at least 2 months after the procedure.
- Superficial peels improve, but do not completely eliminate acne scars.
- You may need to repeat the procedure three to six times for optimal results.

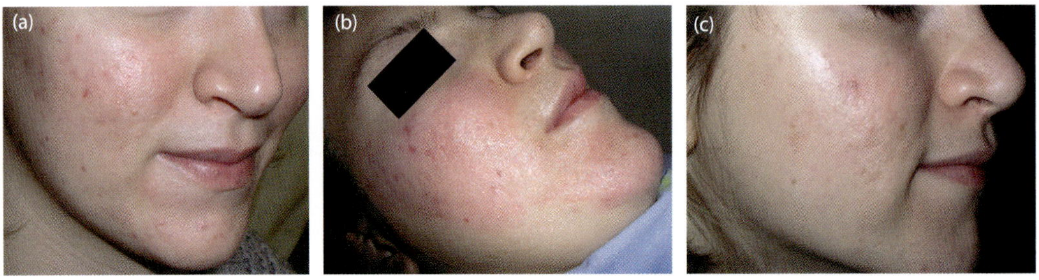

FIGURE 4.6 Patient active acne with macular scars (a) before, (b) during procedure, and (c) after 4 sessions of pyruvic acid peeling. The presence of homogeneous erythema indicates a need for neutralization with 10% sodium bicarbonate solution (see b).

Photographic Documentation

It is essential to obtain good quality pictures before starting the procedure. This provides a means of documentation that is useful for follow up and before/after comparisons [15] (Figure 4.6a–c).

Choice of Agent, Concentration, and Formulation

When choosing a chemical peeling agent, it is vital to tailor the peeling regimen to the individual needs of the patient [14]. The most commonly used SCP agents are glycolic acid, TCA, and JS. Concentrations depend on skin type and thickness, type of scar, and location being treated, as, for example, the periocular and perioral regions require lower concentrations or milder application of the peel.

Suggestions for choice of peeling agent include:

- *Trichloroacetic acid*: Boxcar scars, especially in patients without active acne lesions
- *Glycolic acid*: Macular scars, especially in patients without active acne lesions
- *Pyruvic acid*: Active acne lesions, macular lesions, and/or very superficial boxcar scars
- *Salicylic acid*: Active acne lesions and/or macular scars
- *Jessner's solution followed by trichloroacetic acid*: Active acne lesions, superficial boxcar scars, and/or macular scars

In general, most chemicals utilized for superficial peelings are available as solutions. Select agents are available in gels and pads, which are preferred formulations as they provide slower penetration and are easier to control.

Peeling Tray

Common materials present on the tray include the peeling agent(s), neutralizing solution, alcohol, acetone, cold water, gauze, cotton-tipped applicators, disposable fan brushes, disposable hair caps, zinc oxide cream, and sunscreen. It is imperative to take special precautions and clearly label the peeling agent container to avoid possible confusion with the neutralizing solution or water. Also of importance, always keep the peel agent contained on the side of the patient to avoid inadvertent droppings.

Application

Instruct the patient to wear a disposable hair cap and maintain their eyes closed for the remainder of the SCP procedure. Before the peeling procedure, the skin should be cleaned with an antiseptic cleanser and alcohol or acetone to remove the hydrolipidic film on the skin's surface, as well as any remnants of makeup, sebum, and/or debris [3]. This will allow for optimal penetration of the peeling agent in a homogenous fashion [4]. Apply zinc oxide pads over the lip and eyelid commissures.

The modality of application depends on the formulation. Liquid solutions are best applied using a fan brush, while gel products require cotton tipped applicators or gloved finger application. The contact time varies with the causative agent used and the desired depth of penetration [4].

Initiate peeling agent application starting in areas of thicker skin. Apply the peeling agent on the forehead first, from side to side, two or three times, and then do the same on the cheeks, nose, and chin. The periocular and perioral regions should be treated last. Wrinkles are commonly stretched to allow the acid to penetrate into the folds. To acquire a homogenous peel, repeat the application in regions that do not show erythema or frosting. For best results, apply strong pressure to the skin around the scar during treatment to enhance penetration of the peeling agent in the surrounding skin. This produces uplifting of the atrophic area. For deep boxcar scars, it is important to compress the central region of the scar with a cotton tip [9]. After application of the peeling agent, rinse off or neutralize the treated area with water or sodium bicarbonate [4]. For anti-inflammatory purposes, many dermatologists apply a mild steroid or an emollient cream after rinsing off the peeling agent with cold water. A hand-held fan can be used to reduce patient discomfort at any stage during the treatment [3].

Specific Peel Agent Application Practices

- *Trichloroacetic acid peel*: Apply the TCA in solution or gel until frosting. Use cold water to neutralize the peel [9,16,17] (Figure 4.7a–c).
- *Glycolic acid*: Apply the glycolic acid solution or gel and leave on for 2–3 minutes until diffuse erythema develops. Next, neutralize with 10% sodium carbonate. Avoid development of frosting, as it may be a cause of post-peeling complications [11].
- *Pyruvic acid*: Apply the PA solution or gel and leave on for 3–4 minutes (or until frosting for boxcar scars). Use 10% sodium carbonate solution to neutralize the peeling [18,19].

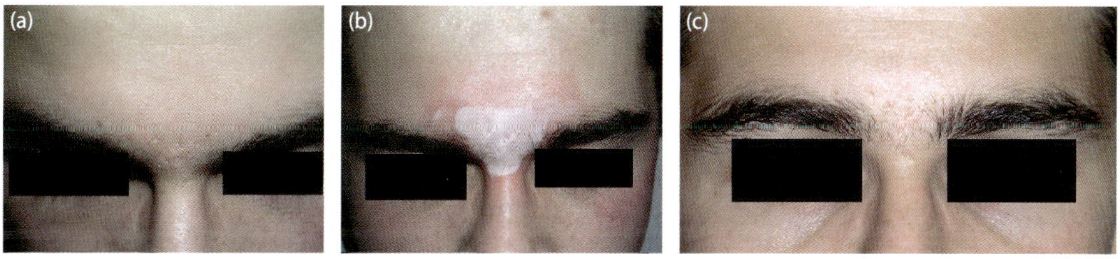

FIGURE 4.7 Boxcar scars and ice pick scars of the glabella (a) before, (b) during, and (c) after four sessions of 30% trichloroacetic acid peeling. The white frosting in (b) indicates that the agent has reached the reticular dermis.

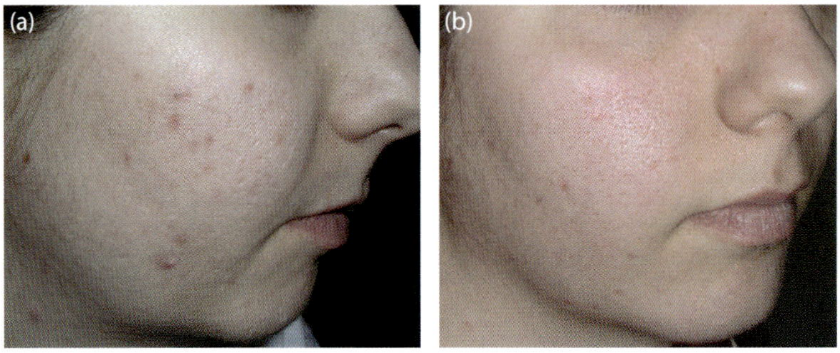

FIGURE 4.8 Active acne with rolling scars (a) before and (b) after three sessions of 25% salicylic acid and three sessions of 25% trichloroacetic acid peel.

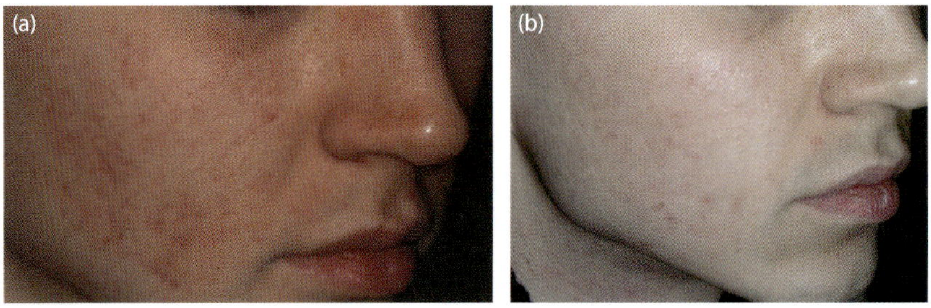

FIGURE 4.9 (a,b) Active acne after combined peeling with Jessner's solution and 25% trichloroacetic acid.

- *Salicylic acid*: Apply the SA and leave on for 2–3 minutes until evaporation of the alcoholic vehicle occurs. Remove the residual SA white power from the treated area with a moisturizing cream. This improves penetration of SA in the skin [20].
- *Combined salicylic acid with trichloroacetic acid peel*: Apply the SA solution first, and leave on for 2–3 minutes until evaporation of the alcoholic vehicle occurs. Remove the residual SA from the treated area with water or with a moisturizing cream. Next, apply the TCA in solution or gel until frosting occurs. The optimal frost is white-pink for macular scars and white-gray for other scars. Use cold water to neutralize the peel (Figure 4.8a,b).
- *Combined Jessner's solution with trichloroacetic acid peel*: Apply the JS first and then follow the same modalities as for the combined salicylic–trichloroacetic peel [21,22] (Figure 4.9a,b).

Immediate Post-Peel Care

The post-peel care regimen consists of 1–2 days of soothing the skin with cooling compresses, 7 days of healing care and hydration, 7 days of avoidance of inflammatory agents and 1 month of careful sun protection. To relieve the burning sensation commonly encountered on the first day, cooling with 1/4 acetic acid compresses is recommended [3].

The patient should be instructed to apply a moisturizing cream three to four times a day for the immediate post-peeling period. Most importantly, inform the patient to avoid sun exposure and use sunblock during and for up to 6 months after the last peeling session. Scratching or intentional removal of scales or crust should be strongly advocated against as it can lead to prolonged erythema and possible inhomogeneous skin pigmentation. A mild skin cleanser can be utilized without rubbing. In case of intense erythema, a low potency topical steroid for 2–3 days can be prescribed.

After 7–10 days, when reepithelization is typically complete, the patient can reassume application of topical products containing 1%–2% SA, 2%–3% PA or 0.05% retinoic acid and 4% topical hydroquinone to prepare the skin for the next procedure. Superficial peels typically require four to six applications, generally 2–4 weeks apart [4]. Patients with active acne lesions can use topical antibiotics and/or benzoyl peroxide.

Key Points for Post-Peel Care

- The patient may complain of burning a few seconds after beginning the procedure.
- The development of diffuse homogeneous erythema indicates epidermal penetration.
- Development of white frost indicates coagulative necrosis of the papillary dermis.
- Development of gray-white frost indicates coagulative necrosis of the reticular dermis.
- The patient will develop diffuse erythema and edema about 1 hour post-procedure.
- Skin desquamation usually develops 3–4 days after peeling.

Side Effects and Complications

Minor Side Effects

Minor side effects are common, yet transitory. These include temporary swelling, burning, itching, dryness, skin hypersensitivity, and transient hypo or hyperpigmentation. Swelling, itching and burning usually do not require treatment and resolve spontaneously in 1 week [14]. In severe cases, a mild topical steroid can be given for 1–2 days. Skin dryness and hypersensitivity may last for 2 weeks and requires frequent application of moisturizing creams. Pigmentary changes may last 3–4 weeks. In these patients, it is very important to completely avoid sun exposure. For hyperpigmented spots, bleaching agents such as 4% hydroquinone and 0.05% retinoic acid can be prescribed.

Superficial peelings may temporarily worsen papulopustular acne. Some patients may even develop active papules and pustules in the immediate post-peeling period. These patients can be treated with systemic antibiotics as in the management of active acne [23,24]. Of note, exacerbation of pre-existing conditions, such as warts, seborrheic or atopic dermatitis and psoriasis may occur [3].

Complications

Complications from SCP are rare, yet possible. Possible complications of SCPs include pigmentary changes, infections, prolonged erythema, allergic reactions, and technical errors [3]. Meticulous care is needed to avoid physician and technical errors, such as dripping acid into the eyes or applying excessively concentrated or inadequate solutions of peeling agent thereby resulting in inhomogeneous penetration. If prophylaxis is not prescribed, reactivation of herpes simplex may occur thereby requiring immediate treatment with systemic antivirals [14].

Permanent complications include corneal damage, atrophic or hypertrophic scars, diffuse or spotted hypo or hyperpigmentation, and patchy inhomogeneous areas of different skin colors. Atrophic scars can be treated with fillers, while hypertrophic scars can be addressed with steroid injections and silicone dressing. Pigmentary changes can be treated with prescription bleaching agents. In patients with inhomogeneous skin pigmentation, a few sessions of 40% PA peeling or 5% retinoic acid peeling can be of help.

Patients must also follow instructions to avoid self-induced complications. Common patient noncompliant behaviors include not using sunblock or intentionally peeling off the scales or crust with hopes of accelerating healing.

Future Directions

Superficial chemical peeling is a safe and effective procedure to improve the appearance and the quality of the epidermis [3]. Wide use of peeling combinations with other treatment modalities for acne scars, such as needling, lasers and fillers, should be explored. Evidence-based studies to evaluate the efficacy of different superficial peelings in active acne and acne scars is strongly desired.

REFERENCES

1. Fabbrocini G, Annunziata MC, D'Arco V et al. Acne scars: Pathogenesis, classification and treatment. *Dermatol Res Pract.* 2010;2010:893080.
2. Peric S, Bubanj M, Bubanj S, Jancic S. Side effects assessment in glicolyc acid peelings in patients with acne type I. *Bosn J Basic Med Sci.* 2011;11(1):52–7.
3. Zakopoulou N, Kontochristopoulos G. Superficial chemical peels. *J Cosmet Dermatol.* 2006;5(3):246–53.
4. Fischer TC, Perosino E, Poli F, Viera MS, Dreno B, Cosmetic Dermatology European Expert Group. Chemical peels in aesthetic dermatology: An update 2009. *J Eur Acad Dermatol Venereol.* 2010;24(3):281–92.
5. Goodman GJ. Management of post-acne scarring. What are the options for treatment? *Am J Clin Dermatol.* 2000;1(1):3–17.
6. Cunliffe WJ, Holland DB, Clark SM, Stables GI. Comedogenesis: Some new aetiological, clinical and therapeutic strategies. *Br J Dermatol.* 2000;142:1084–91.
7. Al-Waiz MM, Al-Sharqi AI. Medium-depth chemical peels in the treatment of acne scars in dark-skinned individuals. *Dermatol Surg.* 2002;28(5):383–7.
8. Gozali MV, Zhou B. Effective treatments of atrophic acne scars. *J Clin Aesthet Dermatol.* 2015;8(5):33–40.
9. Lee JB, Chung WG, Kwahck H, Lee KH. Focal treatment of acne scars with trichloroacetic acid: Chemical reconstruction of skin scars method. *Dermatol Surg.* 2002;28(11):1017–21; discussion 1021.
10. Erbagci Z, Akcali C. Biweekly serial glycolic acid peels vs. long-term daily use of topical low-strength glycolic acid in the treatment of atrophic acne scars. *Int J Dermatol.* 2000;39(10):789–94.
11. Wang CM, Huang CL, Hu CT, Chan HL. The effect of glycolic acid on the treatment of acne in Asian skin. *Dermatol Surg.* 1997;23(1):23–9.
12. Griffin TD, Van Scott, EJ, Maddin S. The use of pyruvic acid as a chemical peeling agent. *J Dermatol Surg Oncol.* 1989;15:1316.
13. Ghersetich I, Brazzini B, Peris K, Cotellessa C, Manunta T, Lotti T. Pyruvic acid peels for the treatment of photoaging. *Dermatol Surg.* 2004;30(1):32–6; discussion 36.
14. Rendon MI, Berson DS, Cohen JL, Roberts WE, Starker I, Wang B. Evidence and considerations in the application of chemical peels in skin disorders and aesthetic resurfacing. *J Clin Aesthet Dermatol.* 2010;3(7):32–43.
15. Goodman GJ, Baron JA. Postacne scarring: A qualitative global scarring grading system. *Dermatol Surg.* 2006;32:1458–66.
16. Brody HJ. Chemical peeling and resurfacing. 3rd edn. St. Louis: Mosby; 2008.
17. Ghersetich ITP, Gantcheva M, Ribuffo M, Puddu P. Chemical peeling: How, when, why? *J Eur Acad Dermatol Venereal.* 1997;8:1.
18. Cotellessa C, Manunta T, Ghersetich I et al. The use of pyruvic acid in the treatment of acne. *J Eur Acad Dermatol Venereol.* 2004;18(3):275–8.
19. Berardesca E, Cameli N, Primavera G, Carrera M. Clinical and instrumental evaluation of skin improvement after treatment with a new 50% pyruvic acid peel. *Dermatol Surg.* 2006;32(4):526–31.
20. Grimes PE. The safety and efficacy of salicylic acid chemical peels in darker racial-ethnic groups. *Dermatol Surg.* 1999;25(1):18–22.
21. Rubin MG. *Manual of Chemical Peels: Superficial and Medium Depth.* J.B. Lippincott Company P, 1995, 79–88.
22. Moy LS, Peace S. Comparison of the effect of various chemical peeling agents in a mini pig model. *Dermatol Surg.* 1996;22:429–432.
23. Tosti AGP, De Padova MP. *Altlas of Chemical Peels.* Springer, 2006.
24. Furukawa F, Yamamoto Y. Recent advances in chemical peeling in Japan. *J Dermatol.* 2006;33(10):655–61.
25. Brody HJ. Chemical peeling: An updated review. *J Cutan Med Surg.* 1999;3:S4-14–S4-20.

5

Medium-Depth and Deep Peeling

Marina Landau

KEY FEATURES

- Differentiation between post-acne sequels and real scars is essential for choosing the right treatment tool.
- Post-acne sequelae can be addressed by superficial and medium-depth peels, while scars require deeper approach or combination modalities.
- Best satisfaction from chemical peels is observed in older patients with scars, since deeper peels address facial aging issues as well.
- The degree of the frosting in a TCA peel correlates with the depth of solution penetration.
- Full-face deep peels are carried out under full cardiopulmonary monitoring and intravenous hydration.

Introduction

Chemical peelings are a procedure used for cosmetic improvement of the skin or for treatment of some skin disorders. Although a few years ago some predicted the disappearance of chemical peels in favor of lasers, quite the opposite has occurred [1]. According to the official website of the American Society of Plastic Surgeons (ASPS), chemical peeling is still the third most popular minimally invasive procedure with an increase of 4% between 2015 and 2016 (similar to Botulinum toxin injections) and an 18% reported increase from 2000 to 2016 (http://www.plasticsurgery.org). To note, in 2012 following the demand for education on chemical peels among professionals, the International Peeling Society was established (http://www.peelingsociety.com).

The popularity of chemical peels is related to their versatility and relative simplicity. During the peeling procedure, a chemical exfoliating agent is applied to the skin to destruct portions of epidermis and/or dermis with subsequent regeneration and rejuvenation of the tissues. The peels are classified as superficial, medium, and deep according to the depth of penetration of the peeling solution. The depth of the peel determines the final outcome, together with the patient's inconvenience during and after the procedure, healing time, and the rate of the potential side effects [2].

Acne is a common disease that affects almost 100% of youngsters [3,4]. Acne settles in the vast of age [5]. Scarring occurs early in the course of acne and may affect to some degree a significant number of patients from both sexes [6]. Minor acne scarring may occur in up to 95% of patients, and significant scarring in 22% [7]. Differences in the cell-mediated immune response are involved in the personal tendency to develop post-acne scarring [8].

Acne scars are socially disabling for the individual, with a significant negative effect to the quality-of-life index [9]. Healthy normal skin is essential for a person's well-being. A recently published study demonstrated that the self-esteem of the patients who underwent chemical peelings for both cosmetic and therapeutic reasons improved significantly after the procedure [10]. This can be possibly explained by the

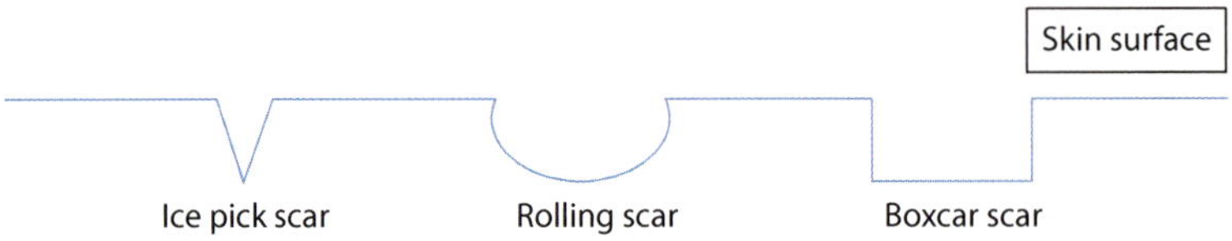

FIGURE 5.1 Atrophic acne scars subtypes.

fact that skin lesions treated with chemical peelings have a significant impact on patients' emotions by influencing their perceived body image, making them feeling embarrassed and unworthy [11].

Acne scars are classified into three categories based on their clinical features: macular, atrophic, and hypertrophic. Macular scars are mainly erythematous or hyper- or hypopigmented macules, without any textural changes [12]. For the purposes of treatment choice, macular scars can be related as superficial post-acne sequels. Due to their superficial character, they are relatively easily addressed by superficial treatments, including superficial peels [13,14].

Hypertrophic scars are linked to uncontrolled proliferation of abnormally arranged collagen fibers in the dermis and are treated by therapies that address these issues, such as corticosteroids or 5-fluorouracil [15–18].

Atrophic scars involve both superficial and deeper layers of the skin. They are the most common type of facial post-acne scars. According to their specific morphology, they can be further subdivided to ice pick, boxcar, and rolling scars [19] (Figure 5.1).

There is no doubt that the treatment of atrophic acne scars presents a challenge for a physician. Combination procedures are often required. Some of them are associated with significant morbidity and longer healing periods. Therefore, proper physician–patient communication is essential for success. Although a wide range of interventions have been proposed to treat atrophic facial scars, a recently published Cochrane Database systematic review on interventions for acne scars failed to find the most effective and safe methods of managing this condition [20]. In this chapter I discuss the role of chemical peels in the treatment of atrophic facial post-acne scarring.

History of Using Chemical Peels for Post-Acne Scarring

As far back as 1905, surgical methods have been used to improve skin that has been scarred by facial acne. One hundred years ago two New York dermatologists, George MacKee and Florentine Karp, began using phenol peels for post-acne scarring [21]. Thereafter, following the development of new medical technologies, other methods have been introduced to treat acne scars [22–38].

Chemical peels, relevant for the treatment of facial atrophic post-acne scarring, include medium and deep peels, their combinations, and the chemical reconstruction of skin scars (CROSS) technique based on in-scar application of a high percentage of trichloroacetic acid (TCA) [21,39–52].

Basic Chemistry

TCA is the most common chemical used in medium-depth peels. TCA ($C[Cl]_3COOH$) is found as anhydrous hygroscopic crystals. TCA is a strong acid with a pKa of 0.26. Its destructive activity is related to the acidity of the solution; therefore, more concentrated solutions of TCA have a more destructive effect on the skin.

The solutions for deep peeling are based on a combination of phenol and Croton oil. Phenol (C_5H_5OH), or carbolic acid, is an aromatic hydrocarbon derived originally from coal tar, but prepared synthetically in a process that utilizes monochlorobenzene as a starting point; 98% phenol appears as transparent crystals, whereas liquefied phenol consists of 88% United States Pharmacopeia solution of phenol in water.

Croton oil is an extract of the seed of the plant *Croton tiglium* and has been commercially prepared as Croton resin since 1932. Its activity on the skin is related to free hydroxyl groups that cause skin vesiculation even in low doses.

Other chemicals in use in deep chemical peel formulas include septisol, water, and vegetable oils (glycerin, olive, sesame).

All the modern phenol formulas are based and modified from a few lay peelers' formulations. Names such as Grade, Coopersmith, Kelsen, and Maschek are the origins of Baker-Gordon's, Brown's, Hetter's, Stone's, Litton's, Exoderm, and other formulas. All of them are based on the aforementioned chemical components in different concentrations. The concentration of phenol ranges from 45% to 80%, whereas the concentration of Croton oil ranges from 0.16% to 2.05%. It is generally accepted that the role of liquid soap is to reduce the skin–surface tension and to improve solution penetration [47–51]. In spite of this, septisol is not included in all of the formulas [52]. Some of the formulas contain oils [47–49]. The role of the oils in the formula has not been clarified yet. Our personal experience shows that oily phenol solution penetrates the skin in a slower and controllable fashion.

Techniques

Medium-Depth Peels

TCA is the most common chemical used in medium-depth peels. Whereas 10%–20% TCA creates superficial skin exfoliation, 35% concentration peels the skin down to the upper dermal layers. Concentrations higher than 35% are not recommended because the results are less predictable and the potential for scarring increases significantly. In order to increase the depth and efficacy of a TCA peel without increasing the concentration of the acid, it has been suggested to combine this chemical with Jessner's solution, 70% glycolic acid or solid carbon dioxide (CO_2). Sandpaper dermabrasion of the scarred areas can be combined with a TCA peel to further improve the outcomes of the peel.

The TCA solution is compounded in a weight-to-volume preparation. Thirty-five grams of TCA crystals are dissolved in water to make a total volume of 100 mL. TCA is stable at room temperature and not light sensitive.

Skin preparation is important before a TCA peel performance. Retinoid (0.25%–0.1%) cream, glycolic acid-based moisturizer, or a hydroquinone-containing preparation is used, starting 2–6 weeks before the procedure. Systemic antiherpertic agent is initiated a day before the peel in patients with herpes simplex history, being continued for 10 days. Before starting the procedure, all patients are photographed and sign a consent form.

Prior to the peeling solution application, a thorough cleaning of the skin is performed with a detergent solution; thereafter, defatting is done using acetone. A TCA peel is usually well tolerated by patients. However, in some cases it can be performed under intravenous sedation, but in most cases a combination of oral sedative such as lorazepam, zolpiderm, alprazolam, or diazepam and an analgesic, such as tramadol, is sufficient.

For a TCA application, cotton Q-Tips or gauzes are dipped in a small container that contains the peeling solution and squeezed properly to avoid dripping the solution onto undesired areas. Using a gauze, a more aggressive abrasive effect is achieved. If TCA is painted by a Q-Tip, a more superficial effect is created. Ready-to-use Q-Tip applicators are usually too compact and do not absorb enough of the peeling solution. My practice is to add a layer of soft cotton on top of ready-to-use Q-Tips. In the treatment of scarred facial skin, we use both tools alternatively during a single treatment according to the damage severity in each area. Whichever tool is used, TCA solution is applied systematically according to the cosmetic units until white frost appears. It should be noted that frost does not immediately appear after the solution application. Patient observation of the skin by the treating physician is required for a properly performed TCA peel. The degree of the final frosting correlates with the depth of solution penetration. Level I has a speckled white frosting with mild erythema and corresponds to superficial penetration. Level II is characterized by an even white-coated frost with background erythema (Figure 5.2). This degree of frosting is usually desirable for medium-depth peels. If level II frosting is not achieved by 2 minutes after a thorough application of the peeling solution, additional layering of TCA should be performed after

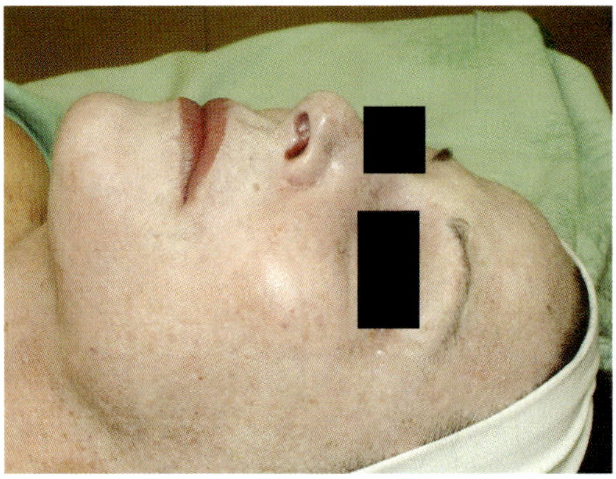

FIGURE 5.2 Level II frosting achieved during 35% peel.

re-dipping the applicator or a gauze. Level III has a solid white opaque frost with little or no background erythema, usually characterizing deep peels, and is not desirable in TCA procedure.

Frosting appearance correlates with an intense burning sensation experienced by a patient. If a patient is not sedated, as frosting develops, cooling of the area using wet, cold compresses provides symptomatic relief and does not neutralize TCA. A patient usually becomes completely comfortable 15–20 minutes after the procedure when the frosting subsides.

After-peel care includes continuous wetting of the skin. During the next few days patients may expect to feel tightening and swelling of the skin together with gradual darkening of the skin color, related to crust development. On day 3 or 5, the crust starts to crack and desquamation begins. At this stage, moisturizing cream can be applied. Full reepithelialization is completed after 5–7 days. At this stage, the patient is advised to wear camouflage makeup and resume normal daily activities. Blunt moisturizer and high-level sun protection are recommended for the next 2–3 weeks. In case post-inflammatory hyperpigmentation is expected, a bleaching preparation based on a combination of retinoic acid and hydroquinone is initiated.

The mechanism of action of medium-depth peels includes the restoration of keratinocyte polarity and an increase in collagen type I content [53].

Ice pick atrophic scars were always considered extremely challenging with no visible improvement being achieved with almost any treatment modality. Focal application of high-concentration TCA has been reported as efficient to treat these specific scars and labeled as CROSS [44–46]. In this technique, 80%–100% weight-to-volume TCA solution is applied by a sharp applicator (wooden tooth stick is optional) directly into the ice pick acne scar without affecting adjacent areas. White frosting appears inside the ice pick scar shortly after application of peeling solution. This procedure can be combined with full-face medium-depth peeling. CROSS treatments can be repeated every 6 weeks until a desirable level of correction is achieved. Histological changes following CROSS techniques have been documented [54].

Combination Peels

Combination peels are performed when a deeper effect on the skin is required yet deep peeling is not considered an option.

a. *Monheit's combination* [55] *of Jessner's solution with 35% TCA*: Classical Jessner's solution is composed of resorcinol (14%), lactic acid (14%), and salicylic acid (14%) in alcoholic solution, and modified Jessner's solution contains lactic acid (17%), salicylic acid (17%), and citric acid (8%) in ethanol. After washing the face, a peeling solution is applied using wet gauze by systematically covering facial cosmetic units. Repeated coats are usually needed until erythema and patchy frost develops. At this stage TCA is applied using Q-Tips or gauzes. Some authors recommend waiting 5 minutes between the Jessner's solution and application of TCA. The after-peel course and care are similar to that of a TCA peel.

b. *Brody's combination* [56]: Icing the skin with solid CO_2 deepens the penetration of TCA and improves the clinical effect. The main indications that this combination should be used are flattened edges of depressed acne scars, actinic and seborrheic keratosis, and fine wrinkles. The depth of the skin icing is determined by the exposure time of the skin to CO_2. Usually the skin is rubbed for 5 (mild exposure) to 15 (hard exposure) seconds. The application of TCA is performed in a normal fashion.

c. *Coleman's combination* [57]: Glycolic acid at 70% is applied usually for 2 minutes and neutralized before further application of TCA. This combination is least likely to produce pigmentation complications.

d. *Combination with dermabrasion*: To improve efficacy of the procedure, the peel can be combined with mechanical dermabrasion [58]. Ready-to-use tip polisher, which is sterile surgical equipment designed originally for cleaning cautery tips during operations, or pre-sterilized sandpaper are used for this purpose. If using the tip polisher, it can be attached to a 10 mL syringe to ease the abrasion process. The abrasion is performed in the most scarred areas, usually being the cheeks. Before the abrasion, local infiltration of the area with adrenaline–lidocaine-containing anesthetic is advised, unless a specific contraindication exists. The abrasion is performed until pinpoint bleeding is induced. Antibiotic ointment is applied in the abraded area immediately after the bleeding stops.

Deep Peels

All patients are required to complete an electrocardiogram and complete a blood count prior to the procedure. Any heart disease requires special precautions, and it is always recommended to work in cooperation with the patient's cardiologist.

Prophylactic systemic antiherpetics is given to patients with history of recurrent herpes simplex, starting a day before the procedure and continuing for 10 days until full reepithelialization is achieved. It is still debatable whether preparation of the skin is required for deep chemical peeling. Standard photography and a consent form are always obtained before the procedure.

Full-face deep peels should be carried out under full cardiopulmonary monitoring with intravenous hydration throughout the procedure. Intravenous sedation or regional blocks make the procedure pain free. A combination of oral sedative such as lorazepam, zolpiderm, alprazolam, or diazepam and analgesic, such as tramadol, can be also considered as optional. Before the peeling, meticulous degreasing of the skin is performed using oil-free acetone-soaked gauze sponges. This step is imperative to obtain even penetration of the solution into the skin.

For application of the peeling solution hand-made cotton-tipped applicators are employed (same as for the TCA peel). The application of phenol solution is accomplished with a semidry applicator. The usual end point is an ivory–white to grey–white color to the skin (Figure 5.3). All the cosmetic units

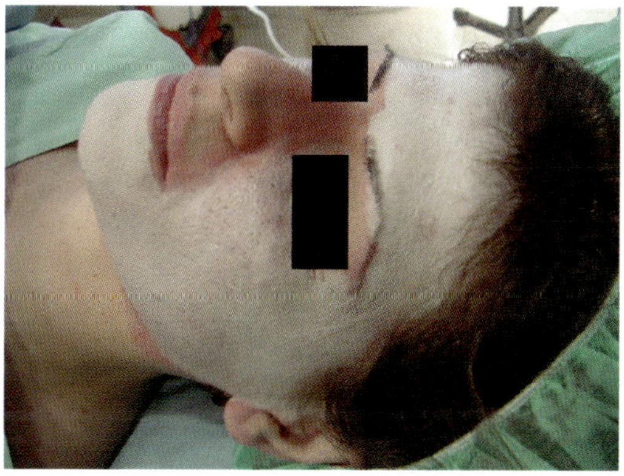

FIGURE 5.3 The application of phenol solution creates an ivory–white to gray–white color to the skin.

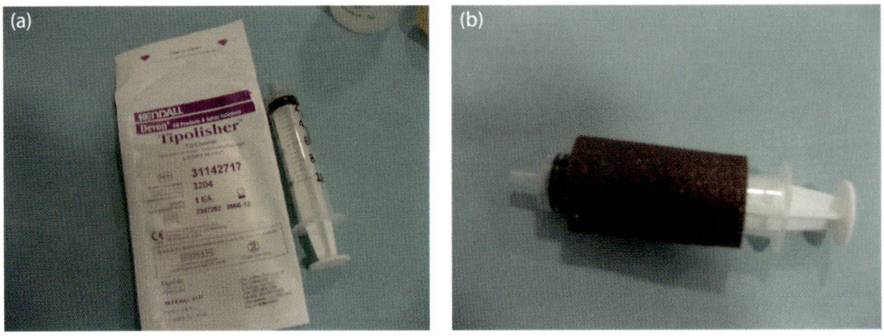

FIGURE 5.4 (a) Tipolisher is sterile surgical equipment designed originally for cleaning cauthery tips during operations. (b) Tipolisher is attached to a standard 10-mL syringe to perform skin abrasion.

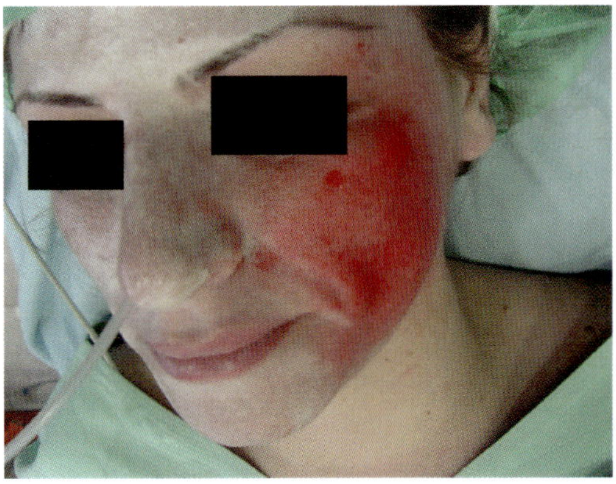

FIGURE 5.5 Bleeding is observed following skin abrasion using Tipolisher.

are gradually covered. While others perform mechanical abrasion of the skin the next day [47,48,51], I perform it immediately after the application of the peeling solution. Sterile Tipolishers or sterilized gentle sandpaper (Figure 5.4) are used to abrade the scarred skin until pinpoint bleeding is observed. Reapplication of the peeling solution coagulates most of the bleeding. The face is covered with impermeable tape mask for 24 hours (Figure 5.5). After 24 hours, the tape mask is removed and the exudate is cleansed with sterile saline. A regional reapplication of peeling solution and re-taping of the scarred areas can be performed again and the tape is left for an additional 4–6 hours and then removed by the patient. The face is covered with bismuth subgallate antiseptic powder for 7 days (Figure 5.6). On day 8, wet soaking with tap water while standing in the shower is used to soften the powder mask and to remove it. The erythema gradually subsides over 2 months. During this time, the use of makeup with a green foundation is encouraged in order to assist the patient in resuming all the daily activities. The third phase of the treatment is regional re-peeling, being performed 6–8 weeks after the original treatment [47–49,51].

Comparison between TCA and Phenol Peels

There is a single study comparing the results of a phenol-based solution with TCA 20% preceded by percutaneous collagen induction (PCI) on atrophic acne scars [42]. While a deep peel was performed once, a TCA–PCI procedure was repeated in four cycles, and therefore was associated with a significantly longer accumulative downtime. Despite an overall similar improvement achieved in both groups, in the TCA–PCI group, a higher degree of improvement was achieved for the rolling scars.

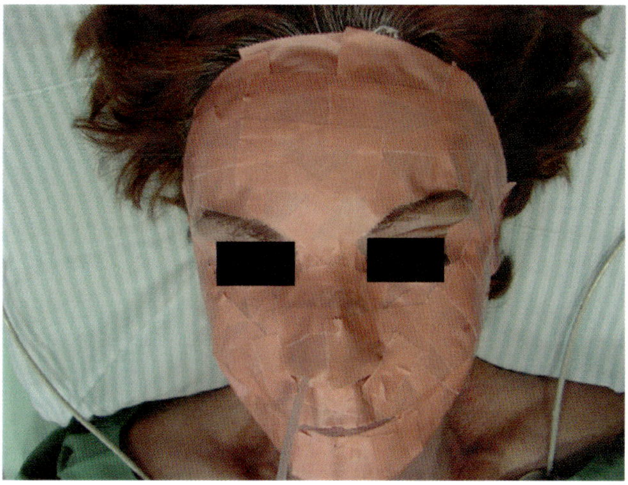

FIGURE 5.6 The face is covered with an impermeable tape mask for 24 hours.

Complications

The list of potential complications of chemical peels includes pigmentary changes, infections, milia, an acneiform eruption, scarring, and cardiotoxicity [59].

1. *Pigmentary changes*: Reactive hyperpigmentation can occur after any depth of chemical peels. Usually lighter complexions have a lower risk of hyperpigmentation, but genetic factors play an important role, and sometimes light-skinned patients hyperpigment unexpectedly. Skin priming using a combination of hydroquinone and tretinoin cream (Kligman's formulation) before the medium-depth peels, and early introduction of this preparation after deep peels, reduces the rate of this complication. Demarcation lines can be avoided if the boundaries of the peeling area are hidden under the mandibular line and feathered gradually to the normal skin. Hypopigmentation after phenol peels is proportional to the depth of the peel, amount of the solution used, number of drops of Croton oil in the solution, inherent skin color, and post-peel sun-related behavior. Hypopigmentation is a major drawback for performing medium and deep peels focally. Intradermal nevi can hyperpigment after deep peels.
2. *Infection*: Bacterial and fungal complications in chemical peels are rare. Patients with a positive history of herpes simplex infection are treated prophylactically with acyclovir or valacyclovir during medium and deep peels until full reepithelialization is achieved. Toxic-shock syndrome has been reported after chemical peels [60].
3. *Milia/epidermal cysts*: Milia or epidermal cysts appear in up to 20% of patients after chemical peels, usually 8–16 weeks after the procedure. Electrosurgery is simple and effective to treat this post-peel complication.
4. *Acneiform dermatitis*: Acneiform eruption after chemical peels is not rare and usually appears immediately after reepithelialization. Its etiology is multifactorial and is related to either exacerbation of previously existing acne, or is due to the over-greasing of newly formed skin. This complication is not uncommon when treating thick sebaceous skin complexions, which is frequently the case in acne-scarred patients. Short-term systemic antibiotics together with the discontinuation of any oily preparations will usually provide satisfactory results. If not effective enough, a short course of oral isotretinoin will be usually satisfactory.
5. *Scarring*: Scarring remains to be the most dreadful complication of chemical peels. The contributing factors are not well understood yet. The most common location of the scars is

in the lower part of the face, probably due to more aggressive treatment in this area, or due to greater tissue movement, or due to eating and speaking during the healing process. Delayed healing and persistent redness are important alarming signs for forthcoming scarring. Topical antibiotics and potent steroid preparations should be introduced as soon as this diagnosis is made.

6. The most important potential complication exclusive to phenol-based peels is cardiotoxicity. Phenol is directly toxic to myocardium. Studies in rats showed a decrease in myocardial contraction and in electrical activity following systemic exposure to phenol [61]. Since fatal doses ranged widely in these studies it seems that individual sensitivity of myocardium to this chemical exists. In humans, sex, age, previous cardiac history, or blood phenol levels are not accurate predictors for cardiac arrhythmia susceptibility. Cardiac arrhythmias have been recorded in up to 23% of patients when a full-face peel was performed in less than 30 minutes. Adequate patient management reduces this complication to less than 7% [62]. No hepatorenal or central nervous system toxicities have been reported in the literature when chemical peels were properly performed.

Outlook and Future Developments

In spite of the high level of improvement achieved using chemical peels, acne scars are still challenging, especially in young individuals. In most cases, a complete smoothening of the skin is impossible, especially on tight skin areas, such the forehead and temples. This is an essential message to be clearly conveyed to a patient before the intervention to build up an appropriate level of expectations. Patients have to be shown pre- and post-treatment photographs and be asked about their expectations (Figures 5.7 and 5.8). All exaggerated expectations should be discouraged. A need for repeating peeling sessions, limited to the most scarred areas, is also discussed.

In general, best results are achieved in older female rather than in young male patients (Figures 5.9 and 5.10). Atrophic scars respond better than ice pick and hypertrophic ones, unless combination with CROSS

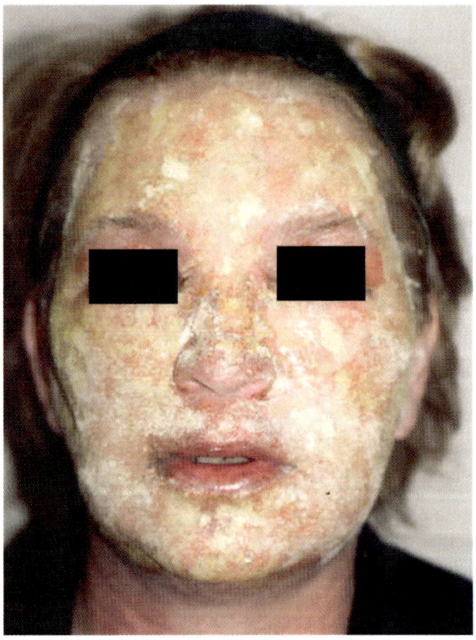

FIGURE 5.7 The face is covered with bismuth subgallate antiseptic powder for 7 days.

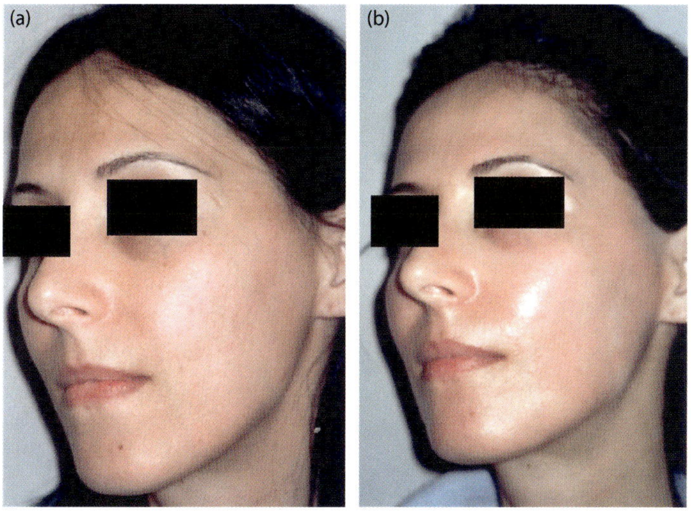

FIGURE 5.8 A 32-year-old woman: (a) before and (b) 4 weeks after a deep peel (Exoderm method) combined with mechanical dermabrasion.

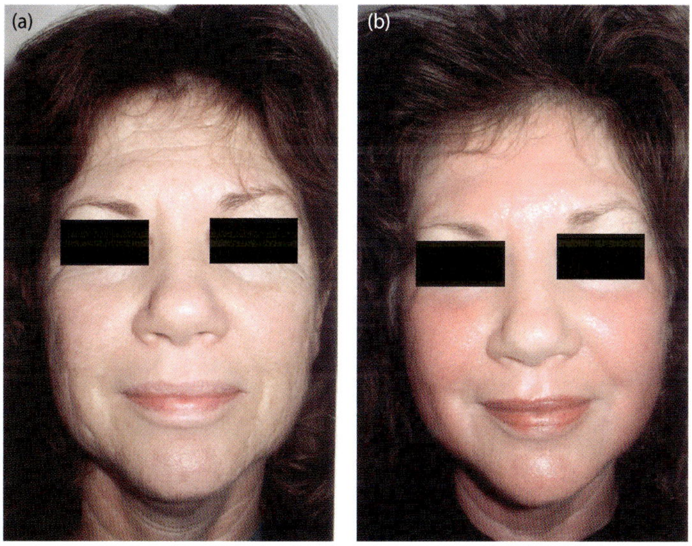

FIGURE 5.9 A 56-year-old fair-skinned woman: (a) before and (b) 2 weeks after a deep peel combined with dermabrasion.

technique is combined. The deeper the procedure, the more significant the result. Therefore, while with a phenol-based peel, a single or double treatment is required, TCA-treated patients are expected to have multiple sessions.

Nonfacial skin is a special challenge. Since the healing process is less effective on this skin, only milder peels are possible. Therefore, the results are usually less adequate.

In my opinion, future developments will include a combination of chemical abrasion of the facial skin with topical application of fractional ablative or non-ablative light technologies. Although promising, these technologies *per se* have not yet provided comparable results to chemical peels. With time, the appropriate combination will be found.

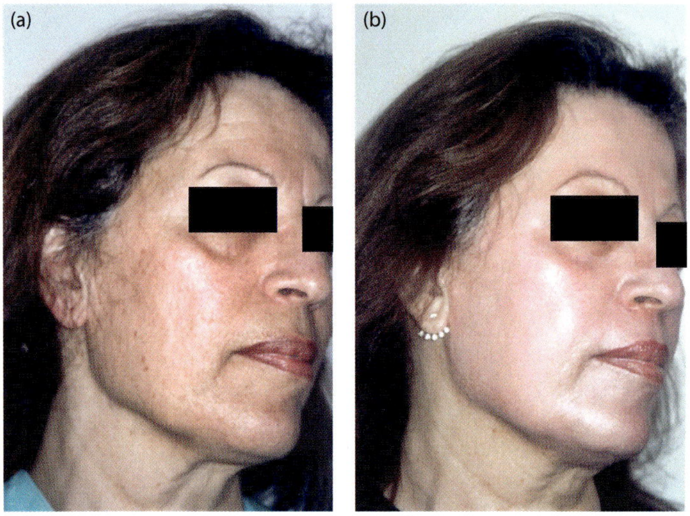

FIGURE 5.10 A 62-year-old Fitzpatrick 4 woman: (a) before and (b) 4 weeks after a deep peel combined with dermabrasion.

REFERENCES

1. Baker TM. Chemical and lasers for skin resurfacing. *Aesthetic Surg.* 1999;19:325–7.
2. Landau M. Chemical peels. *Clin Dermatol.* 2008;26:200–8.
3. Burton JL, Cunliffe WJ, Stafford I, Shuster S. The prevalence of acne vulgaris in adolescence. *Br J Dermatol.* 1971;85:119–26.
4. Rademaker M, Garioch JJ, Simpson NB. Acne in schoolchildren: No longer a concern for dermatologists. *BMJ* 1989;298:1217–9.
5. Cunliffe WJ, Gould DJ. Prevalence of facial acne vulgaris in late adolescence and in adults. *BMJ.* 1979;1:1109–10.
6. Layton AM, Henderson CA, Cunliffe WJ. A clinical evaluation of acne scarring and its incidence. *Clin Exp Dermatol.* 1994;19:303–8.
7. Handog EB, Datuin MS, Singzon IA. Chemical peels for acne and acne scars in Asians: Evidence based review. *J Cutan Aesthet Surg* 2012;5:239–46.
8. Holland DB, Jeremy AHT, Roberts SG, Seukeran DC, Layton AM. Inflammation in acne scarring: A comparison of the responses in lesions from patients prone and not prone to scar. *Br J Dermatol.* 2004;150:72–81.
9. Chuah SY, Goh CL. The impact of post acne scars on the quality of life among young adults in Singapore. *J Cutan Aesthet Surg.* 2015;8:153–8.
10. Kouris A, Platsidaki E, Christodoulous C, Efstathiou V, Markantoni V, Armyra K, Potouridou I, Rigopoulos D, Kontochristopoulos G. Patients' self-esteem before and after chemical peeling procedure. *J Cosmet Laser Ther.* 2017;29:1–3.
11. Bolton MA, Lobben I, Stern TA. The impact of body image on patient care. *Prim Care Companion J Clin Psychiatry.* 2010;12(2):PCC.10r00947.
12. Fife D. Evaluation of acne scars: How to assess them and what to tell the patient. *Dermatol Clin.* 2016;34:207–13.
13. Kurokawa I, Oiso N, Kawada A. Adjuvant alternative treatment with chemical peeling and subsequent iontophoresis for postinflammatory hyperpigmentation, erosion with inflamed red papules and non-inflamed atrophic scars in acne vulgaris. *J Dermatol.* 2017;44:401–5.
14. Sachdeva S. Lactic acid peeling in superficial acne scarring in Indian skin. *J Cosmet Dermatol.* 2010;9:246–8.
15. Ledon JA, Savas J, Franca K, Chacon A, Nouri K. Intralesional treatment for keloids and hypertrophic scars: A review. *Dermatol Surg.* 2013;39:1745–57.

16. Shah VV, Aldahan AS, Mlacker S, Alsaidan M, Samarkandy S, Nouri K. 5-Fluorouracil in the treatment of keloids and hypertrophic scars: A comprehensive review of the literature. *Dermatol Ther.* 2016;6:169–83.
17. Gauglitz G. Management of keloids and hypertrophic scars: Current and emerging options. *Clin Cosmet Investig Dermatol.* 2013;6:103–14.
18. Kant SB, van den Kerckhove E, Colla C, Tuinder S, van der Hulst RRWJ, Piatkowski de Grzymala AA. A new treatment of hypertrophic and keloid scars with combined triamcinolone and verapamil: A retrospective study. *Eur J Plast Surg.* 2018;41:69–80.
19. Jacob CI, Dover JS, Kaminer MS. Acne scarring: A classification system and review of treatment options. *J Am Acad Dermatol.* 2001;45:109–17.
20. Goodman GJ, Baron JA. Postacne scarring: A qualitative global scarring grading system. *Dermatol Surg.* 2006;32:1458–66.
21. Abdel Hay R, Shalaby K, Zaher H, Hafez V, Chi CC, Dimitri S, Nabhan AF, Layton AM. Interventions for acne scars. *Cochrane Database Syst. Rev.*. 2016;(4). Art. No.: CD011946.
22. Mackee GM, Karp FL. The treatment of post acne scars with phenol. *Br J Dermatol.* 1952;64:456–9.
23. Kurtin A. Corrective surgical planing of skin: New technique for treatment of acne scars and other skin defects. *AMA Arch Derm Syphilol.* 1953;68:389–97.
24. Orentreich N. Dermabrasion. *J Am Med Womens Assoc.* 1969;24:331–6.
25. Knapp TR, Kaplan EN, Danieks JR. Injectable collagen for soft tissue augmentation. *Plast Reconstr Surg.* 1977;60:398–405.
26. Forbat E, Ali FR, Al-Niaimi F. The role of fillers in the management of acne scars. *Clin Exp Dermatol.* 2017;42:374–80.
27. Goodman GJ, Van Den Broek A. The modified tower vertical filler technique for the treatment of post-acne scarring. *Australas J Dermatol.* 2016;57:19–23.
28. Halachmi S, Ben Amitai D, Lapidoth M. Treatment of acne scars with hyaluronic acid: An improved approach. *J Drugs Dermatol.* 2013;12:e121–3.
29. Epstein RE, Spencer JM. Correction of atrophic scars with Artefill: An open-label pilot study. *J Drugs Dermatol.* 2010;9:1062–4.
30. Goldberg DJ, Amin S, Hussain M. Acne scar correction using calcium hydroxylapatite in a carrier-based gel. *J Cosmet Laser Ther.* 2006;8(3):134–6.
31. Sadove R. Injectable poly-L-lactic acid: A novel sculpting agent for the treatment of dermal fat atrophy after severe acne. *Aesthetic Plast Surg.* 2009;33:113–6.
32. Sulamanidze MA, Salti G, Mascceti M, Sulamanidze GM. Wire scalpel for surgical correction of soft tissue contour defects by subcutaneous dissection. *Dermatol Surg.* 2000;26:146–50.
33. Garrett AB, Dufresne RG Jr, Ratz JL, Berlin AJ. Carbon dioxide laser treatment of pitted acne scarring. *J Dermatol Surg Oncol.* 1990;16:737–40.
34. Alster TS, West TB. Resurfacing of atrophic facial acne scars with a high-energy, pulsed carbon dioxide laser. *Dermatol Surg.* 1996;22:151–4.
35. Aust MC, Fernandes D, Kolokythas P, Kaplan HM, Vogt PM. Percutaneous collagen induction therapy: An alternative treatment for scars, wrinkles, and skin laxity. *Plast Reconstr Surg.* 2008;121:1421–9.
36. Fabbrocini G, Annunziata MC, D'Arco V, DeVita V, Lodi G, Mauriello C, Pastore F, Monfrecola G. Acne scars: Pathogenesis, classification and treatment. *Dermatol Res Prac.* 2010;(1687–6105). Article ID 893080.
37. Forbat E, Al-Niaimi F. Fractional radiofrequency treatment in acne scars: Systematic review of current evidence. *J Cosmet Laser Ther.* 2016;18:442–7.
38. Faghihi G, Poostiyan N, Asilian A, Abtahi-Naeini B, Shahbazi M, Iraji F, Fatemi Naeini F, Nilforoushzadeh MA. Efficacy of fractionated microneedle radiofrequency with and without adding subcision for the treatment of atrophic facial acne scars: A randomized split-face clinical study. *J Cosmet Dermatol.* 2017;16:223–9.
39. Al-Waiz MM, Al-Shagri AI. Medium-depth chemical peels in the treatment of acne scars in dark-skinned individuals. *Dermatol Surg.* 2002;28:383–7.
40. Puri N. Efficacy of modified Jessner's peel and 20% TCA versus 20% TCA peel alone for the treatment of acne scars. *J Cutan Aesthet Surg.* 2015;8:42–5.
41. Dalpizzol M, Weber MB, Mattiazzi AP, Manzoni AP. Comparative study of the use of Trichloroacetic Acid and Phenolic Acid in the treatment of atrophic-type acne scars. *Dermatol Surg.* 2016;4:377–83.

42. Leheta T, El Tawdy A, Abdel Hay R, Farid S. Percutaneous collagen induction versus full-concentration trichloroacetic acid in the treatment of atrophic acne scars. *Dermatol Surg.* 2011;37:207–16.
43. Lee JB, Chung WG, Kwahck H, Lee KH. Focal treatment of acne scars with trichloroacetic acid: Chemical reconstruction of skin scars method. *Dermatol Surg.* 2002;28:1017–21.
44. Agarwal N, Gupta LK, Khare AK, Kuldeep CM, Mittal A. Therapeutic response of 70% trichloroacetic acid CROSS in atrophic acne scars. *Dermatol Surg.* 2015;41:597–604.
45. Fabbrocini G, Cacciapuoti S, Fardella N, Pastore F, Monfrecola G. CROSS technique: Chemical reconstruction of skin scars method. *Dermatol Ther.* 2008;21(3):S29–32.
46. Nofal E, Helmy A, Nofal A, Alakad R, Nasr M. Platelet-rich plasma versus CROSS technique with 100% trichloroacetic acid versus combined skin needling and platelet rich plasma in the treatment of atrophic acne scars: A comparative study. *Dermatol Surg.* 2014;40:864–73.
47. Fintsi Y. Exoderm chemabrasion: Original method for the treatment of facial acne scars. *Int J Cosm Surg.* 1998;6:111–4.
48. Fintsi Y, Kaplan H, Landau M. Whether to peel or laser for acne scarring and hyperpigmentation. *Int J Cosm Surg.* 1999;7:67–70.
49. Park JH, Choi YD, Kim SW, Kim YC, Park SW. Effectiveness of modified phenol peel (Exoderm) on facial wrinkles, acne scars and other skin problems of Asian patients. *J Dermatol.* 2007;34:17–24.
50. Hetter G. An examination of the phenol-Croton oil peel: Part IV. Face peel results with different concentrations of phenol and Croton oil. *Plast Reconstr Surg.* 2000;105:1061–83; discussion 1084-7.
51. Rullan PP, Lemon J, Rullan J. The 2-day light phenol chemabrasion for deep wrinkles and acne scars: A presentation of face and neck peels. *Am J Cosm Surg.* 2004;21:15–26.
52. Stone PA. The use of modified phenol for chemical face peeling. *Clin Plast Surg.* 1998;25:21–44.
53. Nelson BR, Fader DJ, Gillard M, Majmudar G, Johnson TM. Pilot histologic and ultrastructural study of the effects of medium-depth chemical facial peels on dermal collagen in patients with actinically damaged skin. *J Am Acad Dermatol.* 1995;32:472–8.
54. Yug A, Lane JE, Howard MS, Kent DE. Histologic study of depressed acne scars treated with serial high-concentration (95%) trichloroacetic acid. *Dermatol Surg.* 2006;32(8):985–90.
55. Monheit GD. The Jessner's-trichloroacetic acid peel. An enhanced medium-depth chemical peel. *Dermatol Clin.* 1995;13:277–83.
56. Brody HJ, Hailey CW. Medium-depth chemical peeling of the skin: A variation of superficial chemosurgery. *J Dermatol Surg Oncol.* 1986;12:1268–75.
57. Coleman WP 3rd, Futrell JM. The glycolic acid trichloroacetic acid peel. *J Dermatol Surg Oncol.* 1994;20:76–80.
58. Stagnone JJ. Chemabrasion, a combined technique of chemical peeling and dermabrasion. *J Dermatol Surg Oncol.* 1977;3:217–9.
59. Carvalho Costa IM, Damasceno PS, Carvalho Costa M, Pati Gomez KG. Review in peeling complications. *J Cosmet Dermatol.* 2017;16:319–26.
60. Holm C, Muhlbauer W. Toxic shock syndrome in plastic surgery patients: Case report and review of the literature. *Aesthetic Plast Surg.* 1998;22:180–4.
61. Stagnone GJ, Orgel MB, Stagnone JJ. Cardiovascular effects of topical 50% trichloroacetic acid and Baker's phenol solution. *J Dermatol Surg Oncol.* 1987;13:999–1002.
62. Landau M. Cardiac complications in deep chemical peels. *Dermatol Surg.* 2007;33:190–3.

6

Microdermabrasion and Dermabrasion

Annie Chiu, Deirdre Hooper, and Katherine O. Brag

KEY FEATURES

- Dermabrasion and Microdermabrasion can be utilized to alone or in combination to improve acne scarring.
- Mechanical skin resurfacing involves using a handheld abrading instrument to remove layers of the epidermis, triggering wound healing and collagen remodeling to improve the appearance of acne scars.
- Dermabrasion, a more invasive and technically difficult procedure, involves the removal of skin down to the level of the papillary dermis and is very effective but associated with a higher risk of complications.
- Microdermabrasion, a less aggressive technique, involves abrasion of the superficial epidermis only and can improve milder scarring, especially when combined with simultaneous solution infusion. Most acne scar patients will require multiple treatments in combination with other modalities such as chemical peels and lasers.

Introduction

Mechanical skin resurfacing, which includes dermabrasion and microdermabrasion, involves using a handheld abrading instrument to remove layers of epidermis. The physical exfoliation process injures the skin, thereby triggering the stages of wound healing. By abrading atrophic or hypertrophic skin and inducing inflammation, re-epithelialization, fibroplasia, and collagen remodeling, the appearance of acne scars may improve. Dermabrasion, a more invasive and technically difficult procedure, involves the removal of skin down to the level of the papillary dermis. Microdermabrasion, a less aggressive technique, involves abrasion of the superficial epidermis only.

Dermabrasion

History

Human interest in skin resurfacing has existed for centuries and continues to undergo both innovative and somewhat cyclical modification. In 1500 BC, Ancient Egyptian physicians used sandpaper to flatten scars and sour milk baths to smooth dry, rough skin [1–3]. In 1905, Dr. Kromayer, a German dermatologist, first published an article describing his method of employing skin-planing instruments to improve the appearance of scars [4]. He described pre-treating the skin with local anesthetic and carbon dioxide "snow" to create a more turgid surface upon which to work. He used rotating handheld steel burs to smoothen smallpox and other traumatic scars [4,5]. His technique was expanded upon by Dr. Iverson, an American plastic surgeon, in 1947 when he reported successful removal of a traumatic facial tattoo using carpenter's sandpaper wrapped around a piece of gauze [6]. In 1948, Dr. McEvitt described significant

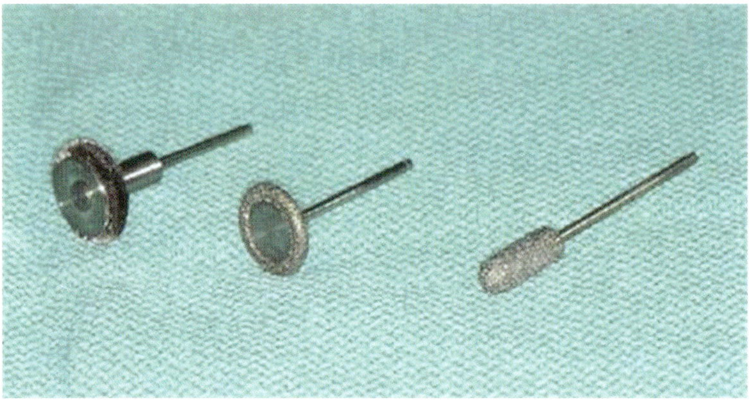

FIGURE 6.1 Commonly used dermabrasion end-pieces. From left to right: wire brush, diamond fraise, cone-shaped diamond fraise. (From Harmon CB, Thiele JJ. In: *Acne Scars*. Tosti A, De Padova MP, Beer K, eds. London: Informa, 2009, with permission [44].)

improvement in the appearance of acne scars using mechanical abrasion [7]. However, it was Dr. Kurtin, a dermatologist in New York City, who dramatically innovated and modernized dermabrasion starting in 1953 [8]. Dr. Kurtin and Noel Robbins worked together to modify a dental device for use in dermabrasion [1,8]. Dr. Kurtin's method involved pre-treating with ethyl chloride, an anesthetic and skin-hardener, then abrading with a motorized steel brush [8]. Robbins later went on to create the diamond fraise, a device still in use today [1]. Figure 6.1 illustrates some commonly used dermabrasion end-pieces.

In 1956, Dr. Burks, another American dermatologist, published *Wire Brush Surgery* in which he described his novel technique of employing a rotating wire brush to treat numerous conditions including rhytides, lentigines, acne keloidalis, and acne scars [9] (Figure 6.2). Then in 1957, he published a study

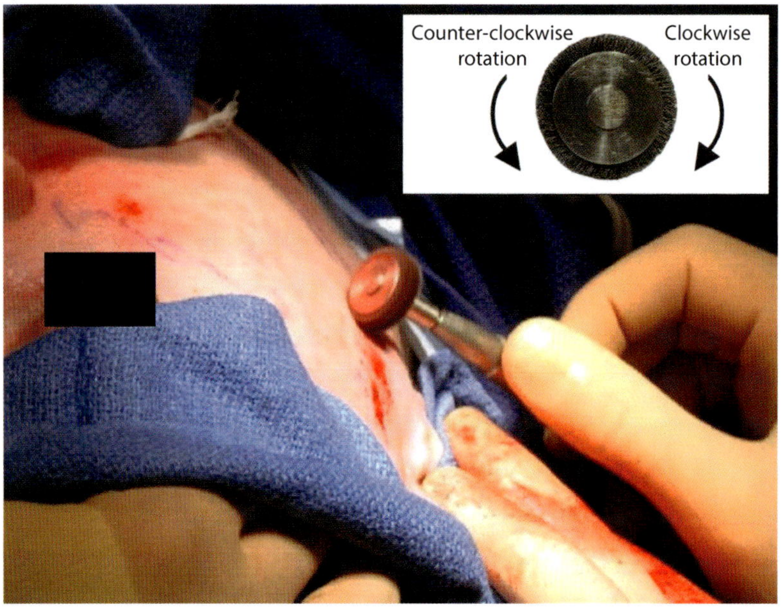

FIGURE 6.2 Demonstration of dermabrasion technique using a wire brush. The instrument is moved in strokes perpendicular to the direction of wire brush rotation. Top right insert: counterclockwise wire brush rotation for a more aggressive approach, and clockwise wire brush rotation for a less aggressive approach. (From Harmon CB, Thiele JJ. In: *Acne Scars*. Tosti A, De Padova MP, Beer K, eds. London: Informa, 2009, with permission [44].)

assessing wound healing after dermabrasion in approximately 1500 patients treated at the Tulane Medical Center in New Orleans [10]. Serial biopsies revealed epidermal regeneration from adnexal structures and remodeled connective tissue [10]. He subsequently reported on the use of microdermabrasion for solar damage [9,10]. Over time, studies further investigated the use and type of refrigerant coolants, applications of dermabrasion ranging from scar to traumatic tattoo treatment, anti-viral prophylaxis in patients with history of herpes labialis, pre-treating the skin with topical retinoid, and exercising caution in patients recently on oral isotretinoin [1]. To this point, dermabrasion was being used to reduce the appearance of scars that had often already achieved maturity at 6–12 months after scar formation. However, in 1988, Dr. Yarborough proposed dermabrading scars in the early post-injury period [11,12]. By treating young and still-evolving scars with dermabrasion, he found that scars could be essentially completely visibly effaced [12].

Pathophysiology

Dermabrasion removes skin layers until pinpoint bleeding is seen, indicating entry into the papillary dermis. By removing the entire epidermis, a partial thickness fresh wound is created and allowed to heal by secondary intention. Cell growth occurs from the wound bed upward, and from the lateral wound edges inward, with skin appendages being a main source of regenerative skin cells during the re-epithelialization process, hence the importance of abrading no deeper than the papillary dermis.

By creating a wound and inducing the three stages of wound healing (inflammation, proliferation, and remodeling), the skin is forced to renew itself, with an end goal of improved texture and coloration [3]. In the inflammation phase, platelets and extracellular matrix molecules form a fibrin clot, which by releasing chemoattractants, draws neutrophils to the wound [13]. Leucocytes adhere to the wound bed and release proinflammatory cytokines and angiogenic growth factors, attracting proliferative cells such as fibroblasts and endothelial cells, to the site [13]. Additionally, early in the healing process, keratinocytes at the wound edge lose cohesivity as they are induced to migrate over the wound bed [13]. Keratinocyte proliferation is stimulated by epidermal and dermal release of keratinocyte growth factor and hepatocyte growth factor [13]. During the proliferative phase, activated macrophages and fibroblasts converge to create granulation tissue [13]. Presence of macrophages and neutrophils also serves a key role in fighting infection at the wound site [13]. In the final remodeling phase, transforming growth factor-β stimulates fibroblasts to become myofibroblasts [3,13]. Myofibroblasts produce more collagen types I and III and over weeks to months, granulation tissue is converted to scar tissue, inflammation subsides, and vascular structures may regress [13–15].

Dermabrasion has been shown, on a histologic level, to increase the density of collagen bundles, increase the amounts of collagen types I and III, promote regular collagen arrangement parallel to the epidermis, and homogenize and organize elastic fibers. These changes underlie the improved skin texture and firmness noted after dermabrasion [14,15].

Indications

Despite the increase in popularity of laser resurfacing and chemical peels, dermabrasion remains the most effective treatment of acne scarring. Both atrophic and hypertrophic scars can be effectively dermabraded (Figure 6.3). For atrophic scars, the indentation itself and the adjacent normal tissue are abraded in order to blend and smooth the skin, creating a more even texture [16]. For hypertrophic scars, the excess scar tissue is abraded and an even plane is restored. Ice pick and boxcar acne scars are more likely to improve with dermabrasion than rolling scars [3,14]. Rolling scars are elongated, wide, ill-defined, and undulating due to scar tissue tethering the dermis to the subcutis [3]. Rolling scars may be better addressed with combination therapy such as subscision or punch excision followed by dermabrasion. Surgical or traumatic scars, burns, tattoos unresponsive to laser, rhinophyma, rhytides, benign adnexal neoplasms, lentigines, and actinic damage can also be treated with dermabrasion [17].

Surgical scars should be treated 6–8 weeks following the inciting operation, as shown by Yarborough and colleagues [11,12]. Numerous studies have confirmed this, particularly as it applies to treatment of Mohs surgery scars [18]. One split-scar model study showed the best outcomes when surgical scars

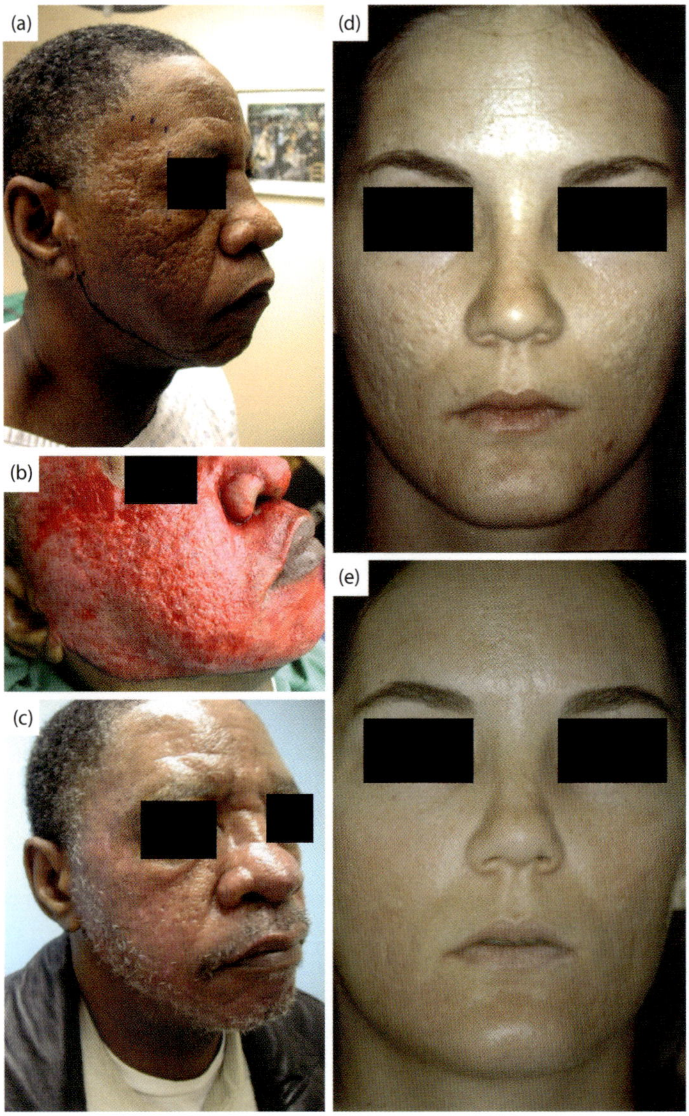

FIGURE 6.3 Dermabrasion for acne scars (a–e). Severe acne scarring in an African American man before dermabrasion (a), immediately after dermabrasion (b) and 4 weeks after dermabrasion (c). Moderately severe acne scarring in a Caucasian woman before dermabrasion (d) and 12 weeks after dermabrasion (e). (From Harmon CB, Thiele JJ. In: *Acne Scars*. Tosti A, De Padova MP, Beer K, eds. London: Informa, 2009, with permission [44].)

were treated at the eighth post-operative week [19]. Interestingly, Emsen found that treatment of burns with manual dermasanding should be done soon after burn injury and reported impressive results after dermasanding facial second degree superficial and partial deep burns in a child one day after the burn had occurred [20]. Hence, when to perform dermabrasion for scars varies by cause—for surgical scars, treatment at 6–8 weeks post-operative produces impressive results, and for burns, earlier is better.

Patient Selection and Pre-Operative Considerations

Before performing dermabrasion, certain measures can be taken to optimize outcomes and promote patient and provider safety. At the initial consultation visit, physicians must clearly explain the details of the procedure as well as the intensity of post-operative wound care. If a patient has a history of poor medical adherence, appointment attendance, or sun protection practices, dermabrasion should not be performed.

Dermabrasion should not be performed in patients with a history of any of the following: dyspigmentation, keloid formation, a bleeding disorder, active Koebnerizing skin disease, active severe rosacea or acne, or isotretinoin use in the last 6–12 months. Exercise caution when considering dermabrasion in patients with a history of immune suppression or chronic illness that may predispose to wound infection or impaired wound healing. In these instances, the decision to proceed must be made on a case-by-case basis. If there is an active infection or open wound in the intended treatment area, dermabrasion should be postponed. Re-treatment of a previously dermabraded area should be done no earlier than 12 months after the prior treatment [3,16].

Physicians may consider placing patients on a topical retinoid for 2–3 weeks before treatment to stimulate faster keratinocyte turnover. If the patient has a history of herpes labialis, anti-viral medication can be prescribed for 2–3 days before dermabrasion as outbreak prophylaxis. Anxious patients may benefit from oral or intramuscular sedation on the day of the procedure [3].

Equipment and Technique

Dermabrasion can be manual or motorized. Manual dermabrasion, also known as dermasanding, uses silicon carbide sandpaper of varying degrees of coarseness to resurface the skin. The paper can be purchased at the hardware store and sterilized in-office, or bought already sterilized and sealed [21]. An equally inexpensive alternative is a cautery-tip scratch pad—scratch pads, given their use in sterile operating room settings, come sterilized and sealed [22,23]. The scratch pad surface abrasiveness is between that of 100- and 60-grit sandpaper [22,23]. However, there is no difference in outcome or ability to reach ideal histologic depth when using the scratch pad versus sandpaper [21,24].

The paper or pad can be held in the physician's hand directly, or wrapped around a syringe barrel or piece of gauze for ease of use [23,25]. The paper or pad is moistened with saline before being applied to the skin. Sandpaper varies in coarseness: fine (#400), medium (#220–320), or coarse grade (#180) [16]. Coarser-grade paper is made of larger grit particles and is better suited to the initial debulking passes over the skin [16]. Finer grade paper is made of smaller grit particles and is better suited to smoothing and feathering after the more aggressive passes have been made [16].

There are many benefits of manual dermasanding. First, the technique is thought to provide better textural blending, especially around the eyes and mouth [16,18,21]. Additionally, there is no blood splattering or aerosolization of particles with manual dermasanding. Sensitive areas, such as eyelids, the vermilion border, and lobules cannot get caught in the device as can happen with mechanized instruments [16,18,21]. Finally, the equipment is inexpensive, easy to set up and operate, and requires no maintenance as it is disposed of with each use [16,18].

Despite resurgence in popularity of manual dermasanding, the development of motorized dermabrasion revolutionized the technique, allowing for faster and less physically demanding resurfacing of larger skin areas. This process requires both a motorized unit and an attachable abrasive tip. The more common power-driven units are the Bell Handengine (Bell International), the AEV-12 hand engine (Ellis International), and the Osada Surgical Handpiece (Osada, Inc.). The most common abrasive tips are the diamond fraise and the wire brush. The fraise is a metal cylinder of varying heights and circumferences encrusted with industrial-grade diamond fragments. The wire brush is a cylinder with protruding circumferential thin metal wires angled in the same direction. The brush is considered the more aggressive modality, achieving deeper abrasion with each pass than the fraise. For this reason, however, caution must be used with a wire brush to maintain an appropriate and consistent level of injury [3,16].

On the day of treatment, patients should present without makeup or jewelry on the intended treatment area. The patient should lie in the supine position. The treatment area should be cleansed, and then degreased using rubbing alcohol to remove any oil, residual makeup, or sunscreen from the skin. Both the patient and provider should wear eye protection. Anesthesia can be achieved with nerve block, local injection, tumescent anesthesia, or cryoanesthesia techniques. The skin should then be sterilized with chlorhexidine, being sure to avoid contact with the eyes and ears. Finally, the area can be covered with sterile drapes. With the motorized technique, pre-treatment of the area with a refrigerant spray provides a hard, consistent surface upon which to work [3,26].

To treat an area, the skin should be stretched between two fingers of the provider's non-dominant hand. The abrasive instrument, held in the provider's dominant hand, should be contacted with the skin and then moved linearly back and forth or in small circular motions over the treatment area. If using a diamond fraise motorized device, the tip should be run over the treatment area perpendicular to the direction of tip rotation. If using a wire brush, the wires protrude at an angle and are all pointing in the same direction. Less aggressive abrasion occurs when the rotation of the tip is in the same direction of the angulation of the wires. More aggressive abrasion occurs when the rotation of the tip is in the opposite direction of the angulation of the wires. Just as with the diamond fraise, the brush should be run over the skin perpendicular to the direction of the brush rotation. With all abrading instruments, the abrasive material should be passed over an area only until pinpoint bleeding is seen, indicating entry into papillary dermis. Areas with pinpoint bleeding should be abraded no further to prevent removal of adnexal structures and scar formation. If fibrous debris is seen, this indicates injury at the level of the reticular dermis. Throughout the procedure, blood and debris should be continuously wiped from the skin with wet cotton towels to keep the surgical site clean and visible. When using sandpaper, any residual silicon carbide particles remaining on the skin must be cleaned off to prevent formation of a pigmented tattoo. The face should be treated by cosmetic subunit with the central face being treated last [3].

Post-Operative Considerations

After the abrasion is complete, the entire surface should be gently wiped with a cotton towel. Then, gauze soaked in lidocaine/epinephrine can be applied to the skin to mitigate any post-operative stinging. Firm pressure should be held to more heavily bleeding areas for at least 10 minutes. A petrolatum-based ointment should then be applied to the treated area and a semipermeable dressing or full-face mask should be put in place. For the first 2–3 days, patients should present to the clinic daily to have the dressing changed. This can be quite painful and may require local anesthesia. Initial close in-office follow-up is essential for infection monitoring, dressing changes, wound-care discussions, and progress evaluation. After the third or fourth post-operative day, patients can start open wound care at home. The area should be soaked in 0.25% acetic acid four to six times daily with gentle debridement using a moistened cotton swab if needed. The acetic acid solution is used for both its antimicrobial and mild debridant properties. After each soak, ointment must be re-applied and a non-occlusive gauze dressing put in place. Patients should be warned that erythema and edema can be very pronounced in the first few hours to days following dermabrasion; nonsteroidal anti-inflammatory drugs and ice packs may alleviate the swelling and discomfort. As healing begins, pruritus may occur and should be treated with an anti-histamine medication to prevent scratching. At approximately the seventh post-operative day, re-epithelialization is nearly complete and the ointment can be exchanged for a thick moisturizer impregnated with SPF30+ sunscreen or physical sunblock [3].

Patients should be informed that erythema in the area may last for 2–4 months as tissue remodeling occurs. Disproportionate erythema or firm, fibrotic induration may indicate hypertrophic scar formation. Strict sun avoidance for 3–6 months after dermabrasion is essential [3].

Complications

Potential complications of dermabrasion include infection, scar formation, dyspigmentation, acne flare, and milia formation. Of these, acne flare and milia formation are the most likely but also the most treatable. Milia formation is a common complication of dermabrasion and typically occurs 3–4 weeks after the procedure. Extraction is an easy and effective means of treatment. Acne can be treated with appropriate medications but irritating or exfoliating topical treatments should be avoided until full re-epithelialization has occurred [3].

Infection and scar formation are the more concerning potential complications. Close post-operative follow-up allows for early detection and treatment of these conditions. Signs of infection include purulence, malodor, ulcerations, and frank abscess. If suspected, empiric antibiotics should be started with appropriate de-escalation depending on bacterial sensitivity if a culture swab is performed. At the earliest signs of scar formation, such as skin hardening or disproportionate erythema in the first 2–3 weeks, the area should be treated with super potent topical steroids. If there is persistent erythema or firm induration at 2–4 months, this may herald hypertrophic scar or keloid formation and demands immediate treatment with intralesional triamcinolone injections. If hyperpigmentation is noted, patients may begin combination treatment with hydroquinone and a topical retinoid as soon as 3–4 weeks after dermabrasion and continue for 4–8 weeks. In patients with darker Fitzpatrick types, hypopigmentation may occur and can be treated with a 305 nm excimer laser (Harmon). This should not be confused with pseudohypopigmentation in which the treated skin appears lighter than adjacent, untreated, sun damaged skin. Again, sun protection is of the utmost importance in minimizing long-term discoloration following dermabrasion. Camouflage makeup can be worn on patients with persistent post-operative dyschromia [3].

Results

If a well-trained dermatologic surgeon performs dermabrasion on the appropriate patient, the outcomes are excellent. Dermabrasion remains the gold standard for treatment of facial acne scarring. The clinical and histologic impact of dermabrasion is well-established. Pre- and post-dermabrasion biopsies revealed that after dermabrasion, there is an increase in dermal collagen bundle density and collagen bundles are arranged parallel to the skin surface [3]. Additional studies have confirmed that dermabrasion leads to increased deposition of collagen types I and III and homogenization of elastic fibers in the dermis [15]. Dermabrasion has been found to be superior to trichloroacetic acid (TCA) peels on a histopathological level [15]. While some argue that fractional ablative laser treatment is safer and produces less erythema than dermabrasion, both modalities have been shown to be equally as effective in treating post-surgical scars [27]. Studies have shown that manual dermasanding and motorized dermabrasion are equally as effective in reducing the appearance of surgical scars but that manual dermabrasion may be better in more sensitive areas, such as around the eyes and mouth, and that motorized dermabrasion may be better for larger surface areas, such as the entire face or an extremity [28,29].

Dermabrasion is a technically difficult procedure with the potential to produce suboptimal results if done too superficially and scarring if done too aggressively. Today, primarily dermatologic and plastic surgeons perform dermabrasion. Physicians should undergo intensive training with a skilled mentor before employing this technique independently as results vary greatly with provider experience and technical ability.

Microdermabrasion

Background

Microdermabrasion is a commonly performed superficial skin resurfacing treatment. In 2002, over one million patients underwent microdermabrasion in the United States [30]. Despite the steady increase in laser therapy resurfacing modalities and availability, microdermabrasion remains a popular aesthetic procedure, with an estimated average of at least 500,000 patients being treated annually [2]. Compared with dermabrasion, ablative laser therapy, and deeper chemical peels, microdermabrasion is relatively quick, inexpensive, non-invasive, and low-risk, all of which contribute to its persistent popularity among patients and providers.

In 1985, the Italian company, Molimed Engineering, created the first negative-pressure microdermabrasion unit. In 1988, Monteleone described using this new technique to treat facial scarring. By the early 1990s, the United States Food and Drug Association granted microdermabrasion devices an exempt status, leading to a surge in device manufacturing and usage. Microdermabrasion devices are now commonly found both in physicians' offices and non-medical aesthetic spas and microdermabrasion remains one of the frequently performed cosmetic procedures in the United States [30].

Pathophysiology

Microdermabrasion is intended to remove superficial layers of the epidermis. Treatment involves direct exfoliation with an abrasive instrument and aspiration of debris with a vacuum instrument. In theory, minor skin injury is being induced by both the abrasion and suction elements of treatment [2,16].

With the appropriate device settings, the stratum corneum, stratum granulosum, and partial stratum spinosum may be exfoliated. With each pass of the abrasive device across the skin surface, approximately 10–15 μm of epidermis are removed [2]. Two passes removes the stratum corneum, and four passes penetrates and partially abrades the stratum granulosum [2]. Microdermabrasion is neither designed nor intended for full-epidermal abrasion, as is the case for dermabrasion. However, the two modalities both seek to trigger the phases of skin healing to produce a more consistent, smooth, evenly pigmented skin surface. Given the superficiality of microdermabrasion, the "wound" created by treatment is thin and relatively bloodless, hence wound repair response is minimal compared with that of dermabrasion [2].

Biochemical and histological impact of microdermabrasion remains controversial. While studies have consistently shown transient changes in biochemical levels and epidermal architecture following microdermabrasion, permanence and depth of these changes appears limited [31–37]. In the days immediately following treatment, a more compacted stratum corneum with improved barrier function develops [2,31]. This is likely why patients and clinicians note improved skin smoothness and firmness in the immediate post-treatment period. These changes, however, appear to last only 1–2 weeks after treatment [30]. Karimipour and colleagues argue there is no change in epidermal barrier function indicated by stable levels of acetyl-conenzyme A (CoA) carboxylase and β-Hydroxy β-methylglutaryl-CoA reductase before and after treatment [32]. Investigations by Tsai et al. and Shim et al. analyzing skin biopsies on post-treatment sites noted superficial dermal edema and increased elastin, respectively [36,37]. Some researchers attribute this to the negative-pressure component of treatment rather than the abrasive component, but this has not yet been proven.

Changes in collagen types, density, and morphology following microdermabrasion have also been reported. Hernandez-Perez and Ibiett reported increased dermal fibrillar collagen, elastin, and rete formation after microdermabrasion in a small patient group [38]. Conversely, others have found increased levels of mediators of collagen production and remodeling but no change in dermal structure following treatment [34,35]. Karimipour and colleagues investigated the biochemical changes induced by microdermabrasion, and found that there were increased levels of wound healing factors including activator protein 1 and nuclear factor kappa B after a single microdermabrasion treatment [32,33]. They also reported increased levels of matrix metalloproteinases, mediators of collagen and extracellular matrix remodeling. However, they did not find an increase in collagen types I or III [32,33].

Patient Selection and Pre-Operative Considerations

Microdermabrasion is most commonly used to treat the following conditions: dry or rough skin, fine lines and wrinkles, solar damage, hyperpigmentation, and acne scarring [2,16,33,39]. Given the superficiality of abrasion with this modality, very shallow acne scars are more likely to improve with microdermabrasion than are rolling or hypertrophic scars. Additionally, acne scar patients considering treated with microdermabrasion should be counseled on variability outcomes and likely need for multiple regularly spaced treatments [2]. Acne scars may be better treated with any combination of microdermabrasion, chemical peels, and laser treatment, or with microdermabrasion with solution infusion [2,16,40–43] (Figures 6.4 and 6.5).

Patients of all Fitzpatrick types can undergo microdermabrasion, as the risk of hyperpigmentation after treatment is low [2]. However, caution is advised when treating patients with Fitzpatrick types IV–VI as hyperpigmentation is more likely in these patients [30]. Patients with an active skin infection at the potential treatment site, a history of keloids, isotretinoin use within the last 6–12 months, a history of a bleeding disorder, active koebnerizing skin disease, active severe rosacea or pustular acne, or poor sun protection practices should not undergo microdermabrasion [2].

Patients with a history of herpes labialis may receive a course of prophylactic anti-viral medication for 2–3 days before microdermabrasion. Patients must be advised to wear sunscreen judiciously throughout

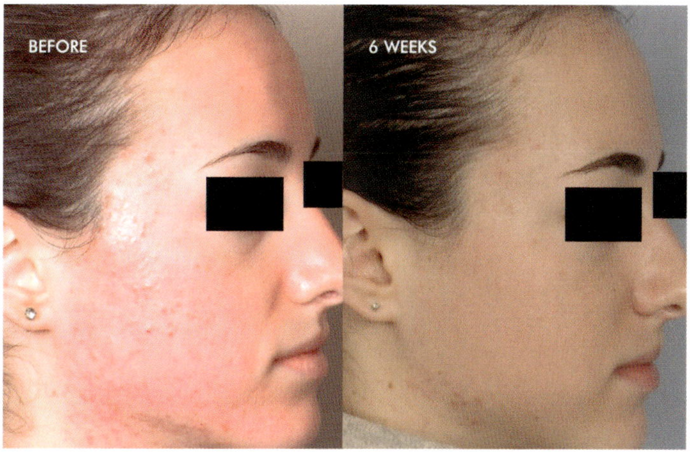

FIGURE 6.4 Results of microdermabrasion with solution infusion. Improvement in the appearance of acne and acne scarring after multiple treatments with microdermabrasion and Dermalinfusion using the SilkPeel device. (Photographs courtesy of Envy Medical.)

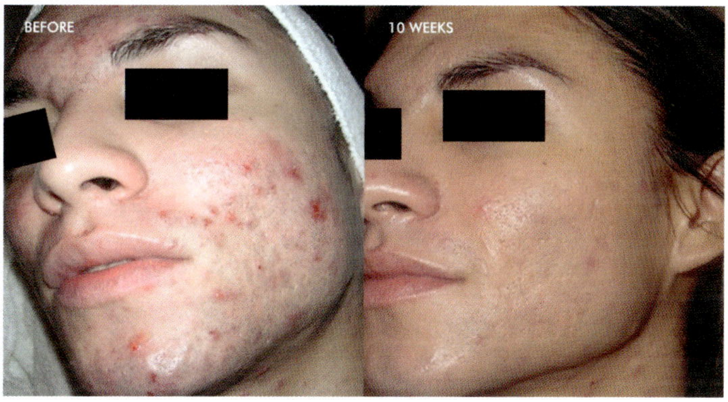

FIGURE 6.5 Results of microdermabrasion with solution infusion. Improvement in the appearance of acne and acne scarring after multiple treatments with microdermabrasion and Dermalinfusion using the SilkPeel device. (Photographs courtesy of Envy Medical.)

the treatment course and should avoid any chemical peels, depilatory treatments, or direct sun exposure to the treatment area starting at least 2 weeks before microdermabrasion [2].

Equipment

There are two essential functions of a microdermabrasion device: negative pressure and exfoliation. The negative pressure component of the device draws the treated skin into the abrasive component, providing firm contact between the skin and abrasive element and also aspirating loose particles and skin debris off of the skin surface. These contents are emptied into a waste container within the device. There are two main types of abrasive elements that are used: flowing crystals or diamond-tipped pads. The most commonly used crystals are aluminum oxide, measuring 100 μm wide (Tan). These very hard and insoluble particles have multifaceted sharp edges, making them effective abrasive elements (Tan). Crystals are blown across the skin and then aspirated back into the device along with cellular debris via negative pressure. Some such devices are the UltraPeel Crystal and UltraPeel II (Mattioli Engineering), MegaPeel Gold (DermaMed International) and ParisianPeel (Aesthetic Technologies). Crystal flow and negative pressure can be adjusted to alter how aggressive treatment is. Slower flow and less negative pressure both decrease the degree of abrasion [2].

Crystal-free devices have become increasingly common, as they circumvent issues associated with using loose crystals, such as residual dusty debris and potential ocular irritation. Diamond-tipped pads of varying coarseness can be attached to a device to achieve different, although still superficial, levels of abrasion. These heads are often reusable with sterilization after each use. Crystal-free devices may incorporate an infusion element in which medicated solutions are applied to the abraded skin. The solutions can target hyperpigmentation (hydroquinone, kojic acid, decapeptide-12), rosacea or acne (erythromycin, salicylic acid), dryness/roughness (glycerin, hyaluronic acid), or photodamage (vitamin C). This technique is called dermal infusion and one such device is the SilkPeel Dermalinfusion (Envy Medical). Another device, the MegaPeel EX (DermaMed International) allows for either crystal or pad modalities to be used. Certain combination devices have incorporated ultrasound or light-emitting diodes into treatment [2].

Technique

On the day of treatment, patients should present without makeup or jewelry on the intended treatment area. The treatment area should be cleansed, and then degreased using rubbing alcohol to remove any oil, residual makeup, or sunscreen from the skin. Both the patient and provider should wear eye protection, especially if a loose crystal-based system is being used. When treating the face, the patient should wear a hairband or surgical cap to keep hair away and improve visibility of the treatment area. No anesthesia is needed. Patients should rest in the supine position [2].

Before beginning, the device settings should be carefully determined. For crystal systems, higher crystal flow rate, higher vacuum pressure, and higher manual downward pressure of the device on the skin increase the depth of abrasion. For diamond-pad devices, coarser grit pads and higher vacuum pressure increase the depth of abrasion. For all devices, more passes over a specific area increases the depth of abrasion. If solution infusion will be incorporated, the appropriate solutions should be chosen. Two solutions for two different conditions can be used with one solution being applied during each of the two treatment passes [2].

To treat an area, the skin should be stretched between two fingers of the provider's non-dominant hand. The device, held in the provider's dominant hand, should be gently contacted with the skin, and, using even pressure, passed slowly over the treatment area parallel to the tension line produced by stretching the skin. It is important to note that with diamond-pad devices, exfoliation does not occur unless the device is moving. Two complete passes over an area are recommended. The second pass should move in strokes perpendicular to those of first pass. Passes are made starting medially and ending laterally. The eyelids and mucosal lips should not be treated. Mild erythema indicates sufficient treatment of an area. If there is pain (beyond mild discomfort), bleeding, petechiae or purpura, the treatment is too aggressive [2].

After treatment, patients must practice judicious sun protection for at least 2 weeks. Patients may note dryness, redness, and tingling lasting for a few days after treatment. Typically, patients undergo one microdermabrasion treatment every 2–4 weeks for six treatments. Maintenance treatments can be done at longer intervals. For certain conditions, especially acne scarring, fifteen or more treatments may be needed to see improvement [2,16,30].

Results

Patients are generally very satisfied with the outcomes of microdermabrasion and report improved skin texture and coloration after one treatment [30]. However, multiple treatments are needed to achieve more noticeable clinical improvement. Studies have shown that patients and lay people but not clinicians noticed reduction in fine lines and wrinkles after eight once-weekly treatments [30]. Improvement in the appearance of sun damaged skin (solar lentigines, dullness, fine lines) and acne with microdermabrasion with the application of topical solutions occurs after at least six microdermabrasion treatments in most reports [2,30,39]. Microdermabrasion with Dermalinfusion of a skin lightening solution may improve post-inflammatory hyperpigmentation after just four treatments [42] (Figure 6.6).

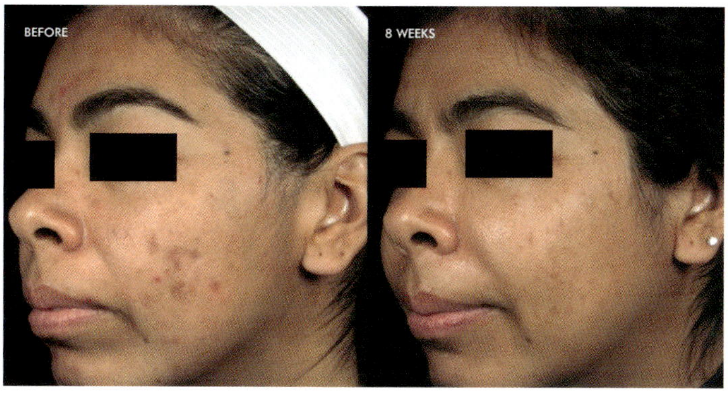

FIGURE 6.6 Results of microdermabrasion with solution infusion. Improvement in the appearance of acne scarring and post-inflammatory hyperpigmentation after multiple treatments with microdermabrasion and Dermalinfusion using the SilkPeel device. (Photographs courtesy of Envy Medical.)

To reduce the appearance of acne scars, more than six treatments are generally needed [2,30]. Tsai et al. found that patients required an average of nine treatments when using aluminum oxide crystal devices to reduce the appearance of all kinds of facial scarring [36]. However, to obtain good-to-excellent results, the study found acne scar patients needed an average of 15 treatments and some patients needed as many as 40 treatments to see results [36]. Another study by El-Domyati and colleagues investigated the clinical and histologic impact of microdermabrasion on melasma, acne scars, and striae distensae after eight treatment sessions [31]. In the melasma group, mild-to-moderate improvement in dyspigmentation was noted clinically and decreased melanization and more regular distribution of melanosomes was noted histologically [31]. In the acne scar group, patients with superficial erythematous acne scars showed the greatest improvement compared with patients with rolling, ice pick, or boxcar scars [31]. Histologically, these patients had more regular collagen bundle arrangement and increased collagen density, but no change in elastic fiber density or arrangement [31]. In the striae distensae group, erythematous lesions responded better than hypopigmented lesions; there was no statistically significant difference in epidermal thickness but again, these patients had more regular collagen bundle arrangement and increased collagen density [31].

Combination resurfacing treatments, such as a combination of microdermabrasion with chemical peeling, or microdermabrasion with laser therapy, may provide better results [40–43]. Lee and colleagues found that the combination of a 595 nm pulsed-dye laser, 755 nm alexandrite laser, and microdermabrasion improved the roughness and brawny discoloration associated with keratosis pilaris [43]. Another study found that both microdermabrasion treatments and salicylic acid treatments increase dermal collagen but that salicylic acid is slightly superior [41]. A combination of microdermabrasion followed by 5% retinoic acid peel was found to improve the clinical appearance of sun damaged skin better than microdermabrasion alone and both were well-tolerated and safe [40].

REFERENCES

1. Lawrence N, Mandy S, Yarborough J. History of dermabrasion. *Dermatol Surg.* 2000;26(2):95–101.
2. Small R, Quema R. Microdermabrasion. In: *Dermatologic and Cosmetic Procedures in Office Practice.* Usatine RP, ed. Saunders, Philadelphia, PA. 2012, 274–85.
3. Harmon C, Thiele J. Dermabrasion for acne scars. In: *Acne Scars: Classification and Treatment.* Tosti A, De Padova MP, Beer K, eds. Boca Raton, FL: CRC Press, 2010, 42–8.
4. Kromayer E. Rotation instruments: A new technical procedure in dermatological small surgery. *Dermatol Z.* 1905;12:26.
5. Kromayer E. *Cosmetic Treatment of Skin Complaints.* New York: Oxford University Press, 1930. (English translation of the second German edition, 1929).
6. Iverson P. Surgical removal of traumatic tattoos of the face. *Plast Reconstr Surg.* 1947;2427–32.

7. McEvitt, WG. Treatment of acne pits by abrasion with sandpaper. *JAMA*. 1950;142:647–8.
8. Kurtin A. Corrective surgical planing of the skin. *Arch Dermatol Syphil.* 1953;68:389.
9. Burks J. *Wirebrush Surgery*. Springfield, IL: Charles C Thomas, 1955.
10. Burks J. Abrasive removal of scars. *South Med J.* 1955;48:452–9.
11. Yarborough J, Beeson WD, Beeson W, McCullough E. *Aesthetic Surgery of the Aging Face.* St Louis, Mo.: CV Mosby Co., 1986, 142–81.
12. Yarborough J. Ablation of facial scars by programmed dermabrasion. *J Dermatol Surg Oncol.* 1988; 33: 14292–4.
13. Eming S. Biology of wound healing. In: *Dermatology.* 3rd ed. Bolognia JL, Jorizzo JL, Schaffer JV, eds. Elzevier, Philadelphia, PA. 2012, 2313–25.
14. Harmon C, Zelickson B, Roenigk R et al. Dermabrasive scar revision: Immunohistochemical and ultrastructural evaluation. *Dermatol Surg.* 1995;21503–8.
15. El-Domyati M, Attia S, Saleh F. Trichloracetic acid peeling versus dermabrasion: A histometric, immunohistochemical, and ultrastructural comparison. *Dermatol Surg.* 2004;30(2):179–88.
16. Monheit G, Chastain M. Chemical and mechanical skin resurfacing. In: *Dermatology.* 3rd ed. Bolognia JL, Jorizzo JL, Schaffer JV, eds. Elzevier, Philadelphia, PA. 2012, 2493–508.
17. Fulton J. Dermabrasion, chemabrasion, and laserabrasion: Historical perspectives, modern dermabrasion techniques, and future trends. *Dermatol Surg.* 1996;22(7):619–28.
18. Zisser M, Kaplan B, Moy R. Surgical pearl: Manual dermabrasion. *JAAD.* 1995;33(1):105–6.
19. Katz B, Oca A. A controlled study of the effectiveness of spot dermabrasion ("scarabrasion") on the appearance of surgical scars. *J Am Acad Dermatol.* 1991;24:462–6.
20. Emsen I. Effect of dermasanding (manual dermabrasion) with sandpaper on appearance of both post-surgical and burn scars. *Aes Plast Surg.* 2007;31(5):608–11.
21. Emsen I. A different and cheap method: Sandpaper (manual dermasanding) in treatment of periorbital wrinkles. *J Craniofac Surg.* 2008;19(3):812–6.
22. Zaimi I, Romanzi A, Gherardini G. Tricks and tips for manual dermabrasion. *Dermatol Surg.* 2016;42(12):1393–4.
23. Landau M. Commentary on tricks and tips for manual dermabrasion. *Dermatol Surg.* 2016;42(12):1395.
24. Kidwell W, Apprey C, Messingham M. A comparison of histologic effectiveness and ultrastructural properties of the electrocautery scratch pad to sandpaper for manual dermabrasion. *Dermatol Surg.* 2008;34(9):1194–9.
25. Pavlidis L, Spyropolou G-A. A simple technique to perform manual dermabrasion with sandpaper. *Dermatol Surg.* 2012;38(12):2016–7.
26. Wilson J, Ayres S, Luikart R. Mixtures of fluorinated hydrocarbons as refridgerated aesthetic. *Arch Dermatol.* 1956;74:310–11.
27. Christophel J, Elm C, Edrizzi B. A randomized controlled trial of fractional laser therapy and dermabrasion for scar resurfacing. *Dermatol Surg.* 2012;38(4):595–602.
28. Poulos E, Taylor C, Solish N. Effectiveness of dermasanding on appearance of surgical scars: A prospective randomized blinded study. *Derm Surg.* 2002;48(6):897–900.
29. Gillard M, Wang T, Boyd C. Conventional diamond fraise versus manual spot dermabrasion with drywall sanding screen for scars from skin cancer surgery. *Arch Dermatol.* 2002;138(8):1035–9.
30. Nahm W, Rotunda A, Han K, Schmidt A, Moy R. Microdermabrasion for treatment of photoaging. In: *Photoaging.* Rigel D, Weiss R, Lim H, Dover J, eds. New York: Marcel Dekker, 2004, 95–110.
31. El-Domyati M, Hosam W, Abdel-Azim E, Abdel-Wahab H, Mohamed E. Microdermabrasion: A clinical, histometric, and histopathologic study. *J Cosmet Dermatol.* 2016;15(4):503–13.
32. Karimipour D, Kang S, Johnson T et al. Microdermabrasion: A molecular analysis following a single treatment. *J Am Acad Dermatol.* 2005;52:215–23.
33. Karimipour D, Karimipour G, Orringer J. Microdermabrasion: An evidence-based review. *Plast Reconstr Surg.* 2010;125(1):372–7.
34. Kirkland E, Hantash B. Microdermabrasion: Molecular mechanisms unraveled, part 1. *J Drugs Dermatol.* 2012;11(9):e2–9.
35. Kirkland E, Hantash B. Microdermabrasion: Molecular mechanisms unraveled, part 2. *J Drugs Dermatol.* 2012;11(9):e10–17.
36. Tsai R, Wang C, Chan H. Aluminum oxide crystal microdermabrasion: A new technique for treating facial scarring. *Dermatol Surg.* 1995;21:539–42.

37. Shim E, Barnette D, Hughes K, Greenway H. Microdermabrasion: A clinical and histopathologic study. *Dermatol Surg*. 2001;27:524–30.
38. Hernandez-Perez E, Ibiett E. Gross and microscopic findings in patients undergoing microdermabrasion for facial rejuvenation. *Dermatol Surg*. 2001;27(7):637–40.
39. Tan M, Spencer J, Pires LM, Amjeri J, Skover G. The evaluation of aluminum oxide cystal microdermabrasion for photodamage. *Dermatol Surg*. 2001;28:745–50.
40. Faghihi G, Fatemi-Tabaei S, Abtahi-Naeini B et al. The effectiveness of a 5% retinoic acid peel combined with microdermabrasion for facial photoaging: A randomized, double-blind, placebo-controlled clinical trial. *Dermatol Res Pract*. 2017;2017:8516527.
41. Abdel-Motaleb A, Abu-Dief E, Hussein M. Dermal morphological changes following salicylic acid peeling and microdermabrasion. *J Cosmet Dermatol*. 2017, 16(4):e9-e14.
42. Bhatia A, Hsu J, Hantash B. Combined topical delivery and dermalinfusion of decapeptide-12 accelerates resolution of post-inflammatory hyperpigmentation in skin of color. *J Drugs Dermatol*. 2014;13(1):84–5.
43. Lee S, Choi M, Zheng Z, Chung W, Kim Y, Cho S. Combination of 595-nm pulsed dye laser, long-pulsed 755-nm alexandrite laser, and microdermabrasion treatment for keratosis pilaris: Retrospective analysis of 26 Korean patients. *J Cosmet Laser Ther*. 2013;15(3):150–4.
44. Harmon CB, Thiele JJ. Dermabrasion for acne scars. In: *Acne Scars*. Tosti A, De Padova MP, Beer K, eds. London: Informa, 2009.

7

Fillers for Acne Scarring

Karin Eshagh and Sabrina Fabi

KEY FEATURES

- The advent of fillers has provided a new host of approaches to atrophic acne scarring which can be a psychologically distressing condition.
- The properties of each filler (i.e. particle size, cross-linking, gel hardness) allow them to target certain types of scars better than others.
- Hyaluronic acid is the most commonly used temporary filler for the treatment of acne scars and can be injected immediately beneath the scars.
- Calcium hydroxylapatite and Poly-L-lactic acid are semi-permanent fillers with a biostimulary effect that increases collagen production. Thus, these fillers can be useful for a greater extent of dermal atrophy.
- Polymethylmethacrylate (PMMA), also known as Bellafill, is the only dermal filler on the market that is approved for the treatment of acne scars. Due to the use of bovine collagen, a skin test is required prior to injection.
- Autologous fat transfer can be useful for acne scarring if attempting to replete significant areas of volume deficit in the face.

Acne and the Impact of Scarring

Acne is one of the most common inflammatory skin diseases, affecting nearly 80% of adolescent boys and girls [1]. Unfortunately, most cases lead to scarring that persists into adulthood, causing psychological distress. While different therapies have previously been used, such as chemical peels or microneedling, the advent of fillers has opened a new field of revolumizing atrophic acne scars, that is, rolling or boxcar type of scars. Many studies have demonstrated that injectable fillers have been effective for the treatment of atrophic scars, and some have evaluated the long-term outcomes.

In this chapter we will focus on the different types of dermal fillers and fat transfer techniques used for the purpose of volumizing atrophic scars. There are several variables that contribute to the unique qualities and clinical effects of fillers, including particle size, degree of high-molecular-weight hyaluronic acid (HA) versus low-molecular-weight HA, HA concentration per mL of gel, cross-linked versus free HA, HA alignment, viscosity, cohesiveness of a gel, extrusion force, gel hardness (G'), or rheological (flow) properties, as measured by stored energy deferred upon passage through a syringe and then restored to an expanded viscoelastic state. Table 7.1 lists the properties of commonly used United States Food and Drug Association (FDA)-approved HA, calcium hydroxylapatite (CaHA), poly-L-lactic acid (PLLA) and polymethylmethacrylate (PMMA) fillers in the United States.

Dermal fillers can be divided into temporary (i.e., HA fillers), semi-permanent (lasting up to 2 years) (i.e., CaHA and PLLA), and permanent (lasting longer than 3 years) (i.e., PMMA), and there is also the option of fat transfer. Given the varying facial deficits, skin thickness among patients, and different biochemical properties of each injectable, certain dermal fillers are best suited for the each type of scar and region of the face.

TABLE 7.1

Commonly Used FDA-Approved HA, CaHA, PLLA, and PMMA Fillers in the United States

Filler Type	Compound	Approved Indications and Other Commonly Used Indications	Author Injection Depth	Syringe and Needle Size
Belotero (Merz Pharma, Greensboro, NC, USA) 22.5 mg/mL: particles are not "sized" and they are not broken apart into smaller particles	Cross-linked HA stabilized by butanediol-diglycidyl ether (BDDE); not completely hydrated in the syringe—will bind water and slightly expand within 24 hours	Temporarily smooth out and fill in moderate-to-severe facial wrinkles and nasolabial folds	Mid-to-deep dermis	1 mL and 30 Gauge 1/2 inch needle
Prevelle Silk (Genzyme Biosurgery, Cambridge, MA, USA) 5.5 mg/mL: particle size of 500 μm (Mentor Worldwide LLC, Santa Barbara, CA, USA, and Genzyme Corportation, Cambridge, MA, USA)	93% cross-linked HA with DVS—completely hydrated in syringe, will not expand after injection	Correction of moderate-to-severe facial wrinkles and folds (such as nasolabial folds). Lasting 4–6 months	Mid-to-deep dermis	1 mL and 30 G 1/2 inch needle
Restylane Silk (Galderma Laboratories, Forth Worth, TX, USA) 20 mg/mL: particle size of 50–220 μm 250,000 gel particles/mL HA	HA gel (20 mg/mL), cross-linked with BDDE, stabilized and suspended in phosphate-buffered saline at pH 7, with 0.3% lidocaine	Correction of moderate-to-severe facial wrinkles and folds (such as nasolabial folds, and for lip augmentation, perioral rhytids). Lasts up to 6 months	Mid-to-deep dermis for facial folds, submucosal for lips	1 mL and 30 G 1/2 inch needle
Restylane and Restylane L (Galderma Laboratories, Fort Worth, TX, USA) 20 mg/mL: particle size of ~259–300 μm 100,000 gel particles/mL	1% cross-linked HA stabilized by BDDE—not completely hydrated in the syringe	Correction of moderate-to-severe facial wrinkles and folds (such as nasolabial folds and submucosal lip augmentation in patients over the age of 21 years). Infraorbital hallows "tear troughs," marionettes, and acne scars. Lasts up to 6–12 months	Subdermal	1 mL and 0.5 mL, and 29 G 1/2 inch needle
Restylane Lyft-L (Galderma Laboratories, L.P., Fort Worth, TX) 20 mg/mL: particle size of ~259–300 μm 100,000 gel particles/mL	1% cross-linked HA stabilized by BDDE—not completely hydrated in the syringe	Cheek augmentation and the correction of age-related midface contour deficiencies in patients over the age of 21 years. Also for the treatment of moderate-to-severe facial wrinkles and folds (such as nasolabial folds and smile lines). Last 6–12 months	Deep subdermal	1 and 2 mL, 27 G 1/2 inch needle
Restylane Refyne (Galderma Laboratories, Forth Worth, TX, USA) 20 mg/mL (manufactured using XpresHAn Technology)	HA with moderate lifting capacity. Sodium hyaluronate concentration of 20 mg/mL in phosphate-buffered saline at pH 7 and contains 3 mg/mL lidocaine hydrochloride	Correction of moderate-to-severe facial wrinkles and folds in patients over the age of 21 years. Lasts up to 12 months	Mid-to-deep dermis	30 G 1/2 inch needle

(Continued)

TABLE 7.1 *(Continued)*

Commonly Used FDA-Approved HA, CaHA, PLLA, and PMMA Fillers in the United States

Filler Type	Compound	Approved Indications and Other Commonly Used Indications	Author Injection Depth	Syringe and Needle Size
Restylane Defyne (Galderma Laboratories, Fort Worth, TX, USA) 20 mg/mL (manufactured using XpresHAn Technology)	HA concentration of 20 mg/mL in phosphate-buffered saline at pH 7 and contain 3 mg/mL lidocaine hydrochloride (differs from Refyne based on more cross-linking and larger calibration size of grid used to extrude gel)	Correction of moderate-to-severe, deep facial wrinkles and folds in patients over the age of 21 years. Lasts up to 12 months	Mid-to-deep dermis	1 mL, 27 G 1/2 inch needle
Juvederm Ultra XC (Allergan, Irvine, CA, USA) 24 mg/mL: particles are not "sized" as they undergo Hylacross technology	9% cross-linked HA stabilized by BDDE (more homogeneous gel than Restylane and Perlane)—not completely hydrated in the syringe	Correction of moderate-to-severe facial wrinkles and folds (such as nasolabial folds). Lasts up to 12 months	Subdermal	1 mL, 0.4 mL, 30 G 1/2 inch needle
Juvederm Volbella XC (Allergan, Irvine, CA, USA) 15 mg/mL: particles are not "sized" as they undergo Vycross tecnhology	15 mg/mL mixture of low- and high-molecular-weight HA, which allows for efficiency cross-linking, resulting in highly cohesive gel and greater hardness w/w 0.3% lidocaine in a physiologic buffer	Improve lip volume and smooth lines around the mouth in adults over age 21 years. Can last for 1 year	Dermis Typical volume used for lips and perioral area is 2.6 mL	30 G 1/2 inch needle
Juvederm Vollure XC (Allergan, Irvine, CA, USA) 17.5 mg/mL: particles are not "sized" as they undergo Vycross tecnhology	17.5 mg/mL mixture of low- and high-molecular-weight HA, which allows for efficiency cross-linking, resulting in highly cohesive gel and greater hardness w/w 0.3% lidocaine in a physiologic buffer	Correction of moderate-to-severe facial wrinkles and folds (such as nasolabial folds). Lasts up to 18 months in people over 21 years of age	Mid-to-deep dermis	27 G 1 inch for lips, or fine wrinkles 30 G 1/2 inch needle
Juvederm Voluma XC (Allergan, Irvine, CA, USA) 20 mg/mL: particles are not "sized" as they undergo Vycross tecnhology	20-mg/mL mixture of low- and high-molecular-weight HA, which allows for efficiency cross-linking, resulting in highly cohesive gel and greater hardness w/w 0.3% lidocaine in a physiologic buffer	Deep (subcutaneous and/or supraperiosteal) injection for cheek augmentation to correct age-related volume deficit in the midface in adults over the age of 21 years. Lasts up to 2 years	Deep subcutaneous, supraperiosteal	1 mL, 25 G 1/2 inch needle, and 27 G 1/2 inch needle
Radiesse-Microsphere (Merz Aesthetics, Inc., Raleigh, NC), microspheres of calcium hydroxylapatite 20–45 μm, microporous with pores of 25–45 μm in size, combined with carboxymethylcellulose carrier gel, water, and glycerin	70% carrier gel, 30% is CaHA microspheres	Treatment of moderate-to-severe wrinkles and folds, and midfacial volumization, chin, prejowl sulcus, and jawline. Subdermal implantation for hand augmentation to correct volume in the dorsum of the hands. Lasts 12–18 months	Subdermal injection or supraperiosteal	1.5, 0.8, 0.3 mL, 27 G

(Continued)

TABLE 7.1 (Continued)

Commonly Used FDA-Approved HA, CaHA, PLLA, and PMMA Fillers in the United States

Filler Type	Compound	Approved Indications and Other Commonly Used Indications	Author Injection Depth	Syringe and Needle Size
Sculptra Aesthetic (Galderma, Dallas, TX, USA) microspheres of PLLA 40–63 μm: particle size 140,000, in a suspension of sodium carboxymethylcellulcse and nonpyrogenic mannitol	Irregular product shape of PLLA as well as heavy molecular weight contributes to slow absorption. Sculptra comes as powder, and once reconstituted with 5–9 mL of sterile water, consists of 367.5 mg of poly-L-lactic acid per 5–9 mL	Use in shallow-to-deep nasolabial fold contour deficiencies and other facial wrinkles such as HIV-related facial lipoatrophy. Lasts up to 25 months	Subcutaneous plane, supraperiosteal	25- or 26-gauge
Bellafill (SUNEVA, San Diego, CA, USA) PMMA microspheres 30–50 μm in diameter	Injectable bovine collagen (sourced from calves) with non-resorbable PMMA microspheres. suspended in a water-based carrier gel composed of 3.5% bovine collagen, 92.6% buffered, isotonic water, 0.3% lidocaine hydrochloride, 2.7% phosphate buffer, 0.9% sodium chloride	Correction of nasolabial folds and moderate-to-severe, atrophic, distensible facial acne scars on the check in patients over 21 years old. Lasts up to 5 years	Dermis. A prior skin test is required to check for hypersensitivity to bovine collagen	0.8 mL syringe, 26 G 1/2 inch needle
Silikon 1000 (Alcon, Fort Worth, TX, USA)	10 mL vial containing 8.5 mL purified silicone oil without preservatives	Indicated for use as a prolonged retinal tamponade in cases of complicated retinal detachment	Dermis	28 G, 1/2 inch needle

w/w: weight/weight.

Temporary Fillers

Collagen

Historically, some of the earlier fillers that were used by practitioners were known as the human- or bovine-derived collagen fillers. Zyderm is a bovine-derived collagen filler. It is injected with a 30- to 32- gauge needle into the superficial papillary dermis, and hence it works well for superficial etched-in lines. Zyderm is not highly favored by injectors as it is short lasting (3–5 months) and requires prior skin testing. Cosmoderm and Cosmoplast are made of collagen derived from human fibrocytes. They are the only FDA-approved dermal fillers that contain human collagen; however, they have been stripped of any antigenic determinants so that skin testing is not required. Unfortunately, flu-like symptoms have been seen in up to 4% of patients treated with the human-derived collagen fillers, and these fillers should not be injected if a patient has had an allergic reaction to lidocaine in the past.

While Cosmoderm is injected into the superficial papillary dermis, Cosmoplast is injected into the mid-to-deep reticular dermis. Also, Cosmoderm is diluted with saline and requires overcorrection [2]. Thus, while Cosmoplast works well for facial lines and the vermilion borders of lips, Cosmoderm can be used over it to treat the remaining fine lines. Today, most practitioners do not use these types of fillers, and there are no studies that recommend their use for acne scars.

Hyaluronic Acid

HA fillers are temporary fillers composed of glycosaminoglycan polysaccharides. They are most commonly used to add volume to the aging face [3]. Non-animal-derived synthetic HA is the most commonly used injectable HA, and is generated from bacterial (*Streptococcus*) fermentation. Once purified, the polymer chains are cross-linked for stability. It is this cross-linking procedure, and its variation both in percentage and technique, that determines the monophasic or biphasic nature of the resulting injectable. When the HA and cross-linking polymers are synthesized by mixing in a single step, they are monophasic monodensified fillers, such as Juvederm Ultra XC, Juvederm Ultra Plus XC, Juvederm Volbella XC, Juvederm Vollure XC, and Juvederm Voluma XC. If additional HA of a different density is added after the initial step, the filler is considered poly-densified, such as Belotero. Biphasic gels are "sized" in a process by which cross-linked HA is pushed through a specially sized screen and broken into pieces, with small-sized pieces making up Prevelle Silk and Restylane Silk, medium-sized pieces made into Restylane, and larger ones made into Restylane Lyft. These particles are suspended in a noncross-linked HA, which acts as a lubricant. HA gels that have the same amount of HA concentration, but vary in the degree of cross-linker added, and then are passed through a sieve for a smaller particle gel, makeup Restylane Refyne and a larger particle gel makeup Restylane Defyne. The most significant difference between the injectable fillers in this category is the size of the particles.

The majority of HA gels are approved for the correction of moderate-to-severe facial wrinkles and folds, such as the nasolabial folds, while some have an indication for lip augmentation and the correction of moderate-to-severe midface volume loss. HA gels are routinely used for many facial indications, including the temple and infra-orbital hallows, jawline and chin volume loss, nasal contour, as well as acne scars (Figures 7.1 and 7.2).

Although they are identified as temporary fillers, the injection of HA fillers into the deep layers of dermis has been shown to stimulate fibroblasts to produce collagen, and this can lead to a permanent benefit with little to no side effects [4]. Interestingly, even as the individual molecules of HA are degraded over time, the remaining molecules are able to bind more water and thus maintain the original volume of the filler until the last molecule has been degraded [2].

In one study, a 39-year-old woman with a combination of rolling-type, boxcar, ice pick, and broad atrophic scars, totaling 58 scars, received treatment with 1.05 mL of HA filler, Juvederm Voluma (20 mg/mL, Allergan Australia, Sydney New South Wales, Australia). A 31-gauge needle on an insulin syringe was positioned at 90° into the deeper dermis of each scar. About 0.02–0.04 mL of product was injected with a gradual tapering retrograde deposition "tower technique" as the needle was withdrawn in order to inject more product closer to the skin surface, creating a pyramid-like pillar of product under the

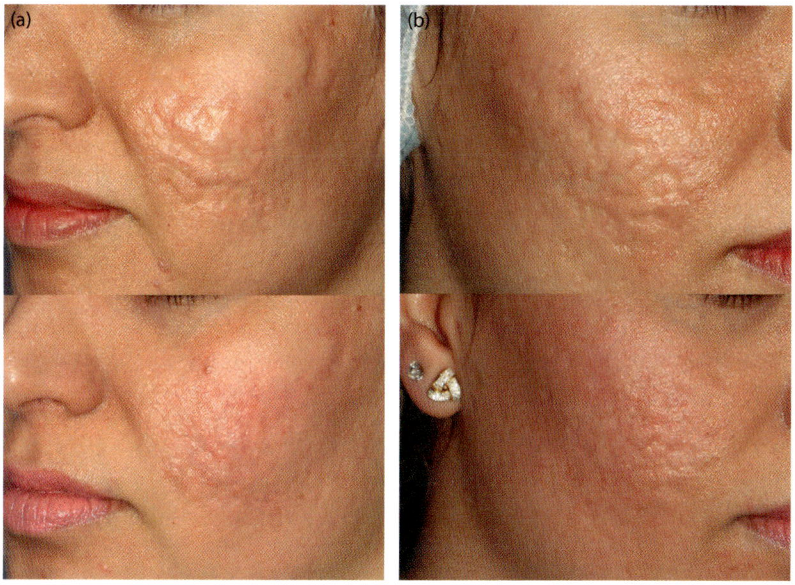

FIGURE 7.1 (a) Left and (b) right view of patient before (top) and after (bottom) a combination of fractionated carbon dioxide with Belotero for the improvement of boxcar scars. (Courtesy of Sabrina Fabi).

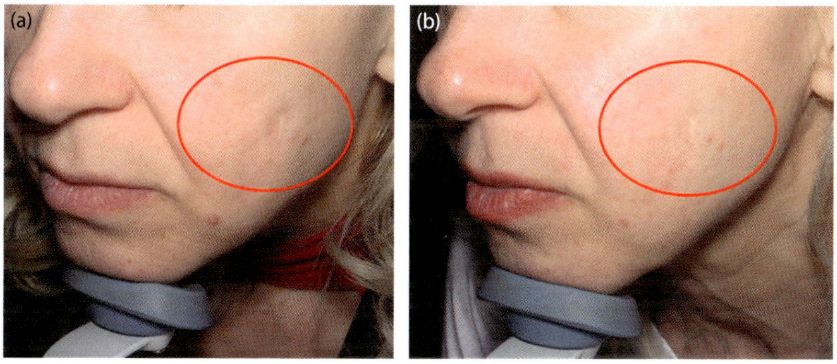

FIGURE 7.2 (a) Before and (b) after treatment with a HA-based filler. (Courtesy of Gabriella Fabbrocini).

skin. The process was repeated again in 2 weeks. One month after the treatment, the patient's number of atrophic scars had been decreased to 10, which is nearly an 83% decrease in the number of atrophic scars. In another study the authors treated a total of five patients in their study (aged between 19 and 40 years), with an average of 48.8 atrophic scars before treatment. After two treatments in a month, the number of scars decreased by 68% to 15.4 scars. The mean volume of filler required for the corrections of scars was 1.144 mL during the first treatment and 0.525 mL during the second treatment [5]. This study demonstrated that Juvederm Voluma was a safe and efficacious tool for the temporary correction of atrophic scars from acne.

In a review paper by Fife [6], HA fillers were preferred for injecting directly under the acne scars, such as rolling scars, whereas volumizing fillers such as PLLA or CaHA, which will be discussed later in this chapter, are better for addressing the deep tissue atrophy that brings attention to the acne scars. The cross-linked HA filler can be injected with a cross-hatching approach or depot injection under the scar. The types of acne scars that respond the best to HA fillers would be broad, rolling scars that are distensible and soft. If there is significant fibrosis under the acne scars, the HA filler should be injected carefully in order to avoid uneven deposition of filler, leading to uneven appearance of nodules and possible extrusion of filler material into the nearby tissue [6].

Semi-Permanent Fillers

Calcium Hydroxylapatite

CaHA is a milky white facial implant comprised of two components: (1) an aqueous gel carrier containing water, glycerin, and sodium carboxymethylcellulose, and (2) the matrix. Once the carrier dissipates, the matrix, composed of CaHA microspheres, provides the augmentation. Nonporous, ceramic CaHA, and macroporous CaHA (which has a highly organized pore structure with pores varying from 10 to 500 μm) permit osseointegration. Nonceramic CaHA cement is widely used in reconstructive surgery to repair bony defects as CaHA is a nonallergenic (inert) bioceramic that is identical to the primary mineral constituent found in bone and teeth. CaHA facial implants (Radiesse and Radiesse +) are microporous, with a particle size of 20–45 μm and pore size of only 2–5 μm, too small to promote fibrovascular ingrowth and bone formation. To date, there are no documented cases of bone formation when CaHA is injected into subcutaneous tissue, nor when injected along the periosteum. CaHA has been found histologically to promote neocollagenesis in the deep dermis and subdermis anywhere from 16 to 78 weeks after injection [7,8].

CaHA is approved for correction of moderate to severe facial wrinkles and folds, such as the nasolabial folds [9] but is routinely used for many facial indications, including the temples, midfacial volume loss, jawline, and chin augmentation. Lip augmentation is a contraindication, as there is a recognized tendency for the CaHA filler to move easily along the orbicularis oris muscle and has a greater propensity to form mucosal granulomas.

In a study by Goldberg et al. [10], 10 patients (aged between 18 and 60 years), with at least one saucerized acne scar, were treated with CaHA (Radiesse; Merz, Raleigh, NC, USA). Using a 27-gauge needle, the dermal filler was injected into the mid-to-deep dermis of the acne scar. The total amount of filler used ranged from 0.1 to 0.3 mL per treatment session and results were evaluated 12 months after injection by a non-treating physician. The authors used 0.8 cc syringes and added 0.1–0.2 cc of lidocaine to dilute the product. Six patients were rated as having 50%–75% improvement in scar appearance, three subjects showed >75% improvement, and one subject showed between 25% and 50% improvement in the saucerized scars [10]. Due to the overall biostimulatory nature and longevity of the product, Radiesse can be considered an effective option for treating certain acne scars [11].

Poly-L-Lactic Acid

PLLA is a biocompatible and biodegradable synthetic polymer of lactic acid. It was initially approved by the FDA in 2004 for human immunodeficiency virus (HIV) lipoatrophy, however, it soon became approved in 2009 as Sculptra Aesthetic (Galderma, Dallas, TX, USA) for cosmetic concerns such as shallow-to-deep nasolabial fold contour deficiencies and other facial wrinkles. PLLA is produced through corn dextrose fermentation and prepared as micronized lipophilic PLLA with an average particle size of 4–63 μm. Each glass vial contains 367.5 mg of PLLA in a suspension of sodium carboxymethylcellulose and nonpyrogenic mannitol. Reconstitution with 7–8 ccs of bacteriostatic water and 1 cc of lidocaine 1% with or without epinephrine 1:100,000 always occurs at least 2 hours prior to injection, but is ideally done overnight [2,12,13]. Technically, the manufacturer recommends sterile water for the reconstitution. However, the vast majority of physicians use preservative (bacteriostatic water) because the preservative makes the injection process less painful for the patient.

Studies have demonstrated a reactive process in the skin after injection with PLLA that leads to increase in collagen and dermal thickness that lasts up to 2–3 years [14], and hence characterizes PLLA as a biostimulating volumizing agent. Unlike the other fillers, PLLA does not have instantaneous effects as it relies on the formation of one's own collagen that begins between 4 and 6 weeks after injection [15]. Optimal areas for PLLA injection include nasolabial folds, medial and later cheeks, and temples. The material is injected into the subcutaneous plane in the nasolabial folds, and medial and lateral cheeks, as well as a supraperiosteally in the temporalis fossa, pyriform fossa, and along the zygoma [2]. Twenty-five- or 26-gauge needles with varying lengths can be used [16]. Since it is often deep tissue atrophy that accentuates the appearance of acne scars, Sculptra or Radiesse can be injected diffusely into the atrophic areas, similar to the technique utilized for correction of HIV-associated lipoatrophy [6]. Certain areas such as the lips, neck, periorbital area, and dorsum of the hand should not be treated with PLLA as there is a higher rate of adverse effects such as small <5 mm subcutaneous papules [17]. Successive treatments should be spaced at least 4 weeks apart in order to avoid overcorrection. After the treatment session, the patient is advised to follow the "5-5-5" rule: massage the treated area for "5" minutes, "5" times daily, and for "5" days.

PLLA has been proposed to be beneficial for the treatment of acne scars since the PLLA stimulates production of collagen in previously atrophic areas, and the act of threading/tunneling during injection is thought to undermine scars [18] (Figures 7.3 through 7.5). In Beer's open-label study [18], 16 individuals (with an average age of 42.7 ± 10.7 years) with an average of 10–16 rolling or ice pick scars received monthly treatment sessions with PLLA for a total of seven treatment sessions at 1-month intervals. During the initial treatment, the median injected volume was 0.725 mL for the entire treatment, and then 0.45 mL per treatment for each of the six monthly follow-up sessions. Prior to each injection session, PLLA was reconstituted with 4 mL sterile water and 1 mL of 1% lidocaine with 1:100,000 epinephrine and left to stand for 2–48 hours before the treatment session. During the injection, the needle was inserted in the deep dermis under the depressed portion of the scar and PLLA was injected until the surface of the scar reached the level of the surrounding skin. Immediately after the procedure, vigorous massaging was performed to prevent subcutaneous papules, and subjects were advised to follow the "5-5-5" rule. After the initial month, there was an average reduction of 20.5% in the number of lesions, which reached a maximum of 46.4% as evaluated on their visit day for the seventh treatment session [18]. Thus, the authors suggest that reductions in size of the acne scars may reach a plateau after six treatments. However, there was an increase in patient satisfaction with each treatment session ($p = 0.0899$). While this study only followed the patients for 6 months after their first treatment, the product may have continued to stimulate collagen productions for many more months. Thus, the limitation of this study is that there was no long-range follow-up arm to demonstrate the longer-lasting results. In this study, the scars had a maximal depth of 3 mm, and were at least as wide as they were deep. The authors do not recommend PLLA for small (1–2 mm) ice pick scars, as these could be better treated with 95% trichloracetic acid.

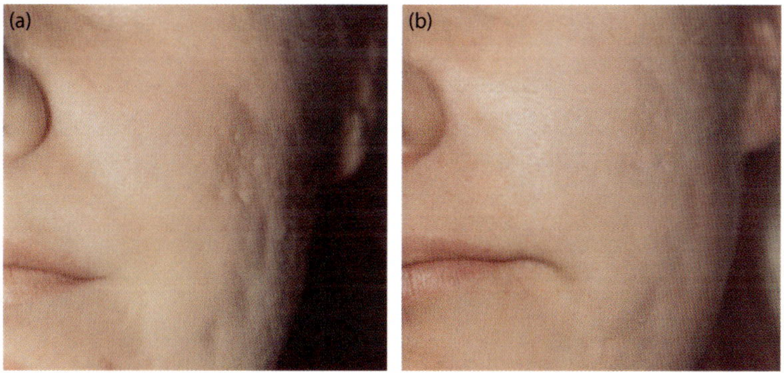

FIGURE 7.3 Acne scars (a) before and (b) after treatment with Sculptra. (From Lowe NJ. *J Eur Acad Dermatol Venereol.* 2006 May;20 (Suppl 1):2–6, with permission [17].)

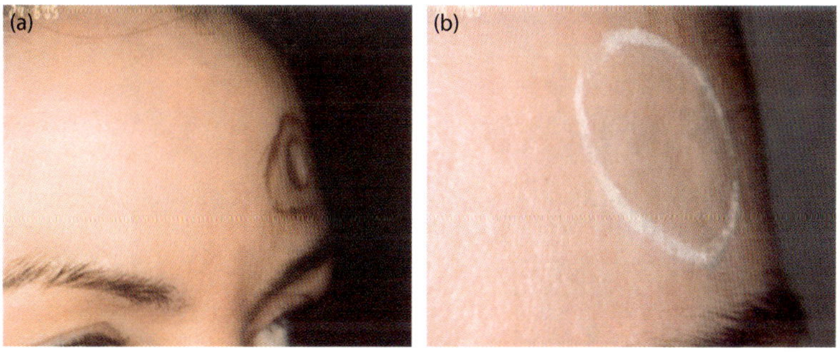

FIGURE 7.4 Atrophic scar (a) before and (b) after treatment with Sculptra. (From Lowe NJ. *J Eur Acad Dermatol Venereol.* 2006 May; 20(Suppl 1):2–6, with permission [17].)

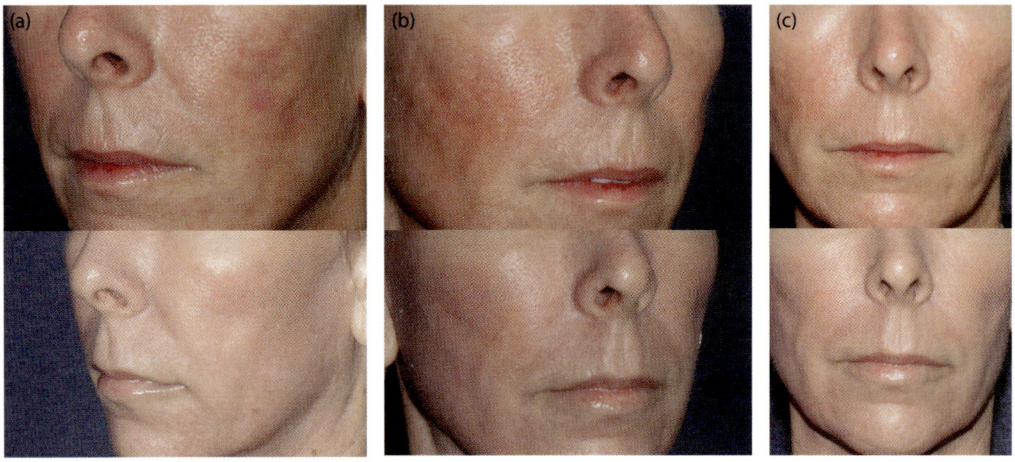

FIGURE 7.5 (a) Left, (b) right, and (c) central views of patient before (top) and after (bottom) two vials of PLLA and one fractionated CO_2/vbeam for scars. (Courtesy of Sabrina Fabi).

In a case study, a 60-year-old Caucasian woman presented with moderate-to-severe deep dermal acne scars with 1- to 3-mm depressions and lipodystrophy of nasolabial folds, which had been previously treated with multiple modalities, such as carbon dioxide laser resurfacing, several dermabrasion treatments, and trichloroacetic acid peels, with only minimal improvement. The patient was treated with PLLA every 4 weeks for a total of seven treatment sessions. The PLLA was reconstituted with 4–7 cc bacteriostatic water and 1% lidocaine simultaneously 24 hours prior to the procedure. For thinner skin areas around the eye, an increased amount of bacteriostatic water was used to increase the dilution of PLLA (6–8 cc) and lessen the chance of nodule formation. For the individual deep dermal acne scars, a lower dilution of PLLA was used (5 cc total) with a smaller gauge, half-inch needle (26-gauge) to insert the product just below the skin. The injections were made just below the scar, however, the injections were a little deeper if there were multiple scars present. The authors did not note how much was injected per scar, however, they mentioned that the amount was based on physician assessment at each visit based on photographic images. The patient noted improvement of acne scars within 6 months of her last treatment, and received a touch-up treatment 14 months after her last injection. The patient reported only mild side effects such as swelling for 24–72 hours and bruising at treatment sites lasting no longer than 7 days [16] (see Figure 7.6).

PLLA has been shown to be effective for replacing dermal volume in boxcar atrophic scars, as demonstrated in a case study by Sadove [19]. In the case study, two women (aged 21 and 45 years) with gross dermal atrophy, dystrophic, and boxcar scars due to severe acne underwent three treatment sessions with injectable PLLA every 6 weeks. At each treatment session, the PLLA was reconstituted with 5 mL of sterile water and allowed to stand for 24 hours. The areas to be treated on the cheeks were first cleaned with alcohol and then anesthetized with 1% lidocaine–epinephrine, injected with a 30-gauge needle. A 23-gauge, 2-inch needle was used to administer the PLLA into the deep dermis, which allowed for a more controlled injection, given the bigger needle size. About 2 mL of PLLA was injected into each cheek area for a total volume of 4 mL per treatment session. For each cheek, 1 mL was use to inject under specific scars until the layer of the treated area was raised to the level of neighboring skin, and 1 mL was dispersed in the skin at the dermal/subcutaneous tissue junction using a layering technique with active motion of the needle in order to prevent pooling of PLLA below the skin. The author did not perform any massage after the injection and discouraged the patients from doing so at home because the injection technique should allow for even distribution of the material. There were no product-related adverse events such as nodules or papules at the 3-year follow-up evaluation for the 21-year-old, and the 6-year follow-up evaluation for the 45-year-old. The author used photographs and physical exam to determine the improvement in contour and color of the treated areas and found that the results were considered excellent at the 1-year follow-up for the 21-year-old, and 4-year follow-up for the 45-year-old woman, with fewer apparent shadows in the skin [19].

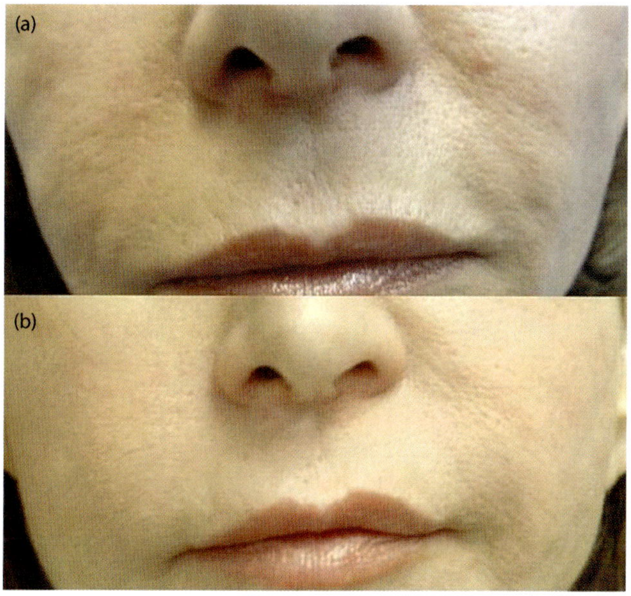

FIGURE 7.6 Mid-cheek and nasolabial folds acne scars (a) before treatment and (b) 1 month after seven treatments with injectable PLLA. (From Sadick NS, Palmisano L. *J Dermatolog Treat*. 2009;20(5):302–7, with permission [18].)

Permanent Fillers

Polymethylmethacrylate

In the initial development stage of PMMA fillers, scientists found that a smaller microsphere size led to a foreign body inflammatory response with giant cell formation. The creation of larger microspheres, 30–50 μm, significantly reduced the rate of granuloma formation to less than 0.01%, and thus came the development of Artefill, which was rebranded as Bellafill (Suneva Medical, San Diego, CA, USA) in 2014 [13]. Artefill is composed of 20% non-resorbable PMMA microspheres suspended in 80% solution of mostly denatured bovine collagen, and was FDA approved for the correction of smile lines. Once the product was rebranded to Bellafill in 2014, it became FDA approved for the treatment of moderate-to-severe, atrophic, distensible facial acne scars on the cheek(s) in patients over 21 years. Bellafill is the only dermal filler in the market that is approved for the treatment of acne scars. Studies have shown a 3% prevalence of hypersensitivity to the bovine collagen, therefore, a skin test is required prior to injection [15,20]. While the bovine collagen leads to volume below the pitted acne scars, the PMMA microspheres create a matrix that stimulates collagen production around the spheres leading to long-term support by autologous connective tissue. Since the microspheres are too large to be phagocytosed by macrophages, they are permanent and, hence, Bellafill is considered an irreversible filler. Additionally, the large size of the microsphere makes the filler unsuitable for thin areas such as the lips and periocular [13].

In a prospective, randomized, placebo-controlled, double-blind, multicenter clinical trial, subjects over 18 years of age (mean age: 44.6 years) were recruited if they demonstrated moderate-to-severe atrophic, distensible acne scarring on the cheeks. In the study 147 subjects (57 men and 90 women) with depressed distensible rolling scars were treated. Ice pick, boxcar, or bound-down acne scars were not included as treatable scars, but could be present in the treatment areas. Prior to enrollment in the study, subjects had to receive a skin test to check for sensitivity to bovine collagen in order to confirm eligibility into the trial. The average number of treated scars with Bellafill was 8.9, with an average initial injection volume of 0.11 mL per scar, and 0.93 mL per subject. About 82.5% of the patients received a touch-up injection, which involved an average injection volume of 0.10 mL per scar and 0.69 mL per subject about 4 weeks after the initial injection. The primary endpoint was based on a blinded investigator who assessed improvement 6 months after initial injection. Improvement was defined as a two-point improvement of at least 50% of treated scars based on the four-point Acne Scar Rating Scale. The primary endpoint was achieved in 64.4% subjects using Bellafill ($p = 0.0005$). Subjects were followed for 12 months after their initial treatment session, and based on ratings from the Subject Global Aesthetic Improvement Scale, over 77% of the Bellafill subjects claimed that their appearance improved from baseline [21].

Bellafill is pre-packaged in a sterile 0.8-mL single-use syringe with a 26-gauge needle and should be injected into the deep dermis or dermal/subdermal junction. One or two touch-up injections can be given as early as 2 weeks after initial injection. The safety of injections of more than 3.5 mL per site has not been determined [22].

Silicone

The unadulterated, purified form of silicone that is used today is known as Silikon 1000 (Alcon Laboratories, Fort Worth, TX, USA). Silikon 1000 is FDA approved for retinal detachment of the eye, but it has been used off-label for HIV-associated lipoatrophy. Historically, there have been unpredictable complications with silicone injections due to overuse or the contamination with mineral oil. However, it is currently supplied as a 10 mL vial containing 8.5 mL purified silicone oil without preservatives, making it less likely to cause granulomatous reactions when appropriate amounts are injected. In order to prevent the risk of migration of the product, the material is injected as a few 0.01 cc microdroplets under each individual scar, at 4–6 week time intervals, and patients usually require two to three treatment sessions [2]. When the product is injected into the dermis as small 0.01 cc microdroplets, controlled fibrosis in the area leads to soft tissue enhancement. One of the indications for injecting sterile, pure, medical-grade liquid silicone is to camouflage shallow acne scars. In order to inject such small amounts of silicone into the desired area, the Becton Dickinson (Franklin Lakes, NJ, USA) 3/10 cc insulin U-100 syringe with a swaged 28-gauge, 0.5-inch (12.7 mm)-long Micro-Fine IV needle is better than other standard syringes [23]. Microdroplets could be deposited at 2- to 5-mm intervals and per session. The treatment volume should be limited to 0.5 mL for small surface areas, such as nasolabial folds. Also, follow-up treatment should not occur earlier than 1 month post-treatment in order to allow for a fibrous tissue reaction around the silicone microdroplets. Post-injection erythema or edema is a common side effect and usually resolves within a few days. Another side effect from injecting the silicone into the dermis is that the inflammatory response to the silicone can lead to post-inflammatory hyperpigmentation or telangiectasias.

Autologous Fat Transfer

Adipose Tissue

Beginning in the early 1900s, autologous fat transfer to correct facial folds demonstrated some benefit; however, the long-term effects were unpredictable and variable [24,25]. According to Peer [26], there was a 45% reduction in the weight of the fat after 1 year, which demonstrates the importance of blood supply in the recipient tissue area [26]. Soon, with the advent of liposuction around the 1970s, more cases of fat transfer were performed for the cosmetic enhancement of facial features. Fat can be extracted from the adipose tissue of various parts of the body during a liposuction procedure using a blunt-tipped microcannula, which is then isolated from the rest of the infranatant. It is recommended to overcorrect by 30%–50% during injection of the face as there will be an expected amount of resorption [27]. Additionally, some authors recommend injecting the fat directly into the muscle for better vascularization [2]. The inflammatory reaction that ensues produces fibrotic tissue, which has been seen in biopsied samples and may explain the process of volume restoration [27]. Due to the excessive scarring in cases of severe acne, leading to the skin tethering down and volume loss of the midface, fat transfer can help to replete the significant areas of volume loss in the face. Thus, the role of fat transfer in acne scarring is for more deep volume augmentation, which then allows the practitioner to focus on the more superficial component of acne scarring [28].

Conclusion

In conclusion, a wide-range of fillers can be used with varying success for different post-acne type of scars (Table 7.1). While certain fillers, such as HA fillers, can specifically be injected immediately beneath each acne scar, other volumizing fillers such as PLLA or CaHA have to be injected in a more widespread fashion to address the extensive dermal atrophy. Since patients with post-acne scarring tend to have different types of scars, they can benefit from the use of various fillers. Until today, only one filler has been FDA approved for moderate acne scarring of the cheeks, and that is Bellafill. As practitioners become more comfortable with the use of other fillers for treating acne scars, future studies may approve non-permanent fillers for the treatment of post-acne scarring.

REFERENCES

1. Dréno B. Recent data on epidemiology of acne. *Ann Dermatol Venereol.* 2010;137(Suppl. 02):S49–51.
2. Narins RS, Bowman PH. Injectable skin fillers. *Clin Plast Surg.* 2005;32(2):151–62.
3. Gold MH. Use of hyaluronic acid fillers for the treatment of the aging face. *Clin Interv Aging.* 2007;2:369–76.
4. Wang F, Garza LA, Kang S et al. *In vivo* stimulation of *de novo* collagen production caused by cross-linked hyaluronic acid dermal filler injections in photodamaged human skin. *Arch Dermatol.* 2007;143:155–63.
5. Goodman GJ, Van Den Broek A. The modified tower vertical filler technique for the treatment of post-acne scarring. *Australas J Dermatol.* 2016;57(1):19–23.
6. Fife D. Practical evaluation and management of atrophic acne scars: Tips for the general dermatologist. *J Clin Aesthet Dermatol.* 2011;4(8):50–7.
7. Marmur ES, Phelps R, Goldberg DJ. Clinical, histologic and electron microscopic findings after injection of a calcium hydroxylapatite filler. *J Cosmet Laser Ther.* 2004;6(4):223–6.
8. Tzikas TL. Evaluation of the Radiance FN soft tissue filler for facial soft tissue augmentation. *Arch Facial Plast Surg.* 2004;4(6):234–9.
9. Solish N. Calcium Hydroxylapatite With Integral Lidocaine Provides Improved Pain Control for the Correction of Nasolabial Folds. *J Drugs Dermatol.* 2016;15:8.
10. Goldberg DJ, Amin S, Hussain M. Acne scar correction using calcium hydroxylapatite in a carrier-based gel. *J Cosmet Laser Ther.* 2006;8:134–6.
11. Jacovella PF. Use of calcium hydroxylapatite (Radiesse) for facial augmentation. *Clin Interv Aging.* 2008;3(1):161–74.
12. Lorenc ZP, Greene T, Gottschalk RW. Injectable poly-L-lactic acid: Understanding its use in the current era. *J Drugs Dermatol.* 2016;15(6):759–62.
13. Attenello NH, Maas CS. Injectable fillers: Review of material and properties. *Facial Plast Surg.* 2015;31(1):29–34.
14. Mest DR, Humble GM. Duration of correction for human immunodeficiency virus-associated lipoatrophy after retreatment with injectable poly-L-lactic acid. *Aesthetic Plast Surg.* 2009;33:654–6.
15. Greco TM, Antunes MB, Yellin SA. Injectable fillers for volume replacement in the aging face. *Facial Plast Surg.* 2012;28(1):8–20.
16. Sadick NS, Palmisano L. Case study involving use of injectable poly-L-lactic acid (PLLA) for acne scars. *J Dermatolog Treat.* 2009;20(5):302–7.
17. Lowe NJ. Dispelling the myth: Appropriate use of poly-L-lactic acid and clinical considerations. *J Eur Acad Dermatol Venereol.* 2006;20(Suppl 1):2–6.
18. Beer K. A Single-center, open-label study on the use of injectable poly-L-lactic acid for the treatment of moderate to severe scarring from acne or varicella. *Dermatol Surg.* 2007;33:S159–67.
19. Sadove R. Injectable poly-L-lactic acid: A novel sculpting agent for the treatment of dermal fat atrophy after severe acne. *Aesthetic Plast Surg.* 2009;33(1):113–6.
20. Haneke E. Polymethyl methacrylate microspheres in collagen. *Semin Cutan Med Surg.* 2004;23(4):227–32.
21. Joseph JH, Eaton LL, Cohen SR. Current concepts in the use of Bellafill. *Plast reconstr Surg.* 2015;136(5 Suppl):171S–9S.

22. Bellafill for acne scars. *Med Lett Drugs Ther.* 2015;57(1471):93–4.
23. Benedetto AV, Lewis AT. Injecting 1000 centistoke liquid silicone with ease and precision. *Dermatol Surg.* 2003;29(3):211–4.
24. Jatana KR, Smith SP Jr. The scientific basis for lipotransfer: Is it the ideal filler? *Facial Plast Surg Clin North Am.* 2008;16(4):443–8, vi–vii.
25. Coleman SR. Structural fat grafting: More than a permanent filler. *Plast Reconstr Surg.* 2006;118(3, Suppl.):108S–20S.
26. Peer LA. Loss of weight and volume in human fat grafts: With postulation of a "cell survival theory." *Plast Reconstr Surg.* 1950;5:217–30.
27. Ali MJ, Ende K, Maas CS. Perioral rejuvenation and lip augmentation. *Facial Plast Surg Clin North Am.* 2007;15(4):491–500, vii.
28. Goodman GJ. Post acne scarring: A review. *Journal of Cosmetic and Laser Therapy.* 2003;5(2):77–95.

8

Skin Needling in Acne Scars

Gabriella Fabbrocini, Marianna Donnarumma, and Maria Vastarella

KEY FEATURES

- Skin needling is a dermatologic treatment performed to achieve percutaneous collagen induction, which is effective at improving depressed acne scarring.
- This dermal damage induces the release of growth factors that stimulate the production of new collagen and elastin in the upper dermis.
- The number of treatments that are required varies depending on the individual collagen response on the condition of the tissue, and the desired results, and it will be determined by the dermatologist whether two to six treatments are needed.

Skin needling is a dermatologic treatment performed to achieve percutaneous collagen induction (PCI), which is effective at improving depressed acne scarring and smoothing wrinkles, as well as reducing the appearance of stretch marks. It is carried out using a skin roller that causes multiple tiny pinpoint puncture wounds to the dermis. This dermal damage induces the release of growth factors that stimulate the production of new collagen and elastin in the upper dermis. Skin needling creates dermal damage without the removal of the healthy epidermis, which happens with other resurfacing techniques [3].

History

Simonin published his results in *Baran's Cosmetic Dermatology* in 1994, but his ground-breaking technique, which he named electroridopuncture, remained largely unknown to the wider medical community [1]. In 1995, Orentreich and Orentreich described "submission" as a way of building up connective tissue below retracted scars and wrinkles [2]. Fernandes treated wrinkles of the upper lip by inserting a 15-gauge needle into the skin and then tunneling under the wrinkles in various directions, parallel to the skin surface [4–6]. In 1997, Camirand and Doucet described their experience on patients with facial hypochromic scars that he tattooed with a skin-color pigment [7]. After 1–2 years, they noticed that even though the pigment was long gone, it was replaced by actual melanin, while the scars were immensely improved in texture, appearance, and color. So he thought that the drilling of scars with the tattoo gun caused improvement and the repigmentation of the scar. PCI results from the natural response to the injury of the skin, even though the wound is minute and mainly subcutaneous. They understood that puncturing the scar with a tattoo gun alone, without pigment, would in a way break down the scar collagen, cause realignment and stimulate melanogenesis.

Fernandes et al. thought that the needle needed to penetrate relatively deeply to stimulate the production of elastin fibers oriented from the deep layers of the dermis to the surface, and he experimented with a special tool for PCI, consisting of a rolling barrel with microneedles, at regular intervals [4–6].

Pathophysiology

PCI provokes the natural response to wounding of the skin, even though the wound is minute and mainly subcutaneous. Needle penetration into the skin promotes the normal wound healing that develops in three stages [8,9].

1. The inflammation starts very soon after the injury: Platelets are activated to release chemotactic factors, which cause an invasion of other platelets, leucocytes, and fibroblasts. After the platelets have been activated by exposure to thrombin and collagen, they release numerous cytokines. This process involves a complex concatenation of numerous factors that are important in recruiting fibroblasts into the wounded area: fibroblast growth factor (FGF), platelet-derived growth factor (PDGF), transforming growth factor (TGF)-α, TGF-β, connective tissue-activating peptide III, and neutrophil-activating peptide.
2. About 5 days after skin needling, neutrophils are replaced by monocytes. They remove cellular debris and release several growth factors, including PDGF, FGF, TGF-α, and TGF-β, which stimulate the migration and proliferation of fibroblasts and the production and modulation of the extracellular matrix. Keratinocytes, the main cells in this case, change in morphology and become mobile to cover the gap in the basement membrane and start producing all the components to reestablish the basement membrane with laminin and collagen types IV and VII. A day or two after PCI, the keratinocytes start proliferating and act more to thicken the epidermis than close the defect. Initially after PCI, the disruption of blood vessels causes a moderate amount of hypoxia. The low-oxygen tension stimulates the fibroblast to produce more TGF-β, PDGF, and endothelial growth factor. Procollagen messenger ribonucleic acid is also upregulated, but this cannot cause collagen formation because oxygen is required, which occurs only when revascularization occurs. Prevascularization occurs quite soon after needling. TGF-β is a powerful chemotoxic agent for fibroblasts that migrate into the wound at about 48 hours after injury and start producing collagen types I and III, elastin, glycosaminoglycans, and proteoglycans. Collagen type III is the dominant form of collagen in the early wound healing phase and becomes maximal 5–7 days after injury. The collagen is laid down in the upper dermis just below the basal layer of the epidermis. Although the injury in skin needling extends deeper than the adnexal structures, because the epithelial wounds are simply cleft, myofibroblast wound contraction may not play a part in the healing. A number of proteins and enzymes are important for fibroplasia and angiogenesis that develop at the same time. Anoxia, TGF-β, FGF, and other growth factors play an important part in angiogenesis. Fibroblasts release insulin-like growth factor, which is an important stimulant for proliferation of fibroblasts themselves, endothelial cells, neovascularization, and is one of the main active agents for the growth hormone. Integrins facilitate the interaction of the fibroblasts, endothelial cells, and keratinocytes.
3. Tissue remodeling that is mainly regulated by fibroblasts continues for months after the injury. The remodeling phase starts and continues for several months: Collagen type III is laid down in the upper dermis, just below the basal layer of the epidermis, and is gradually replaced by collagen type I. The matrix metalloproteinases (MMPs 1, 2, and 3) are essential in this process.

Technique

Preparation Phase

Patients should use a topical product that contains α- and ω-hydroxy acids; ω-hydroxy acids should be used for at least 3 weeks before the skin needling session begins. If the stratum corneum is rough, a series of mild trichloroacetic acid (TCA) peels (2.5%–5% TCA) will get the surface of the skin prepared for needling and improve clinical results because they can stimulate neocollagenesis.

Day of Treatment

The facial skin is disinfected and then a topical anesthetic is applied and left for 60 minutes. The treatment is then carried out by rolling the needling tool over the interested areas four times in four different directions: horizontally, vertically, and diagonally, right and left [10].

The tool used for our patients is a device with needles of 1.5–2.0 mm in length; this induces a quick and uniform bleeding over the entire treated area. Actually there are a number of skin rollers available for professional and home use that come in many different needle lengths, diameters, and numbers, which can make it very confusing for their users. The number of needles on a roller is the least important feature, as repeated rolling causes numerous dermal injuries. Needle diameter is very important because we want to maximize the dermal injury without creating a new scar. In our experience, a 0.25 mm needle diameter is of the maximum size that can be used without causing a new scar in the skin. Smaller-diameter needle skin rollers can be used but do not maximize the dermal injury and, therefore, will be slower to produce results. Needle length is also a critical issue. The target when we needle the dermis is a layer in the upper dermis called the intermediate reticular dermis. This dermal layer contains the highest number of stem cells that are able to produce new collagen. The epidermis (the outer layer of the skin) varies in depth from 0.05 mm on the eyelids to 1.5 mm on the soles of the feet. The epidermis of the face (other than the eyelids) varies from 0.3 to 1 mm in depth and, therefore, a 0.75–2-mm long needle is more than adequate to reach the intermediate reticular dermis. The needles used should have a length of 1.5 mm and a diameter of 0.25 mm. Depending on the applied pressure (pressing too hard is not necessary for excellent results and, if you are needling the face, do not use the rolling barrel on the eyelids or lips), they penetrate the scar tissue between 0.1 and 1.3 mm.

Rolling consists in moving, with some pressure, four times in four directions: horizontally, vertically, and diagonally, right and left. This ensures an even pricking pattern, resulting in about 250–300 pricks per square centimeter. The microneedles penetrate through the epidermis but do not remove it; thus, the epidermis is only punctured and will rapidly heal (Figure 8.1).

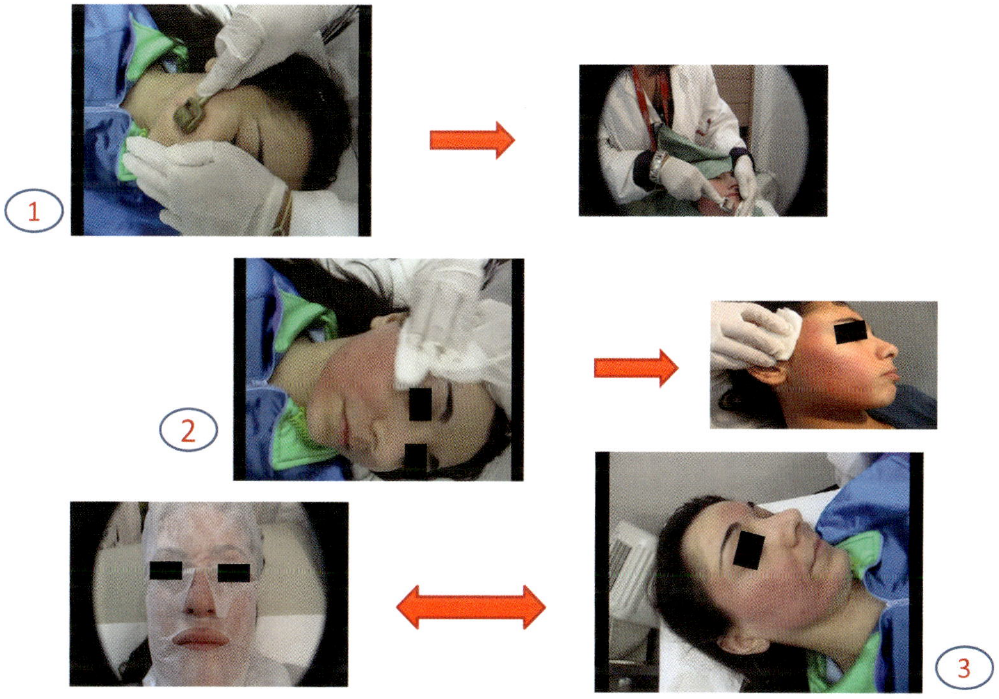

FIGURE 8.1 Skin needling procedure for acne scars: The skin is punctured in multiple directions applying a constant pressure.

Automatic needling can give a standardized pressure to the whole surface treated with a better effect on collagen and elastin rejuvenation. Since the needles are set in a roller, every needle initially penetrates at an angle and then goes deeper as the roller turns. Finally, the needle is extracted at the converse angle; therefore, the tracts are curved, reflecting the path of the needle as it rolls into and then out of the skin, or about 1.3 mm into the dermis.

The epidermis and particularly the stratum corneum remain "intact," except for these tiny holes, which are about four cells in diameter. The treatment times can range from 10 to 60 minutes, depending on the size of the area being treated. Obviously, the skin bleeds for a short time, but that shortly ends. The skin develops multiple microbruises in the dermis that initiate the complex cascade of growth factors that results in collagen production.

The number of treatments required varies depending on the individual collagen response, on the condition of the tissue and on the desired results. Most patients require around three treatments approximately 4 weeks apart.

Post-Treatment Care

Immediately after the treatment, the skin looks bruised, with minimal bleeding. It's a good practice to apply cold compresses.

Finally, it is important that for the first 24 hours after a treatment, the patient doesn't use any skin products that aren't noncomedogenic or specifically designed to be used with microneedling, such as makeup, sunscreen, sunblock, tanning lotion, a facial peel, or any skin care product that contains irritating and toxic ingredients. It's also important to avoid using alcohol-based products immediately after the treatment because they will make the skin very dry.

Normal skincare can be recommenced once the treatment area is completely healed. It is very important to continue using topical vitamin A and C in cream form for at least 6 months post-procedure to ensure the production of healthy collagen and elastin. Patients should be prompted to use only tepid water because the skin will be more sensitive to heat. While the water is running over the face or body, the patient should gently massage the treated skin until all serum, blood, or oil is removed. The importance of a thorough but gentle washing of the skin, a few hours after the procedure, cannot be stressed enough.

The patient should avoid direct sun exposure for at least 15 days. As the skin has a memory and will seek to return to its previous state, it's recommended to repeat skin-needling treatments over a period of 1–2 years.

Days 1 and 2: The tissue may be tender, red, and bruised, with a slight lymph discharge from the treated areas, itching may occur and the "needled" tissue may exhibit the appearance of "cat scratches."

Day 3: The treated areas can present a crust.

Days 4–5: The redness and crusting have diminished.

Days 5–7: The skin is injured.

Clinical Results

Results generally start to be seen after about 6 weeks but complete improvement can take at least 3 months to occur and, as the deposition of new collagen takes place slowly, the skin texture will continue to improve over a 12-month period. Clinical results vary between patients, with some achieving 90% improvement in scarring and others less than 50% (Figures 8.2 and 8.3). However, all patients achieve some improvements. The number of treatments that are required varies depending on the individual collagen response on the condition of the tissue, and the desired results, and it will be determined by the dermatologist whether two to six treatments are needed. Most individuals will require around three treatments approximately 4 weeks apart. Our experience has shown that after only two sessions of treatment the level of severity

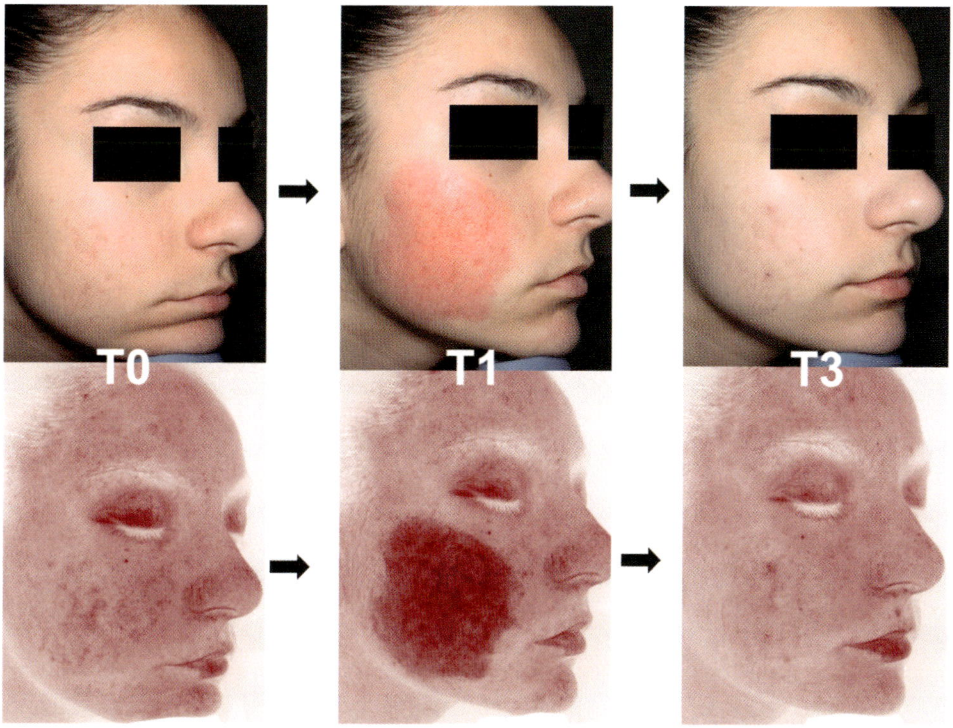

FIGURE 8.2 Acne scars before the first treatment; immediately after the treatment and at 2 months from the treatment.

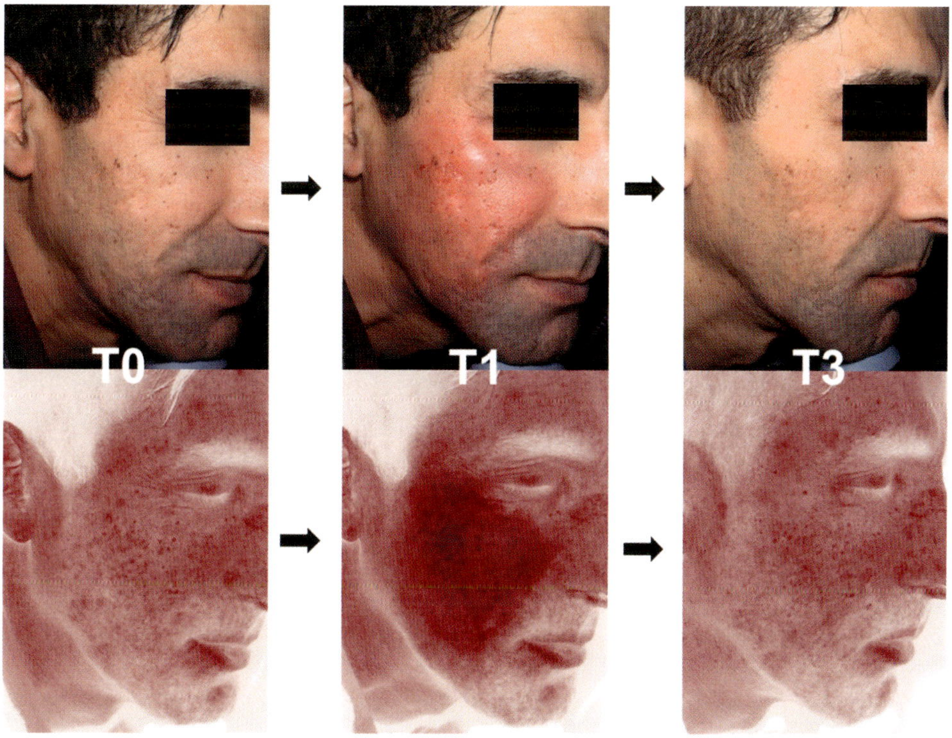

FIGURE 8.3 Acne scars before the first treatment; immediately after the treatment and at 2 months from the treatment.

of rolling scars in all patients is largely reduced: The digital photographic comparison of lesions before and after PCI CIT highlighted that (independently of the grading of lesions) in each group of patients as skin became thicker, the relative rolling scar depth was significantly reduced. Moreover, the degree of irregularity of skin texture, while analyzing surface microrelief of cutaneous casts, showed a 25% reduction (average; in both axes) before and after PCI CIT. Besides, no patient showed visible signs of the procedure or hyperpigmentation.

Different studies report that 6 months after collagen-induction therapy, histology shows a dramatic increase of new collagen and elastin fibers [11–13]. Although difficult to estimate, there is at least 400 and 1,000% more collagen and elastin post-procedure. Recently, Aust et al. showed a considerable increase in collagen and elastin deposition at 6 months post-operation. The epidermis demonstrated a 40% thickening of stratum spinosum and normal rate ridges at 1 year post-operation [6].

The modifications registered by confocal microscopy show that the technique can induce an increase in the number of fibrous bundles, a better distribution of collagen, a higher organization and distribution of melanocytes, and an increase in the density and size of the hair follicles. All these data suggest that skin collagen induction can be a suitable technique for the treatment of acne scars, and confocal microscopy can better define the induced modifications and the improvement of the scars.

Contraindications and Adverse Effects

Some clinical conditions can be considered as absolute contraindications to a skin-needling procedure:

- treatment with isotretinoin within the last 3 months
- presence of open wounds, cuts, or abrasions to the skin
- radiation treatment within the last year
- a current outbreak of herpes simplex or any other infection or chronic skin condition in the area to be treated
- areas of the skin that are numb or lack sensation
- pregnancy or breast feeding
- a history of keloid or hypertrophic scars or poor wound healing

The observation of all the pre- and post-operative precautions and respect of contraindications reduce the risk of adverse effects, which are minimal with this type of treatment and typically include minor flaking or dryness of the skin, with scab formation in rare cases, milia, and hyperpigmentation, which can occur only very rarely and usually resolves after a month. Edema and erythema are the most frequent sequelae. Recovery may take 24 hours or up to a few days. Most patients are able to return to work the following day. Recovery time depends on the treatment level and the length of the needles.

Side Effects, Complications, and Their Management

- Immediately after this procedure the skin is more sensitive to sunlight. It is important to prevent hyperpigmentation by avoiding direct sunlight after treatment for 1 week. The patient has to apply SPF30+ sunscreen when they go outside.
- The skin will feel tender to touch: A facial scrub should be used until the skin is completely recovered.
- After treatment the skin will feel dry. It is important not to use skin toner or to apply topical product with irritation ingredients such as glycolic/salicylic/TCA, and not to use a topical product with toxic ingredient such as hydroquinone.
- The skin will have lost moisture. Avoid invasive treatment (laser/chemical peel/microdermabrasion) until the skin is recovered.

- Adverse events are also known with the procedure. The common ones being potential erythema and irritation, dry skin, and tender skin, which usually subsides within a few days.
- Complications are post-inflammatory hyperpigmentation, erythema, aggravation of acne, and reactivation of herpes systemic hypersensitivity, allergic granulomatous reactions and local infections following the use of a nonsterile instrument. Allergic contact dermatitis to materials used in the needles has also been observed.
- The management of these complications are different for everyone. In case of hyperpigmentation, skin should be treated with a solution of glycolic acid (50%) or hydroquinone creams combined with sunscreen or laser therapy. In the case of an infection, an antibiotic therapy has to be prescribed: either topical therapy with mupirocin 2% ointment, three-times daily for 10 days, alternatively fusidic acid, and, in severe cases, systemic therapy with amoxicillin and clavulanic acid, twice daily for 6 days. If aggravation of acne occurs it is possible to consider local or systemic antibiotic therapy, depending on the gravity of the situation.

REFERENCES

1. Schnitzler L, Adrien A. Cutaneous electric stimulation in aging. *Electroacupuncture of wrinkles following the procedure of Ph. Simonin Rev Fr Gynecol Obstet.* June 1991;86(6):461–6.
2. Orentreich DS, Orentreich N. Subcutaneous incisionless (subcision) surgery for the correction of depressed scars and wrinkles. *Dermatol Surg.* 1995;21:543–9.
3. Jacob CI, Dover JS, Kaminer MS. Acne scarring. A classification system and review of treatment options. *J Am Acad Dermatol.* 2001;45:109–17.
4. Fernandes D. Minimally invasive percutaneous collagen induction. *Oral Maxillofac Surg Clin North Am.* 2005;17:51–63.
5. Fernandes D, Signorini M. Combating photoaging with percutaneous collagen induction. *Clin Dermatol.* 2008;26:192–9.
6. Aust MC, Fernandes D, Kolokythas P et al. Percutaneous collagen induction therapy: An alternative treatment for scars, wrinkles, and skin laxity. *Plast Reconstr Surg.* 2008;121(4):1421–9.
7. Camirand A, Doucet J. Needle dermabrasion. *Aesthetic Plast Surg.* 1997;21:48–51.
8. Cohen KI, Diegelmann RF, Lindbland WJ. *Wound Healing. Biochemical and Clinical Aspects.* Philadelphia: WB Saunders Co, 1992.
9. Fabbrocini G, Fardella N, Monfrecola A. Needling. In: *Acne Scars: Classification and Treatment.* Antonella Tosti, Maria Pia De Padova, Kenneth Beer, eds. Informa Health. 2010.
10. Fabbrocini G, De Padova M. Combination of chemical peels and needling for acne scars. In: *Color Atlas of Chemical Peels.* Antonella Tosti, Pearl E. Grimes, Maria Pia De Padova, eds. Springer. 2012.
11. Fabbrocini G, De Vita V, Fardella N et al. Skin needling to enhance depigmenting serum penetration in the treatment of melasma. *Plast Surg Int.* 2011;2011:158241.
12. Fabbrocini G, Fardella N, Monfrecola A et al. Acne scarring treatment using skin needling. *Clin Exp Dermat.* 2009;34(8):874–9.
13. Fabbrocini G, De Vita V, Monfrecola A, De Padova MP, Brazzini B, Teixeira F, Chu A. Percutaneous collagen induction: An effective and safe treatment for post-acne scarring in different skin phototypes. *J Dermatol Treat.* April 2014;25(2):147–52.

9

Hyaluronic Acid, Platelet-Rich Plasma, and Polylactic Reasorbable Threads in Acne Scars

Gabriella Fabbrocini, Marianna Donnarumma, and Maria Vastarella

KEY FEATURES

- Hyaluronic acid is indicated for the treatment of atrophic acne scars: box scars, ice pick and rolling scars with an involvement of 30% of the face area.
- PRP is indicated for the treatment of boxcar, ice pick, and rolling scars with an involvement of more than 30% of the face area. Usually associated with other treatments (skin needling and laser).
- Polylactic reasorbable threads are indicated for the treatment boxcar and rolling scars with an involvement of less than 30% of the face area or single acne scars.

Hyaluronic Acid

Introduction

Hyaluronic acid (HA) is a glycosaminoglycan composed of alternating D-glucuronic acid and N-acetyl-D-glucosamine monosaccharide residue. These are cross-linked to form long, unbranched chains, which form an anionic biopolymer. Due to its combination of properties, endogenous HA contributes turgor and elasticity to the dermis.

When injected into facial skin it provides immediate and short-term augmentation, and it appears to induce longer-term effects by stimulating collagenesis by native fibroblasts [1,2]. HA has been prepared in different forms, which vary in viscosity and formulation to make the most of its utility and range of applications. HA's viscoelastic properties are a function of the length of the molecular chains of the polymer, cross-linking, concentration, and particle size.

Medium-viscosity HA is best for moderate lines and wrinkles, such as glabellar lines and nasolabial folds, and it is injected into the mid-to-deep dermis. Finer HA formulations are available for correction of fine facial lines, such as perioral and periorbital wrinkles, and are injected in the superficial dermis [3,4]. Specialized formulations are designed to be injected into the lip, while others are indicated for restoring volume lost due to natural aging. Given the properties, superficial injection, and microdosing delivery technique, a low-viscosity HA gel could be an excellent candidate product for the treatment of depressed acne scars [5].

Functions

The natural dermal function of HA in the skin is to fill the interstitial space, with its highly hydrophilic structure, thus avoiding the collapse of the reticular fibers and promoting the mesenchymal and immunocompetent cell viability and motility. Cross-linking creates a water-insoluble gel, stabilizing the molecule.

It also regulates also the turnover of the keratinocytes by means of the two main HA-receptors: CD44 and RHAMM (the receptor for HA-mediated motility); furthermore, it inactivates the free radicals and the reactive oxygen species (ROS) produced by ultraviolet rays [6].

The physiologic role of this polymer can be artificially restored by the injection at different dermal and subdermal levels of cross-linked acid chains, that give to skin a very appealing softness and turgor, with an half life of 4–6 months accordingly with the polymerization degree via liver degradation.

HA-based fillers act by directly adding dermal or subdermal volume, which can be further augmented by in-tissue water attraction by HA. Moreover, native hyaluronic acid promotes cell proliferation and extracellular matrix synthesis and modulates the diameter of the collagen fibers.

Indications

- Atrophic acne scars: boxcar, ice pick, and rolling scars
- Atrophic acne scars with an involvement of 30% of the face area

Modalities of Implant

Low-viscosity HA gel, available in 12 or 20 mg/mL, is injected with a metered dose injector that deposits 10 μL per injection site. To improve acne scars our experience shows that a subdermal injection with a retrograde short straight line technique (needle 30G) can be an option of treatment. It consists in series of tiny, fine-needle injections into the mid to deep dermis (the underlying layer of the skin).

- 20 mg/mL HA for boxcar and ice pick scars
- 12 mg/mL HA for rolling scars

These micro injections will focus on acne scars. During the procedure, some people experience a certain level of discomfort. Each treatment session usually takes around 15–20 minutes. Treatment can be repeated after every 20 days (Figure 9.1).

After Treatment

Low-viscosity HA is a treatment course for gradual skin quality improvement. Some of its effect will be immediately noticeable after a single treatment, but for best results a minimum of three treatments is required, each with a period of 3–4 weeks in between (Figure 9.2). After treatment the skin can swell and show light bruising. This will disappear within several days.

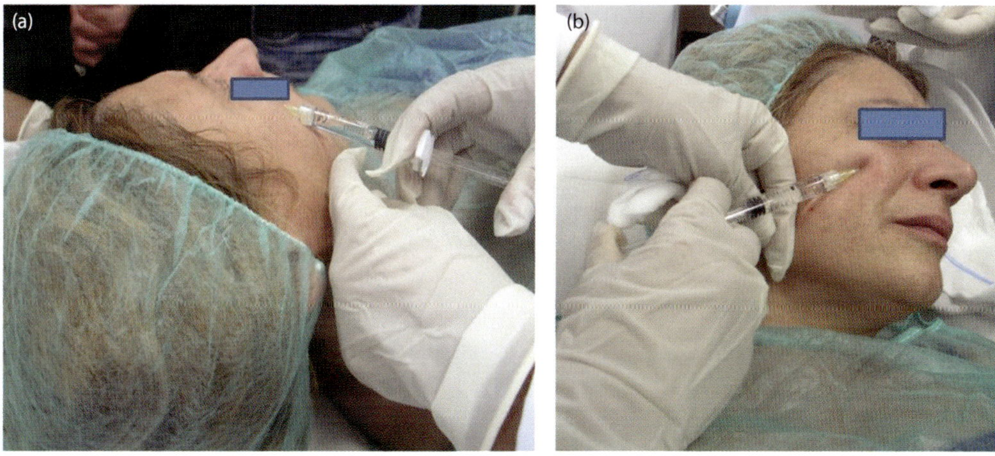

FIGURE 9.1 (a,b) Treatment with HA low viscosity.

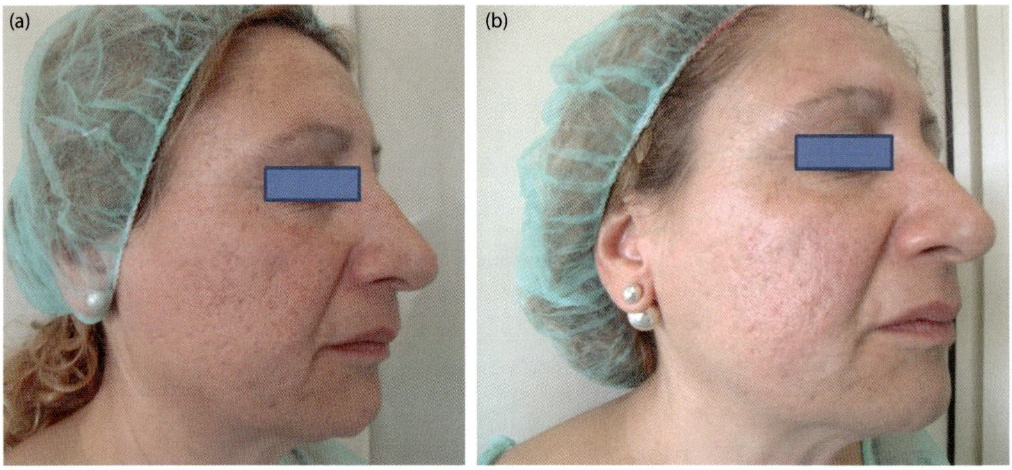

FIGURE 9.2 (a) Pre- and (b) immediately post-treatment with filler.

Advantages

HA has become the leading dermal filler due its combination of low allergenicity, high biocompatibility as demonstrated in ocular and intra-articular uses, and longevity. Being a natural component of the soft tissues, no severe allergic reactions have been reported [7]. It can be used on all skin types regardless of the phototype, and it can be done in every season of the year.

Disadvantages

Injection of HA low viscosity does not work well for deep pitted scars like ice pick scars.

Clinical Results

On the base of our experience patients showed a significant improvement in the texture of the skin and clinical imaging showed a global improvement of all scars, both in number and width. The quantitative evaluation of the scars shows a significant improvement both with Goodman and Baron scale and through the Global Aesthetic Improvement Scale (Figures 9.3 and 9.4).

Moreover the efficacy has been proved by confocal microscopy. After treatment, the skin is more refracting and we observed an improved collagen distribution and organization, and an increase of hair follicle density and size [8].

Contraindications

- Severe allergies with a history of anaphylaxis
- Severe allergies to Gram-positive bacteria such as *Streptococcus*
- Bleeding disorders
- Hypersensitivity to amide local anesthetics

Complications

Most side effects of intradermal injections are mild and transient, and include pain and intermittent swelling, edema, erythema, and ecchymosis at the injection site. Technique-related side effects are irregular facial contour and lasting beading caused by a superficial injection of filler to skin necrosis caused by vascular occlusion. Foreign body granuloma caused by HA injection has been also reported.

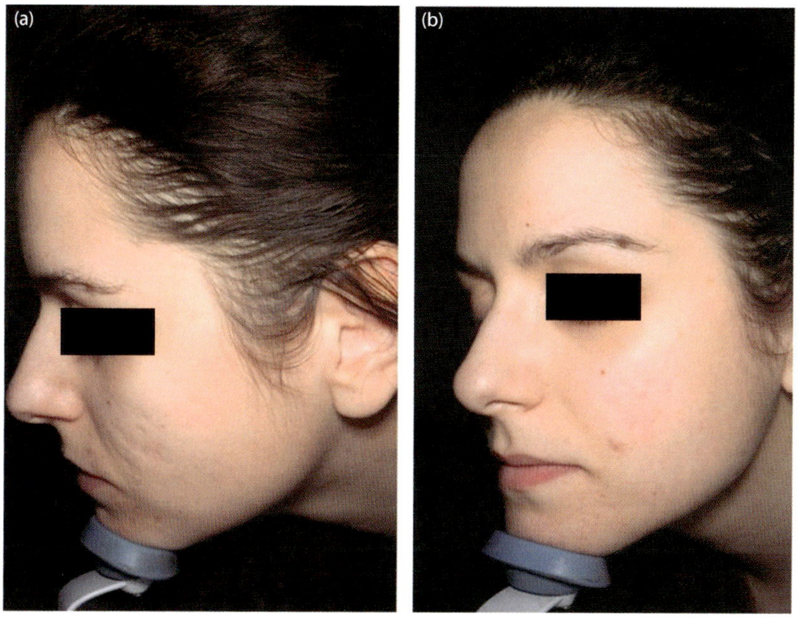

FIGURE 9.3 (a) Pre- and (b) post-treatment with filler.

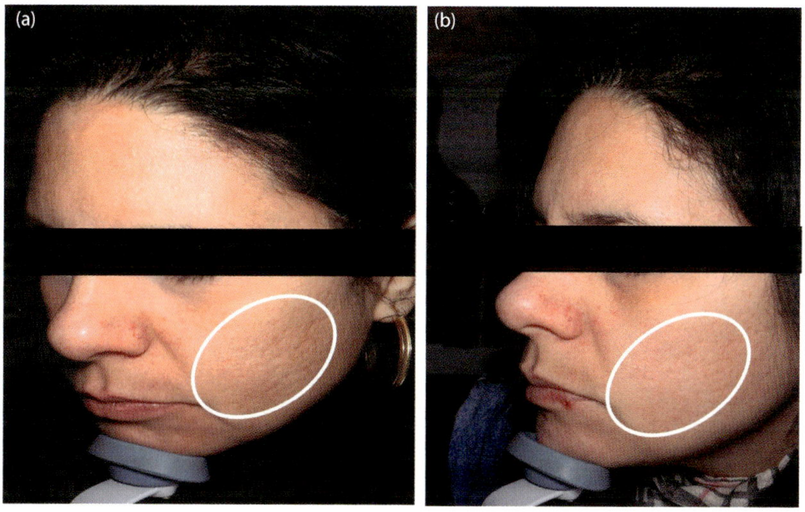

FIGURE 9.4 (a) Pre- and (b) post-treatment with filler.

When HA fillers are placed too superficially into the dermis of patients with a Fitzpatrick 1 or 2, a bluish discoloration, caused by the Tyndall effect, may occur. All these complication are very rare.

Platelet-Rich Plasma in Acne Scars

Introduction

Platelet-rich plasma (PRP) is an autologous preparation of platelets in concentrated plasma full of growth factors, chemokines, and cytokines. PRP therapy is an old therapy and used extensively in specialities of dermatology, orthopedics, and dentistry. PRP is generally well tolerated; with few reported complications, further study may be justified in the context of organized trials.

History

PRP was developed in the 1970s and first promoted by M. Ferrari in 1987 as an autologous transfusion component after an open heart operation to elude excessive transfusion of homologous blood products [9].

In 1990 an autologous fibrin sealant (fibrin glue) obtained by polymerization of fibrinogen with thrombin or calcium chloride was introduced as a topical hemostatic, while the first preparation of an autologous PRP product from a small quantity of blood was described in 1999 [10].

In the beginning, it was used in dental, and oral and maxillofacial surgery. Now PRP has many different applications, from sports medicine to cosmetics, orthopedic surgery, and ophthalmology [11,12]. Publications that study PRP efficacy have increased in the last few decades. Recently it has been used for a various number of dermatological indications including wound healing, fat grafting, alopecia, scar revision, and dermal volume augmentation [13].

Pathophysiology

PRP is an autologous concentration of human platelets contained in a small volume of plasma. Platelets produce numerous growth factors that can stimulate the proliferation of stem cells and the replication of mesenchymal cells, fibroblasts, osteoblasts, and endothelial cells.

PRP is composed by several different growth factors: platelet-derived growth factor (PDGF), transforming growth factor (TGF)-α, vascular endothelial growth factor (VEGF), insulin-like growth factor 1 (IGF-1), epidermal growth factor (EGF), basic fibroblast growth factor (bFGF), TGF-β1, and platelet-activating factor (PAF) (Figure 9.5). The secretion of these growth factors begins within

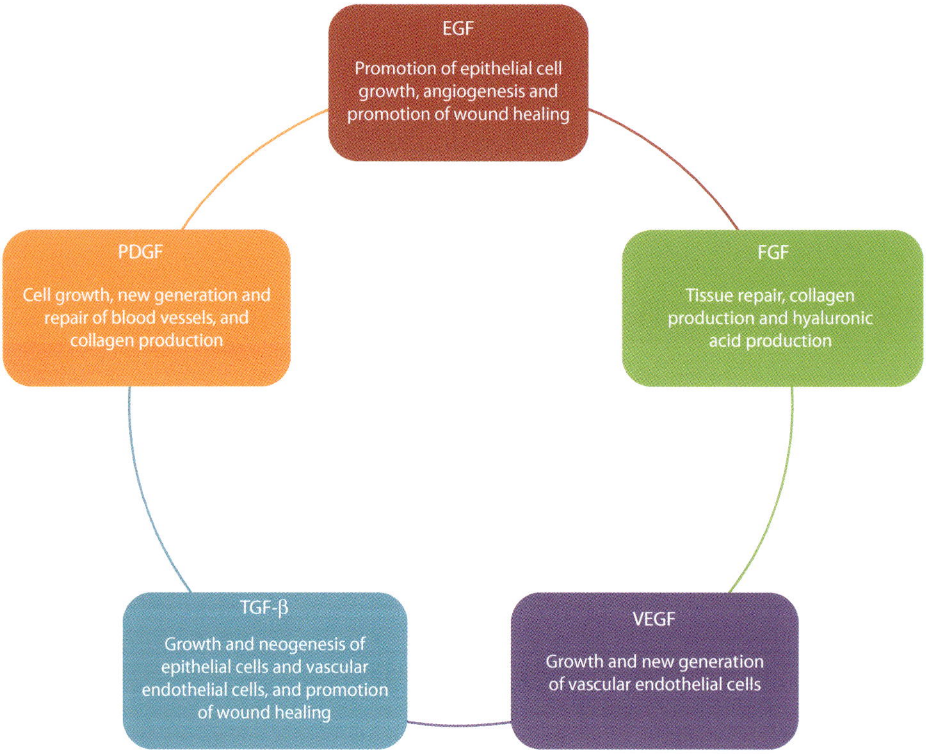

FIGURE 9.5 Main growth factors present in PRP. (From Lovreglio R et al. In: *Nonsurgical Lip and Eye Rejuvenation Techniques.* Fabbrocini G, De Padova MP, Tosti A, eds. Springer, 2016, with permission.)

10 minutes after clotting and more than 95% of the presynthesized growth factors are secreted within 1 hour. The addition of thrombin and calcium chloride actives platelets in PRP and induces the release of factors from α-granules.

Different cells such as adult mesenchymal stem cells, osteoblasts, fibroblasts, endothelial cells, and epidermal cells typically express membrane receptors to growth factors present in PRP. Growth factors binding their receptors can induce cellular proliferation, matrix formation, osteoid production and collagen synthesis.

It is important to underline that the PRP growth factors are not mutagenic because they do not enter the cell or nucleus; therefore, PRP does not induce tumor formation.

Due to the presence of high concentrations of these growth factors, PRP has been used in a wide variety of surgical procedures and clinical treatments, including the treatment of problematic wounds and maxillofacial bone defects, cosmetic surgeries, and gastrointestinal surgeries [14,15].

Indications

- Atrophic acne scars: boxcar, ice pick, and rolling scars
- Atrophic acne scars with an involvement of more than 30% of the face area
- Usually associated with other treatments (skin needling and laser)

Advantages of PRP

- Angiogenic
- Antibacterial properties
- Stimulates the formation of connective and epithelial tissue
- Osteogenesis stimulators
- Security and non-toxic tissue injury
- Can be autologous

Contraindications

Absolute Contraindications

- Platelet dysfunction syndrome
- Critical thrombocytopenia
- Hemodynamic instability
- Septicemia
- Local infection at the site of the procedure
- Patient unwilling to accept risks

Relative Contraindications

- Consistent use of nonsteroidal anti-inflammatory drugs within 48 hours of procedure
- Corticosteroid injection at treatment site within 1 month
- Systemic use of corticosteroids within 2 weeks
- Tobacco use
- Recent fever or illness
- Cancer, especially hematopoetic or of the bone
- Hemoglobin level < 10 g/dL
- Platelet count $< 105/\mu L$

Preparation of Autologous Platelet Gel

Preparation

The phases of the working procedure of platelet gel therapy are: collection of blood into a test tube, cell enrichment, activation, quality control test.

Collection into a Test Tube

PRP is obtained from a sample of patients' blood drawn at the time of treatment. A 40 cc venous blood draw will yield 7–9 cc of PRP depending on the baseline platelet count of an individual, the device used, and the technique employed. The blood draw occurs with the addition of an anticoagulant, such as acid citrate dextrose (ACD) to prevent platelet activation prior to its use. PRP is prepared by a process known as differential centrifugation. In differential centrifugation, acceleration force is adjusted to sediment certain cellular constituents based on different specific gravities.

There are many ways of preparing PRP. It can be prepared by the PRP method. In the PRP method, an initial centrifugation to separate red blood cells (RBCs) is followed by a second centrifugation to concentrate platelets, which are suspended in the smallest final plasma volume. Whole blood (WB) is initially collected in tubes that contain anticoagulants. The first spin step is performed at constant acceleration to separate RBCs from the remaining WB volume. After the first spin step, the WB separates into three layers: an upper layer that contains mostly platelets and white blood cells (WBCs), an intermediate thin layer that is known as the buffy coat and that is rich in WBCs, and a bottom layer that consists mostly of RBCs. For the production of pure PRP, the upper layer and the superficial buffy coat are transferred to an empty sterile tube. For the production of leucocyte-rich PRP, the entire layer of buffy coat and a few RBCs are transferred. The second spin step is then performed. The "g" for the second spin should be just adequate to aid in the formation of soft pellets (erythrocyte platelets) at the bottom of the tube. The upper portion of the volume that is composed mostly of PPP (platelet-poor plasma) is removed. Pellets are homogenized in 5 mL of plasma to create the PRP with a high concentration of leucocytes.

PRP Method

1. Obtain WB by venipuncture in ACD tubes
2. Do not chill the blood at any time before or during platelet separation
3. Centrifuge the blood using a soft spin
4. Transfer the supernatant plasma containing platelets into another sterile tube (without the anticoagulant)
5. Centrifuge tube at a higher speed (a hard spin) to obtain a platelet concentrate
6. The lower third is PRP and upper two thirds is PPP. At the bottom of the tube, platelet pellets are formed
7. Remove PPP and suspend the platelet pellets in a minimum quantity of plasma (5–7 mL) by gently shaking the tube

Buffy-Coat Method

1. WB should be stored at 20–24°C before centrifugation
2. Centrifuge WB at a high speed
3. Three layers are formed due to its density: The bottom layer consisting of RBCs, the middle layer consisting of platelets and WBCs, and the top PPP layer
4. Remove supernatant plasma from the top of the container
5. Transfer the buffy-coat layer to another sterile tube
6. Centrifuge at a low speed to separate WBCs or use leucocyte filtration filter

Commercially Available PRP Kits

There are many PRP systems commercially marketed, which facilitate the preparation of ready-to-apply platelet-rich suspensions in a reproducible manner. All operate on a small volume of drawn blood (20–60 mL) and on the principle of centrifugation. These systems differ widely in their ability to collect and concentrate platelets depending on the method and time of its centrifugation. As a result, suspensions of different concentration of platelets and leucocytes are obtained. Differences in the concentrations in platelets and WBCs influence the diversity of growth factor concentration. It is difficult to assess which kit for PRP preparation is better and which is worse.

PRP devices can be usually divided into lower (2.5–3 times the baseline concentration) and higher (5–9 times the baseline concentration) systems.

Cell Enrichment

In our experience, in order to prepare a gel that is a homogeneous mass of an adequate volume and yet remains manageable, the platelet concentration needs to be 750,000–1,000,000/μL. With this concentration of platelets, the gel forms in about 5–7 minutes. Once the PRP has been obtained, a full blood count is performed and, on the basis of the platelet count, the PRP is diluted or concentrated under sterile conditions.

Activation

The production of autologous thrombin, used as the activator, involves the following steps: collection of another blood sample (in ACD or sodium citrate), centrifugation of the sample for 10 minutes at 3000 rpm, collection of the plasma supernatant in a new test tube (under sterile conditions), addition of 0.2 mL of calcium gluconate for every 1 mL of plasma, incubation at 37°C for 15–30 minutes, collection of the supernatant containing the precursors of thrombin (under sterile conditions), and freezing and storage at 30°C until needed. In order to produce the gel, the platelet concentrate is placed in a sterile plate and then the activators are added—that is, 1 mL of autologous thrombin and 1 mL of calcium gluconate for every 10 mL of PRP. At this point, the mixture is left to incubate at room temperature. If the coagulation process takes longer than expected, the preparation can be incubated for about 5 minutes at 37°C to facilitate the reaction.

The platelet concentrate must be sterile. The blood components must be prepared according to the principles of Good Manufacturing Practice. Each procedure must undergo quality control tests, including: determination of the volume, platelet count, count of contaminating WBCs, and an assay of fibrinogen levels.

Clinical Uses of PRP

After centrifugation, the platelet and fibrin component of the blood (the top layer) is extracted and reinjected into the area of concern.

In dermatology and cosmetic medicine, PRP has been used to treat:

- Venous and arterial leg ulcers
- Diabetic foot ulcers
- Pressure ulcers (bedsores)
- Skin graft donor sites
- First- and second-degree thermal burns
- Superficial injuries, cuts, abrasions, and surgical wounds
- Hair loss disorders—PRP has been shown to reinvigorate dormant hair follicles and stimulate new hair growth

- Post-traumatic scars—PRP combined with centrifuged fat tissue and fractional laser resurfacing improves the cosmetic appearance of scars
- Facial rejuvenation—PRP injections can treat wrinkles, photodamage, and discoloration in conjunction together with other treatment modalities

PRP Preparation

Blood is drawn and an anticoagulant is added. The mixture is centrifuged and separated into three layers: PPP, PRP, and RBCs. To make PRP, the RBCs are discarded and centrifuged again. The majority of the PPP is discarded, and the end product consists mostly of PRP with a small amount of PPP. Thrombin or calcium chloride is added as a platelet activator.

Skin Needling and PRP: Procedures

Skin needling is used to achieve percutaneous collagen induction in order to reduce skin imperfection. To date, skin needling has mostly been proposed as an effective method of treating scars and wrinkles. Microneedles penetrate through the epidermis, which is only punctured and heals rapidly. Skin needling triggers a cascade of growth factors that stimulate directly the maturation phase of wound healing, so the penetration of the microneedle in the skin does not create a wound in the classic sense, but causes fine wounds and the wound healing process is cut short, as the body is somehow "fooled" into believing that an injury has occurred.

Skin needling can provide a clear channel for topical agents to be absorbed more effectively through the top layer of skin such as the PRP.

Technology

First, the facial skin was disinfected, then a topical anesthetic (EMLA) was applied for 60 minutes. Skin needling was carried out by using a highly specific tool, a 10-mm-wide rolling barrel, equipped with 96 needles in four rows. The needles had a length of 1.5 mm and a diameter of 0.25 mm. Depending on the applied pressure, they penetrated the scar tissue between 0.1 and 1.3 mm. The barrel was rolled over the areas affected by acne scars in four directions: horizontally, vertically, and diagonally, right and left. The left side of the face was treated by the needling technique alone. PRP was applied first on the right side (Figure 9.6) and then the needling tool was rolled.

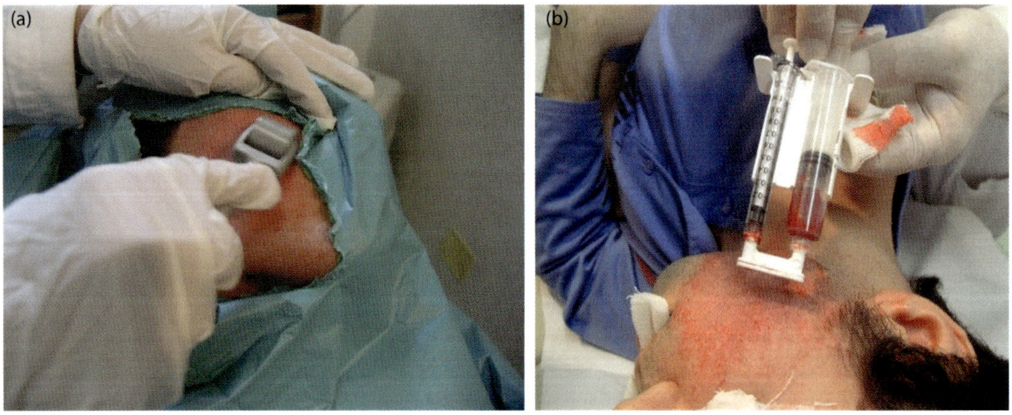

FIGURE 9.6 (a) Needling followed by (b) PRP injection. (With kind permission from Springer Science+Business Media: *Nonsurgical Lip and Eye Rejuvenation Techniques*, The nonsurgical thread lift for facial rejuvenation, 2016, 85–96, Lovreglio R, Fabbrocini G, Delfino M.)

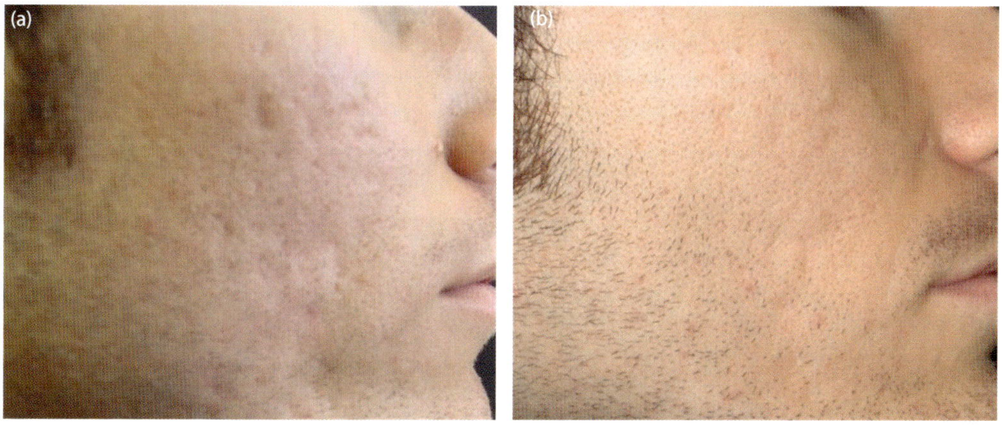

FIGURE 9.7 Acne scars before (a) and 6 months after treatment (b) with needling associated to PRP.

Clinical Follow-up

- Normally, the skin-aging program consists of three sessions of needling a month apart from each other, and the first follow-up is done after one month from the third session, then from 3 to 6 months after the last session.
- Patients were instructed to use topical therapy with emollients and soothing cream for 48 hours after each session. In addition, sun exposure was avoided by using sunscreens of SPF30+ during the daytime.

Clinical Results

In our experience the combined use of skin needling and PRP is more effective in improving acne scars than skin needling alone. Clinical patients achieve some improvements in the smoothness of the skin and in the depth and dimension of the scars. The number of treatments required varies depending on the individual collagen response on the condition of the tissue and desired results, and it will be determined by the dermatologist whether two to six treatments are needed (Figure 9.7).

Resorbable Threads in Acne Scars

Introduction

Barbed suture lifting is a minimally invasive surgical technique widely used for facial rejuvenation. These procedures can lift lax skin.

The treatment by absorbable threads is an innovative technique useful for supporting and stretching up the face and body tissues. The recent introduction of absorbable barbed sutures can be a good alternative to more invasive procedures.

Due to their ability to stimulate tissue regeneration through fibroblast activation, absorbable threads have been proposed for the treatment of acne scars.

A worldwide variety of barbs with differences in costs and in types of material can be split into two types.

1. Polydioxanone (PDO)
2. L-lactide-ε-caprolactone

Professor Marlen Sulamanidze in the late 1990s inserted bidirectional barbed sutures, manufactured with a non-absorbable polymer (polypropylene), into the subcutaneous plane of the face [16].

However, the complication of non-absorbable threads that remain permanently in the facial soft tissue was very low. For this reason, new, absorbable, barbed suture designs have become available.

In 2008, he launched to the world market three lines of reasorbable wire: Nano, Excellence, and Light Lift. He invented the first thread using permanent traction threads in polypropylene by means of a non-invasive lifting technique [17–20].

Technology

It is a surgical outpatient treatment carried out with or without local anesthesia according to the medical evaluation of the case. Threads are inserted subcutaneously through a micro-hole, along precise lines of skin tension, by means of a thin needle or a needle-pipe blunt tip (the tip shape reduces the local trauma), exerting a slight traction to lift the relaxed tissues. The threads adhere to the skin due to the presence of special anchors (plugs). The effect is achieved because the lift-thread insertion follows geometric traction where nothing is left to chance, and in fact the treatment requires, in addition to a certain manual skill, a flawless knowledge of anatomy.

Indications

- Atrophic acne scars: boxcar and rolling scars
- Atrophic acne scars with an involvement of less than 30% of the face area
- Single acne scars

PDO Threads

Nature

The PDO is a polymer of polylactic p-dioxanone, a bioabsorbable material and antimicrobial already used in surgery and biocompatible with the dermis.

Features

Biocompatible, antimicrobial absorption by hydrolytic action within 6–8 months, medical use, surgery.

The PDO absorbable threads (thickness: 0.05—0.19 mm, and length: 3–16 cm) are positioned inside of a needle (26-, 29-, or 30-gauge).

Functions

The biostimulant PDO threads implanted in the dermal layer are able to stimulate the fibroblasts, activating an increased synthesis of collagen [21].

The shift of the skin tissue through the thread proved to be a fundamental mechanism in the cutaneous tissue repair processes of acne scars.

The cell is stimulated by the presence of several transduction systems mechanically placed at the level of the cell membrane, the best known of which is the integrin. The mechanical stimulus exerted on the outer extracellular matrix determines through integrin some intracellular biological changes that can activate specific genes.

The fibroblasts are particularly sensitive to mechanical stimuli, and when subjected to mechanic stimulation they activate genes for the production of collagen and other proteins.

Duration

After approximately 6–8 months, the threads have been completely reabsorbed, naturally and harmlessly, by hydrolytic action. However the mechanical support is stable for 6–8 months, and generates a significant endogenous stimulation whose benefits will last much longer.

Thread with l-lactide-ε-caprolactone

Feature

Threads with polylactic acid are biocompatible and fully resorbable. The caprolactone allows the gradual absorption of polylactic acid and ensures the mechanical strength and the elasticity of the threads. Moreover their capacity of biostimulation can restore luminosity and color.

Function

The microcirculation capillaries of the proximal threads increase in number as the peripheral and the vessel lumen are more dilated. Studies have shown that for the entire period post-insertion the vessels remain dilated with a constant hyperemia, maintaining trophism of the treated area with the formation of new collagen, fibrin and elastin. The fibroblasts of the fibrotic tissue created with the placing of the threads are functionally active; this can be seen from the increasing nucleus and cytoplasm, with a spread of chromatin. The connective tissue layer, in which the thread is implanted, treated with blue dye, toluidine, contains an increased number of mast cells, and at the same time they show a concentration to the vascular channels of microcirculation. The mast cells in their granules contain hyaluronic acid, a polysaccharide complex, which is a structural component of the papillary dermis granular layer of the epidermis and is also available in the superficial vessels of the skin. There is evidence that the reduction of the amount of hyaluronic acid affects the immune status of the skin, and that its inner dermal injection improves the structure of the skin. During the 40 days after planting, the smooth thread is surrounded by a thin capsule of connective fibrosis tissue [22–25].

The reabsorption process begins after about 180 days post-implantation and is completed after a year.

Technique

The threads are inserted subcutaneously through a micro-hole, along main lines of the scars exerting a slight traction to lift the atrophic scars tissues. The number of wires implanted may vary according to the material of the thread used and to the form, chosen by the operator. To place an individual thread, the surgeon guides the straight needle through the incision and into the subcutaneous plane. For some anatomic locations, it is advantageous to bend the needle to more easily allow it to follow the dynamic face lines. The needle is advanced in this plane in a zig-zag movement along the marked trajectory. Once anchored, this zig-zag placement of the suture limits retrograde motion along the suture and results in an implanted suture that is longer than the drawn trajectory. This maximizes the number of barbs in the subcutis and theoretically provides more stability of the translocated skin. Movement of the needle and suture through the subcutis is generally well tolerated by patients. If the straight needle moves superficially to this plane it is immediately apparent as linear dimpling of the overlying skin. If the needle enters into the deep subcutis or approaches the muscle fascia or periosteum, the patient will report the sensation of pain or pressure. At any point, the straight needle may be partially or completely removed and repositioned. Anesthesia is not necessary and it will be sufficient to cool the treated area with dry ice [26,27].

Contraindications

- Current acute acne or skin diseases
- Systemic infections
- Allergic anamnesis
- Treatment with immune suppressors
- Uncontrolled hypertension or anticoagulant regimes
- Recurrent herpes simplex (requires antiviral prophylaxis)

- Predisposition to form keloids
- Pregnancy or lactation
- Coagulation disorders
- Autoimmune disease

Advantages

Designed to be less invasive, it can reduce acne scars more quickly and with less risk than the conventional approach. And while thread lifts generally produce noticeable results almost immediately and with less risk and inconvenience than more intensive procedures, thread lift costs are quite reasonable compared with traditional options. It is an innovative technique in the field of aesthetic medicine; the process has very little pain but improves the skin tone and its aspect.

Disadvantages

Limitations of these implants have included the protrusion of sutures through the skin, asymmetry of cosmetic effect, often require correction with additional sutures, and limited durability of effects.

Post-Treatment

The down-time lasts for 3–4 days. Mild complications such as swelling, bruising, and subjective feelings of "tightness" usually resolve within 1–3 weeks.

Since this technique may be released with intense pressure, patients must initially avoid strenuous exercise or movements that could dislodge the tightened skin from the hundreds of barbs along the sutures. Non-peer-reviewed data from the manufacturer demonstrates that in laboratory rats these sutures develop a fibrous capsule that becomes well integrated into the dermis and subcutaneous tissue over several months. A similar process in human skin can lead to a long-lasting cosmetic effect. The actual long-term durability of the tightening effects of these sutures is unknown. Early adopters of this procedure have demonstrated maintenance of cosmetic effects at 6 months.

After the intervention the patient will have to:

- Disinfect the points where sutures were introduced with antiseptic solutions for 3 days
- Not take hot liquids and solids for 3 days
- Not take alcoholic beverages for 2–3 weeks
- Limit mimic activity for 7 days
- Limit gym, sauna, swimming, and direct solar exposure for 3–5 weeks
- Take antibiotics for 3–5 days if more suture packs are required for surgery
- Sleep supine with a cushion side-by-side if the surgery was on the face, neck or abdomen

Results

Clinical patients achieve some improvements in the smoothness of the skin, and in the depth and dimension of the scars. The number of treatments required varies depending on the individual condition of the tissue and desired results, and will be determined by the dermatologist (Figure 9.8).

After Treatment

Rapid lifting of the treated acne scars is visible already at the end of the treatment. The patient can re-start their normal activities at the end of treatment.

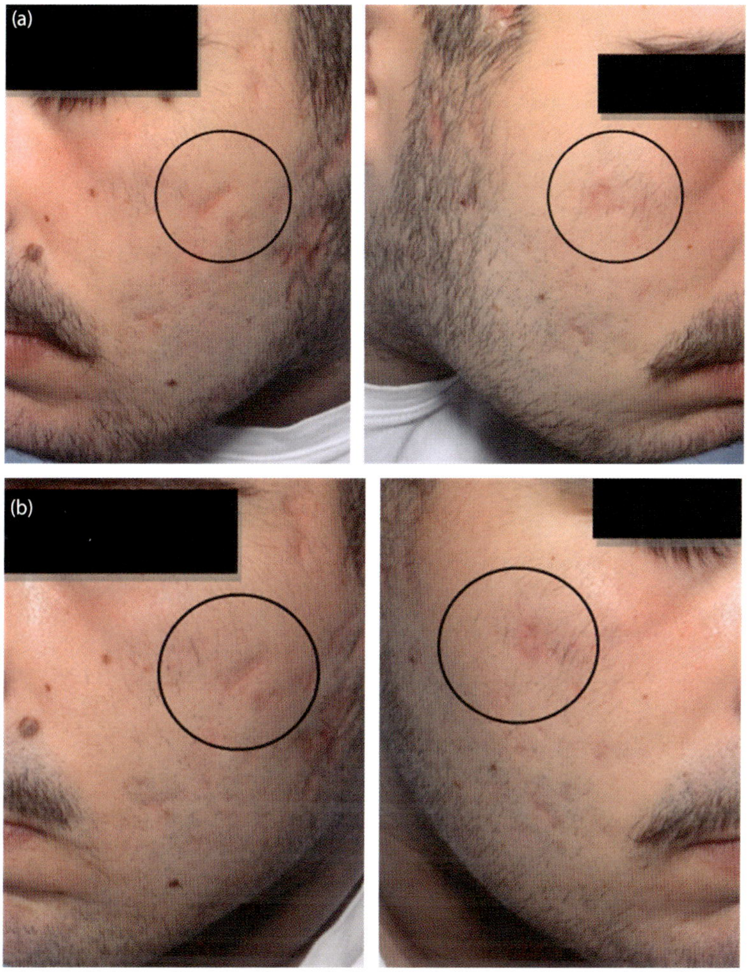

FIGURE 9.8 Acne scars before (a) and two months after treatment with PDO threads (b).

After 2 Months

Marked improvement after 1–2 months. The skin gets better in the skin tone as well. It improves the appearance of acne scars.

Adverse Reactions and Management of Complications

The most common adverse reaction is edema and erythema for 24–48 hours after treatment and hematomas at implant hardening small transients. High sensitivity in the treated area usually disappears within 1–3 days following treatment. In extreme cases, the threads can be extracted after 20 days by a small incision and extraction with a clamp.

REFERENCES

1. Ribè A, Ribè N. Neck skin rejuvenation: Histological and clinical changes after combined therapy with a fractional non-ablative laser and stabilized hyaluronic acid-based gel of non-animal origin. *J Cosm Laser Therapy*. 2011 August;13(4):154–61.
2. Williams S, Tamburic S, Stensvik H, Weber M. Changes in skin physiology and clinical appearance after microdroplet placement of hyaluronic acid in aging hands. *J Cosmet Dermatol*. 2009;8(3):216–25.

3. Montes JR. Volumetric considerations for lower eyelid and midface rejuvenation. *Curr Opin Ophthalmol.* 2012;23(5):443–9.
4. Berardesca E, Farinelli N, Rabbiosi G, Maibach HI. Skin bioengineering in the noninvasive assessment of cutaneous aging. *Dermatologica.* 1991;182(1):1–6.
5. Halachmi S, Ben AD, Lapidoth M. Treatment of acne scars with hyaluronic acid: An improved approach. *J Drugs Dermatol.* 2013;12(7):e121–3.
6. Toole BP, Yu Q, Underhill CB. Hyaluronan and hyaluronan-binding proteins. Probes for specific detection. *Methods Mol Biol.* 2001;171:479–85.
7. Distante F, Pagani V, Bonfigli A. Stabilized hyaluronic acid of non-animal origin for rejuvenating the skin of the upper arm. *Dermatol Surg.* 2009;35(Suppl. 1):389–93; discussion 394.
8. Micheels P, Besse S, Sarrazin D. Visual, ultrasonographic, and microscopic study on hyaluronic acid-based gel. *J Drugs Dermatol.* 2016;15(9):1092–8.

Platelet-Rich Plasma

9. Ferrari M, Zia S, Valbonesi M. A new technique for hemodilution, preparation of autologous platelet-rich plasma and intraoperative blood salvage in cardiac surgery. *Int J Artif Organs.* 1987;10:47–50.
10. Zhu JT, Xuan M, Zhang YN et al. Fibrin glue: The perfect operative sealant? *Transfusion.* 1990;30(8):741–7.
11. Simion Labusca L, Cionca D. Clinical review about the role use of platelet rich plasma for the treatment of traumatic and degenerative musculoskeletal disorders. *Ortho & Rheum Open Access J.* 2016;2(3):555–589.
12. Sampson S, Gerhardt M, Mandelbaum B. Platelet rich plasma injection grafts for musculoskeletal injuries: A review. *Curr Rev Musculoskelet Med.* 2008;1(3–4):165–74.
13. Everts P, Knape J, Weirich G et al. Platelet-rich plasma and platelet gel: A review. *JECT.* 2006;38:174–87.
14. Leo MS, Kumar AS, Kirit R, Konathan R, Sivamani RK. Systematic review of the use of platelet-rich plasma in aesthetic dermatology. *J Cosmet Dermatol.* 2015;14(4):315–23. Review.
15. Graziani F, Ivanovski S, Cei S et al. The in vitro effect of different PRP concentrations on osteoblasts and fibroblasts. *Clin Oral Implants Res.* 2006;17(2):212–9.
16. Sulamanidze MA, Fournier PF, Paikidze TG, Sulamanidze GM. Removal of facial soft tissue ptosis with special threads. *Dermatol Surg.* 2002;28(5):367–71.
17. Sulamanidze MA, Paikidze TG, Sulamanidze GM, Neigel JM. Facial lifting with "APTOS" threads: Featherlift. *Otolaryngol Clin North Am.* 2005;38(5):1109–17.
18. Sulamanidze MA, Sulamanidze G. Facial lifting with Aptos methods. *J Cutan Aesthet Surg.* 2008;1(1):7–11.
19. Sulamanidze MA, Sulamanidze G. APTOS suture lifting methods: 10 years of experience. *Clin Plast Surg.* 2009;36(2):281–306, viii.
20. Sulamanidze MA, Sulamanidze G, Vozdvizhensky I, Sulamanidze C. Avoiding complications with Aptos sutures. *Aesthet Surg J.* 2011;31(8):863–73.
21. Sun DH, Jang HW, Lee SJ, Ryu HJ. Outcomes of polydioxanone knotless thread lifting for facial rejuvenation. *Dermatol Surg.* 2015;41(6):720–5.
22. Silva-Siwady JG, Diaz-Garza C, Ocampo-Candiani J. A case of Aptos thread migration and partial expulsion. *Dermatol Surg.* 2005;31(3):356–8.
23. Giampapa VC, Di Bernardo BE. Neck recontouring with suture suspension and liposuction: An alternative for the early rhytidectomy candidate. *Aesthetic Plast Surg.* 1995;19(3):21–3.
24. Lycka B, Bazan C, Poletti E, Treen B. The emerging technique of antiptosis subdermal suspension thread. *Dermatol Surg.* 2004;30(1):41–4.
25. Sasaki GH, Cohen AT. Meloplication of the malar fat pads by percutaneous cable-suture technique for midface rejuvenation: Outcome study (392 cases, 6 years' experience). *Plast Reconstr Surg.* 2002;110(2):635–54.
26. Lovreglio R, Fabbrocini G, Delfino M. The nonsurgical thread lift for facial rejuvenation. In: *Nonsurgical Lip and Eye Rejuvenation Techniques.* Fabbrocini G, De Padova MP, Tosti A, eds. Springer, 2016, 85–96.

Polylactic Resorbable Threads

27. Villa MT, White LE, Alam M, Yoo SS, Walton RL. Barbed sutures: A review of the literature. *Plast Reconstr Surg.* 2008;121:102e–8e.

10

Fractional Photothermolysis in Acne Scars

Gillian Beer, Patrick M. Zito, Adrianna Gonzalez, and Kenneth R. Beer

KEY FEATURES

- Acne scarring is a severe cosmetic concern for many adolescents as well as adults.
- Fractional photothermolysis treats only fractions of the skin.
- Several fractional laser devices are available and each varies as to the type of laser source, treatment settings, spot sizes and treatment depth.
- The choice of which fractional device should be used is dependent on the type and depth of the scarring as well as the patient's skin type and tolerance for risk.
- There are many new laser developments on the horizon, including new fractional CO_2 laser systems that require no anesthesia and are well tolerated.

Introduction

The use of lasers to treat acne scars has been available for decades. Initially, the use of pulsed dye lasers was advocated to reduce the redness associated with acne scars. However, as technology advanced, it became evident that vast improvements in the shape and depth of acne scars (Figure 10.1) could be obtained by using fractional photothermolysis. Initially developed by Manstein et al., fractional photothermolysis is a technology that removes fractions of the skin by causing microscopic areas of thermal damage [1]. Fractional ablative removes fractions of skin while fractional non-ablative heats columns of skin. The intact skin then aids in the healing process via extrusion of necrotic debris. With fractionated thermolysis, the thermal injury spans the epidermis and superficial dermis. The stratum corneum can be relatively spared depending on the energy setting utilized [2]. Ultimately the energy level used determines the depth and diameter.

Since realizing its role in skin resurfacing, both fractional ablative and non-ablative lasers have been used to treat acne scars, in addition to scars from surgical and traumatic injuries. In addition, the utilization of various adjunctive treatments such as growth factors, stem cells, and other types of lasers in combination with fractional thermolysis have ushered in a new era of treatments for acne scars.

Whereas early treatments for acne scars included subcision, trichloroacetic acid (TCA) peels and surgical correction, newer fractional lasers offer the promise of safety and efficacy in which acne scars may be significantly improved.

Since the last edition of this book, newer research and improved technology have brought the use of lasers to the forefront in the treatment of acne scars. This chapter will review newer data as well as consider some future directions. Consideration will be given to the role of ablative fractional resurfacing, non-ablative fractional resurfacing and combinations of these treatments with other modalities.

Fractional Ablative Resurfacing

CO_2 laser resurfacing has been used to treat the skin for more than 20 years. While the early lasers were used to treat photoaging, they have since been used to treat scars resulting from trauma, surgery, burns and acne. Ablative resurfacing utilizes light-based energy to destroy columns of skin. Surrounding the

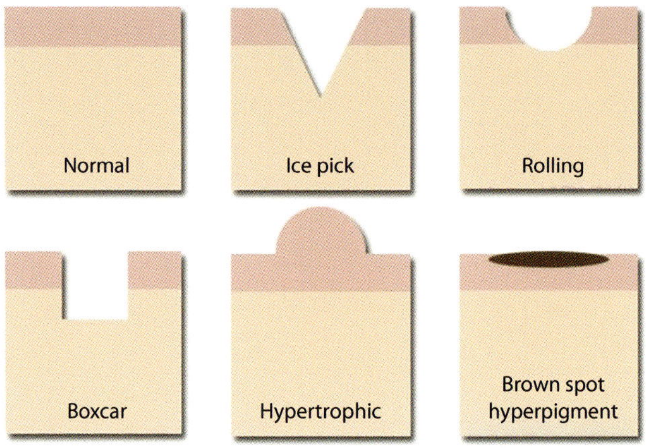

FIGURE 10.1 Classification of acne scars. (Adapted from Jacob et al. *J Am Acad Dermatol.* 2001;45(1):109–17 [3].)

ablative zone is a zone of thermally coagulated tissue. Following injury a reparative process occurs that produces new collagen, elastic fibers and epidermis.

Newer versions of the CO_2 utilize fractionated laser beams rather than non-fractionated devices. By doing so, columns of cells remain intact. These non-treated columns help to rejuvenate the skin. When utilized on acne scars, the formation of new collagen and epithelium can improve their appearance. During the past few years, the use of lasers to treat acne scars has had several improvements. By employing combinations of modalities, the treatment of acne scars has significantly improved.

There are many manufacturers of CO_2 lasers. Each has its own benefits and risks. Many excellent manufacturers produce CO_2 lasers and each has its own settings. In Dr. Beer's office, the Lumenis CO_2 laser is used, and settings mentioned will be provided for that device. For some superficial scars, the Active FX hand piece is used. It has a 1.3 mm spot size that matches the size of many small acne scars and this spot size can be delivered in a variety of patterns and densities. This allows the laser to be adjusted so that different amounts of energy can be delivered to different densities.

The Active FX creates "a shallow, broad crater that can extend into the superficial papillary dermis" [4]. After anesthesia is obtained, settings of between 85 and 125 mJ may be used with a density of between 2 and 4. Different shapes and sizes for the beam pattern are employed depending on the size and distribution of the scars. When using the Active FX, Ramsdell advocates settings for the face of approximately 100–125 mJ with density settings of between 2 and 4 with a higher density used for acne scars [4].

Following this procedure, new collagen and epithelium will grow with a significant effect on scars. Deeper scars may be treated with the DEEP FX handpiece, which has a beam size of 0.12 mm. When using this device, DEEP FX settings of between 15 and 22.5 will produce narrow, deep columns of damage that will be repaired with new collagen, elastic and epithelium. The depth of this modality has been demonstrated to be 416 um at 15 mJ, which correlates nicely to the depth of many acne scars [5].

The ideal interval between treatments has been the subject of great debate. One group of authors has compared treatments done at 1 month with treatments done at 3 months [6]. Patients selected for this treatment had CO_2 laser treatments performed for acne scars. The laser used was the Lumenis Ultra Pulse with the DEEP FX at 17.5–22.5 mJ at a density of 3. This was followed by an Active FX treatment with a setting of 100 mJ and a density of 3. After treatment, there were similar results in both groups with no difference in adverse events. Although there was a small sample (13 people) the data suggest that both groups improved with the laser treatment. This study confirms the efficacy of CO_2 laser for acne scars.

Combination Treatments for Acne Scarring

One combination that includes several modalities employs 20% TCA, subcision and fractional CO_2 laser resurfacing [7]. This combination was used on 114 patients who had mostly rolling acne scars. Following these treatments, 90% of the patients treated were "satisfied" with their results. This study was not blinded and used a simple four-point scale rather than image analysis to determine improvement. However, the fact that 90% of patients saw an improvement is significant.

Another combination treatment that looked at the role of lasers for the treatment of acne scars compared autologous fat grafts with platelet-rich plasma (PRP) with or without a fractional CO_2 laser [8]. These authors used autologous grafts with PRP to treat atrophic acne scars in 30 patients and measured the degree of improvement with the FACE-Q scale. The FACE-Q scale is a patient reported outcome (PRO) instrument used to measure the satisfaction of facial procedures. It is composed of 40 plus scales and checklists designed to measure adverse effects, appearance, health-related quality of life. PRP was harvested using the RegenLab THT tube. Using a CO_2 laser with this combination provided no advantage compared with the group that did not receive laser. The authors concluded that both groups benefited from the micrograft/PRP with no benefit from the laser.

Ramsdell advocates the use of punch excisions prior to treatment of ice pick scars with CO_2 laser. For this treatment, the ice pick scars (Figure 10.1) are anesthetized with 1% lidocaine and small punch biopsies (2–3 mm) are used to cut the scar. Using forceps, the scar is elevated and then secured into place so that it has a flat surface with the adjacent skin. After about 7–10 days the suture may be removed and CO_2 laser is used to resurface the area using the settings outlined previously. With this combination, significant improvements in recalcitrant scars may be achieved.

PRP in conjunction with CO_2 laser has also been used to treat acne scars. One study compared 16 patients with acne scars treated with CO_2 laser [9]. During the treatment, laser was performed on both sides and then one half of the face was treated with PRP while the other was treated with injections of saline. The authors concluded that the both sides had similar outcomes with scar improvement but that the side treated with PRP had significantly more adverse events in the form of longer duration of erythema and edema.

Fractional Non-ablative

Fractional non-ablative lasers are useful for the treatment of acne scars. For patients that have superficial acne scars or do not have the time for a fully ablative procedure, non-ablative resurfacing is a great alternative. Typically, these devices are used for superficial scars in a series of treatments spaced out over the span of a few weeks or months. Non-ablative lasers do not vaporize the skin. Instead, they heat the tissues and stimulate reparative mechanisms to remodel. The injury caused by the laser is less than that associated with an ablative laser and results in faster healing.

Non-ablative laser treatments have been used for treating acne scars in dark skin. One study evaluated the use of nonablative laser for Fitzpatrick type IV–VI [10]. These authors treated skin type IV–VI patients with acne scars using non-ablative fractional lasers (Figure 10.2).

In order to qualify for the study, subjects needed to have at least five acne scars. Scars had to be symmetric to qualify to be treated. The investigators used a 1550-nm Fraxel laser using different density settings (200 versus 393 microthermal treatment zones [MTZ]) but the same fluence (40 mJ) to treat patients at intervals of 4 weeks. Patients who completed the four treatments noted an improvement in the appearance of the scars for both settings with a minimal difference between the densities used. They concluded that this laser was safe and effective for treating acne scars. However, they noted a high incidence of hyperpigmentation following the procedure. This adverse event was significantly higher at the higher density settings.

Fractional Ablative vs. Fractional Non-ablative

It is well known that fractional ablative resurfacing offers significant improvements in acne scars. However, this treatment has been associated with multiple adverse events including persistent erythema, scarring, infection and pigment changes. Researchers have studied if the risks of complications are worth the improvement in acne scars. One group of authors compared ablative fractional CO_2 with ablative CO_2 (non-fractionated), Er:YAG and fractional erbium 1550 nm [11]. Researchers within this group conducted a retrospective review of 58 patients who were treated for acne scars. Settings used for the ablative

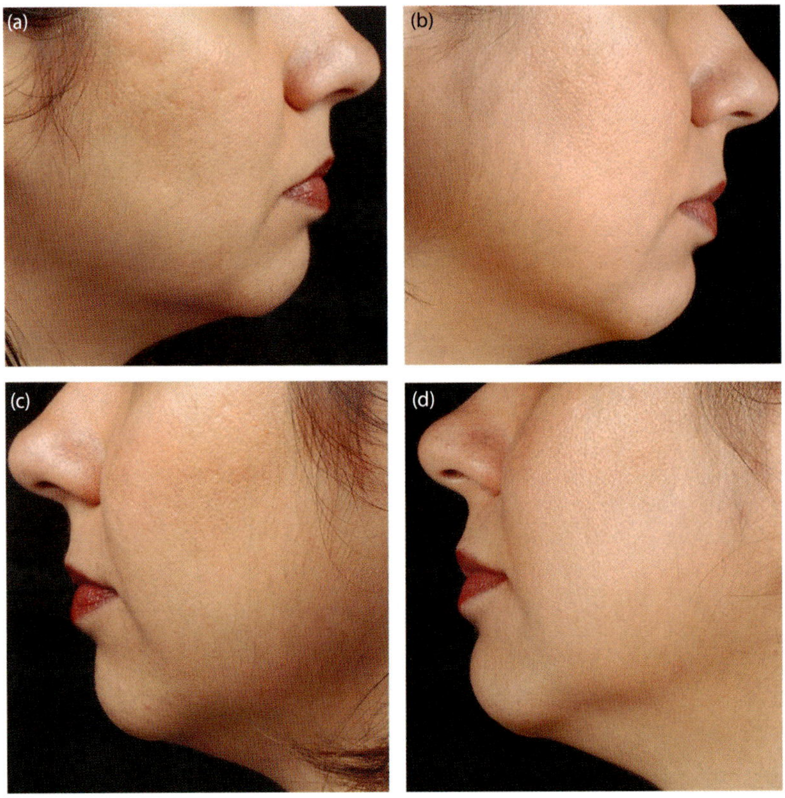

FIGURE 10.2 Before and after treatment from baseline to 24 weeks of a South Asian woman, Fitzpatrick skin Type IV. (a) Right cheek at baseline. (b) Right cheek at week 24 – 12 weeks after four treatments at lower density settings, 40 mJ, 11% coverage. (c) Left cheek at baseline. (d) Left cheek at week 24 – 12 weeks after four treatments at higher density settings, 40 mJ, 20% coverage. (From Alexis AF et al. *Dermatol Surg*. 2016;42(3):392–402. With permission. [10])

fractional laser were "50 mJ, power of 30 W and density of 150 spots/cm^2." A total of three to five sessions were performed. For the non-ablative fractional laser, settings were as follows: "30 mJ/MTZ and at a total density of 2500 MTZ/cm^2. Treatment levels varied from 4 to 6." Each patient was treated with between three and five treatments. Er:YAG and non-fractionated CO_2 lasers were also used in this study but are no longer in common use, so they are not detailed here. These authors found that all groups benefited from the treatments although some had to be repeated after 6–12 months. The data suggests that the ablative fractional laser is about as effective as the non-fractionated CO_2 laser with significantly less erythema. Interestingly, those that received non-ablative fractional resurfacing had significantly less improvement and were less satisfied than the patients treated with ablative lasers. Based on this study, it seems reasonable to utilize ablative fractional resurfacing as a primary mode of treatment for moderate-to-severe acne scars. These authors believe that three treatments with 2-month intervals are the best treatment for these types of acne scars.

Summary

Treatment of acne scars can be complex, requiring a balanced understanding of skin types, classification of acne scar, depth of scars, settings of lasers, and understanding the interaction of ablative and non-ablative lasers on various skin types. Non-ablative and ablative fractionated lasers have a role in the treatment of acne scars. Different modalities are being combined with fractionated lasers such as PRP and TCA peels but more studies are needed before definitive recommendations can be made. Current studies are difficult to compare with each other due to different parameters of the study. For this reason, with regard to Asian patients, it appears that a greater number of treatments with lower settings offer efficacy at a lesser risk of post inflammatory hyperpigmentation [12]. In Fitzpatrick skin types IV–VI, non-ablative fractional resurfacing is an effective and treatment for acne scars; however, precautions must be taken to avoid hyperpigmentation [10]. Utilization of lower temperatures and conservative measures to prevent post-inflammatory hyperpigmentation should be used.

REFERENCES

1. Manstein D, Herron GS, Sink RK, Tanner H, Anderson RR. Fractional photothermolysis: A new concept for cutaneous remodeling using microscopic patterns of thermal injury. *Lasers Surg Med.* 2004;34(5):426–38.
2. Laubach HJ, Tannous Z, Anderson RR, Manstein D. Skin responses to fractional photothermolysis. *Lasers Surg Med.* 2006;38(2):142–49.
3. Jacob CI, Dover JS, Kaminer MS. Acne scarring: A classification system and review of treatment options. *J Am Acad Dermatol.* 2001;45(1):109–17.
4. Ramsdell WM. Fractional carbon dioxide laser resurfacing. *Semin Plast Surg.* 2012;26(3):125–30.
5. Oni G, Robbins D, Bailey S, Brown SA, Kenkel JM. An *in vivo* histopathological comparison of single and double pulsed modes of a fractionated CO(2) laser. *Lasers Surg Med.* 2012;44(1):4–10.
6. Bjorn M, Stausbol-Gron B, Braae Olesen A, Hedelund L. Treatment of acne scars with fractional CO_2 laser at 1-month versus 3-month intervals: An intra-individual randomized controlled trial. *Lasers Surg Med.* 2014;46(2):89–93.
7. Taylor MB, Zaleski-Larsen L, McGraw TA. Single session treatment of rolling acne scars using tumescent Anesthesia, 20% trichloracetic acid extensive subcision, and fractional CO_2 laser. *Dermatol Surg.* 2017;43(Suppl 1):S70–4.
8. Tenna S, Cogliandro A, Barone M et al. Comparative study using autologous fat grafts plus platelet-rich plasma with or without fractional CO_2 laser resurfacing in treatment of acne scars: Analysis of outcomes and satisfaction with FACE-Q. *Aesthetic Plast Surg.* 2017;41(3):661–6.
9. Faghihi G, Keyvan S, Asilian A, Nouraei S, Behfar S, Nilforoushzadeh MA. Efficacy of autologous platelet-rich plasma combined with fractional ablative carbon dioxide resurfacing laser in treatment of facial atrophic acne scars: A split-face randomized clinical trial. *Indian J Dermatol Venereol Leprol.* 2016;82(2):162–8.
10. Alexis AF, Coley MK, Nijhawan RI et al. Nonablative fractional laser resurfacing for acne scarring in patients with Fitzpatrick skin phototypes IV–VI. *Dermatol Surg.* 2016;42(3):392–402.
11. You HJ, Kim DW, Yoon ES, Park SH. Comparison of four different lasers for acne scars: Resurfacing and fractional lasers. *J Plast Reconstr Aesthet Surg.* 2016;69(4):e87–95.
12. Wat H, Wu DC, Chan HH. Fractional resurfacing in the Asian patient: Current state of the art. *Lasers Surg Med.* 2017;49(1):45–59.

11

Non-Ablative and Ablative Devices in Acne Scars

Vic A. Narurkar

KEY FEATURES

- Non-ablative and ablative laser.
- Acne scars.
- Combination therapies.

Introduction

Acne scars are polymorphous and require a multidimensional approach to successful treatments. Scars can be atrophic, hypertrophic, sharply marginated, incongruous, distensible and non-distensible. Surface anomalies could include erythema, hypopigmentation and hyperpigmentation. The advent of lasers, light sources and radiofrequency has added significantly to the treatment and management of post-acne scarring. It is imperative to understand the indications for the class of devices to create a successful algorithm in incorporating devices for the treatment of post-acne scarring. This chapter will review the various light sources, non-ablative and ablative lasers, and radiofrequency devices for acne scarring.

Flash Lamp-Pulsed Dye Laser at 585 and 595 nm

The flash lamp-pulsed dye laser (FPDL) was one of the first lasers utilized to treat hypertrophic and erythematous scars [1,2]. The primary target of the FPDL is oxyhemoglobin. Therefore, the primary objective of using this device is to improve the erythema, which is often prominent in early acne scars. In addition to erythema, improvement in the texture of scars has been observed, leading to the hypothesis that a non-ablative mode of dermal remodeling and collagen production is involved. Higher fluencies of FPDL are indicated for hypertrophic scars and lower fluencies for atrophic scars. The FPDL has also been shown to have a coincidental improvement of active acne, although this has been a hotly debated topic. The mechanisms for acne clearance involve collateral damage to sebaceous glands and destruction of *Propionibacterium acnes*. Transforming growth factor (TGF)-β1 messenger ribonucleic acid has been shown to be increased in patients after FPDL treatments. TGF-β is known to be a potent stimulus for neocollagenesis and also promotes resolution of inflammation, which may explain the dual benefits of FPDL in active acne resolution/erythema resolution and long-term improvement in acne scars. Three to five sessions with FPDL spaced 4–6 weeks apart are usually necessary (Figure 11.1).

Broadband Light Sources with Filters (Intense Pulsed Light)

Broadband light uses selective filters, the majority of which are in the visible light range. Hence, it was appropriate to utilize these devices in a similar manner to the FPDL for the non-ablative treatment of acne

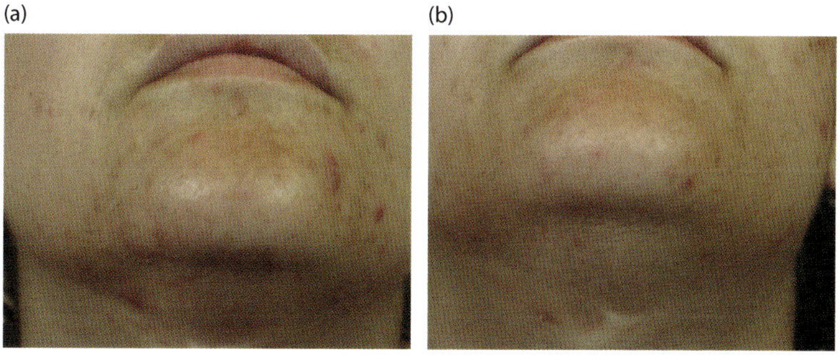

FIGURE 11.1 Distensible erythematous acne scars (a) before and (b) after three treatments with 585 nm flash lamp-pulsed dye laser.

scarring [3]. As with FPDL, three to five treatment sessions are usually necessary and the indications are similar to those with FPDL—primarily subtle atrophic and hypertrophic scars, with the primary goal being the improvement of visible erythema. Coincidental improvement of active acne has also been reported.

Photopneumatic Therapy

Photopneumatic therapy utilizes lower wavelength photons in the 420–500 nm range as broadband light sources compared with traditional visible light filters in broadband light [4]. A concurrent vacuum is applied at the time of light delivery, allowing for dermal targets to be closer to the surface, allowing for more efficient light delivery. These devices primarily treat active acne, as the target is *Propionibacterium acnes*. Subtle improvements in shallow non-distensible and erythematous scars, similar to those with FPDL and intense pulsed light (IPL) are also seen (Figure 11.2). It is also possible that stretching the skin with the vacuum may create some mechanical forces that may lead to long-term dermal remodeling.

Long-Pulsed 1064 nm Lasers

The long-pulsed (LP) 1064 nm lasers were originally developed for hair reduction in darker skin tones. Coincidental improvement in skin texture and tone was observed in hair reduction patients, leading physicians to utilize these lasers for the treatment of post-acne scarring. The primary chromophore for the LP 1064 nm laser is water, with some absorption by hemoglobin, although significantly less than that by FPDL and IPL sources. Therefore, similar to the other non-ablative devices, the LP 1064 is also indicated

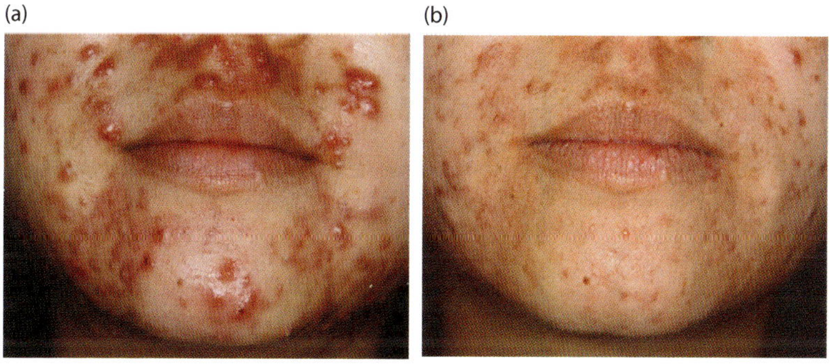

FIGURE 11.2 Concurrent improvement of active acne and distensible erythematous acne scars (a) before and (b) after five treatments with photopneumatic therapy.

for a subtle improvement of distensible non-erythematous acne scars [5,6]. The inherent wavelength of these devices also makes them a better option for treating darker skin tones. It is imperative to utilize lower fluencies and excellent cooling with these devices, as higher fluencies and poor cooling could actually promote scarring. Histology shows neocollagenesis, similar to that seen with other non ablative devices. Treatment intervals are 2–4 weeks apart and necessitate three to five treatment sessions.

Q-Switched 1064 nm Lasers

The Q-switched 1064 nm lasers employs an optomechanical shutter, allowing for nanosecond delivery of laser pulses at the 1064 nm wavelength. The laser was originally developed for the treatment of decorative tattoos of blue–black ink. The mechanism of tattoo removal is primarily photoacoustic, while the mechanism for dermal remodeling for acne scars is a combination of photoacoustic effects and absorption by water, leading to dermal collagen remodeling [7]. This is the safest laser in darker skin tones and does not require contact cooling. Lower fluencies are indicated for acne scarring, in comparison with decorative tattoo removal. Three to five treatment sessions, spaced 4–6 weeks apart are necessary.

Picosecond 755 and 1064 nm Lasers

The most recent advance in lasers for acne scars utilize picosecond pulse duration lasers of 755 and 1064 nm [8,9]. Picosecond lasers utilize primarily photoacoustic versus photothermal energy. The predominance of photoacoustic energy reduces risks of thermal injury and therefore increases safety, especially in darker skin tones. Holographic beam splitters in a picosecond domain and diffractive lens arrays in a picosecond domain create primarily dermal effects leading to neocollagenesis.

1320 nm Laser

The 1320 nm was the first laser to be studied specifically for non-ablative resurfacing of rhytids. The mechanism was to utilize the 1320 nm wavelength, which has deep penetration into the dermis, bypassing the epidermis and protecting the epidermis with cryogen cooling. The results with rhytids have generally been disappointing, but the results with non-distensible acne scarring have been better [10].

1450 nm Diode Laser

As with the 1320 nm laser, the 1450 nm diode laser was originally developed for non-ablative resurfacing of rhytids. A coincidental observation of the 1450 nm laser was its effect on the sebaceous gland, causing thermal necrosis [11]. Hence, lesions of active acne vulgaris improved after a series of treatments. The non-selective absorption of water and the deeper penetration permitted the concurrent dermal remodeling and neocollagenesis, allowing this laser to also be utilized for scarring.The deeper penetration allowed for the treatment of more significant scarring, unlike some of the other non-ablative devices such as FPDL, IPL and 1064 nm lasers. Atrophic, as well as flat and hypertrophic scars can be treated successfully. A series of three to five treatments, spaced 4–6 weeks apart is indicated. The concurrent improvement of acne is also a bonus. The main limiting factor of the 1450 nm diode laser is the significant discomfort, necessitating the use of strong topical anesthetics.

1540 and 1550 nm Non-Ablative Fractional Lasers

The most significant advance in the treatment of acne scarring is the development of non-ablative fractional laser resurfacing in the mid-infra red region [12,13]. These lasers were originally developed

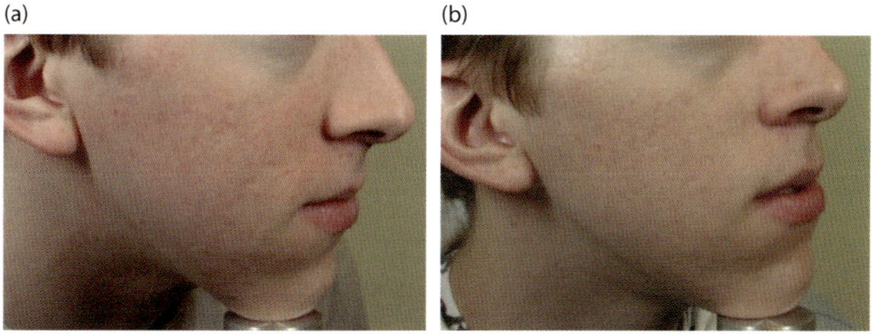

FIGURE 11.3 Polymorphous acne scars (a) before and (b) after five treatments with 1550 nm non-ablative fractional laser resurfacing.

for skin resurfacing for photodamage because ablative laser resurfacing had significant risks while non-ablative laser resurfacing produced minimal results. While these lasers offer excellent results in resurfacing for mild-to-moderate photodamage, the most impressive results are seen with post-acne scarring. The chromophore is water and the depth of penetration is up to 1 mm and beyond in the dermis. The laser energy is delivered in a fractional array of microbeams, either in a stamped fashion (1540 nm laser) or a random pattern (1550 nm). The fractional mode of delivery creates microscopic areas of injury. Treatment densities and fluencies can be adjusted based on the extent of acne scarring, anatomic location and skin tone. All skin colors can be treated with safety. The fractional mode of energy delivery reduces bulk heating, which has been the major source of complications in both ablative and non-ablative lasers. All types of acne scars—ice pick, rolling, boxcar, distensible, non-distensible and erythematous can be treated successfully (Figure 11.3). Moreover, hypopigmented scars can also be treated successfully with non-ablative fractional laser resurfacing. The need for adjuvant treatments of ice pick and bound down scars (e.g., subcision) has been reduced considerably since the advent of fractional laser resurfacing. Three to seven sessions, spaced 4–6 weeks apart are indicated.

Ablative 2940 and 10600 nm Fractional Lasers

The development of ablative 2940 and 10600 nm lasers [14] was promoted due to the need for fewer treatments in skin resurfacing compared with non-ablative lasers and to reduce risks with traditional ablative laser resurfacing at these wavelengths. These devices are relatively new and there is limited data on the efficacy with acne scarring. The 2940 nm wavelength shows the greatest affinity for water but with higher fluencies needed for ablation still produces greater bleeding. The 10600 nm wavelength is best utilized with higher fluencies, allowing for deeper penetration. There have been some reports of impressive improvements with the fractional 10600 nm ablative laser for acne scars with fewer treatments than with the non-ablative fractional lasers [15].

Radiofrequency with Microneedling

Microneedling with radiofrequency creates thermal zones of injury without targeting the epidermis [16]. The delivery of radiofrequency energy via microneedle source involves the use of insulated microneedles that prevent electrothermal damage from occurring anywhere in the dermis except at the tip of the needle. The depth of the needles can be adjusted from 0.5 to 3.5 mm based on depth of injury. Neocollagenesis occurs presumably through release of growth factors. Since the epidermis is spared, healing is accelerated and there is lower risk of post-inflammatory hyperpigmentation, especially in darker skin types.

TABLE 11.1

Summary of Laser and Light-Based Devices for Acne Scars

Device	Mode	Type of Acne Scars for Optimal Treatment
585 nm, 595 nm flash lamp-pulsed dye laser	Non-ablative	Erythematous and distensible scars
Broadband light, photopneumatic therapy	Non-ablative	Erythematous, hyperpigmented and distensible scars
Long-pulsed 1064 nm laser	Non-ablative	Distensible acne scars, subtle pitted scars
Q-switched 1064 nm laser	Non-ablative	Distensible acne scars, subtle pitted scars
1320 nm laser	Non-ablative	Distensible acne scars, subtle-to-moderate pitted and boxcar scars
1450 nm laser	Non-ablative	Distensible acne scars, subtle-to-moderate pitted and boxcar scars
1540 and 1550 nm lasers	Fractional non-ablative	Polymorphous scars
2940 and 10600 nm lasers	Fractional ablative	Polymorphous scars
2940 and 10600 nm lasers	Ablative	Polymorphous scars

Traditional 2940 and 10600 nm Ablative Lasers

Traditional ablative laser resurfacing employs 2940 or 10600 nm wavelengths. These devices have lost popularity due to prolonged healing and recovery, and with the case of 10600 nm ablative laser resurfacing, significant risks of hypopigmentation. The traditional 10600 nm ablative laser offered advantages over the traditional 2940 nm ablative laser due to greater hemostasis. The advent of longer pulsed 2940 nm lasers now can produce better hemostasis. For acne scarring, the ablative 2940 nm may offer advantages over 10600 nm due to deeper penetration, thereby allowing the treatment of a wider variety of acne scars [17–19].

Combination Therapies

Table 11.1 summarizes the monotherapy approach for the treatment of acne scars. It is evident that, as with facial rejuvenation, the approach to acne scarring requires a multimodal approach. This is especially true for ice pick scars, deep scars and communicating scars. Punch excision is often necessary if scars are extensive and ice pick in nature, although the need for this has been considerably reduced with the advent of non-ablative fractional laser resurfacing. Subcision is indicated when scars are bound down and have communicating sinus tracts. Dermal fillers are indicated when there is still atrophy despite treatment with devices.

Conclusions

A variety of devices are successful in treating post-acne scarring. The non-ablative devices include the FPDL, IPL, LP 1064 nm laser, QS 1064 nm laser, 1320 nm laser and 1450 nm laser. These non-ablative devices are best for subtle, shallow acne scarring and acne-associated erythema. The 1320 and 1450 nm may offer additional benefits for more extensive scarring. The non-ablative fractional lasers include the 1540 and 1550 nm laser and are considered the gold standard for acne scarring, treating the widest variety of polymorphous acne scars and diminishing the need for punch excisions and subcisions. The ablative fractional lasers include the 2940 and 10600 nm lasers have been introduced more recently and may offer similar results to non-ablative fractional lasers, but with fewer treatments. Traditional ablative lasers include the 2940 and 10600 nm lasers, and, while effective for post-acne scarring, carry significant recovery and risks. Devices are best employed in acne scarring in combination with subcision, punch excisions and dermal fillers for complete treatment.

REFERENCES

1. Railan D, Alster TS. Laser treatment of acne, psoriasis, leukoderma and scars. *Semin Cutan Med Surg.* 2008;27(4):285–91.
2. Lee DH, Choi YS, Min SU, Yoon MY, Suh DH. Comparison of 585 nm pulsed dye laser and a 1064 nm Nd:YAG laser for the treatment of acne scars: A randomized split faced study. *J Am Acad Dermatol.* May 2009;60(5):801–7.
3. Sawcer D, Lee HR, Lowe NJ. Lasers and adjunctive treatments for facial scars: A review. *J Cutan Laser Ther.* 1999;1(2):77–85.
4. Shamban AT, Enokibori M, Narurkar V, Wilson D. Photopneumatic technology for the treatment of acne vulgaris. *J Drugs Dermatol.* 2008;7(2):139–45.
5. Keller R, Belda Junior W, Valente NY, Rodrigues CJ. Nonablative 1064 nm Nd:YAG laser resurfacing of facial atrophic acne scars: Histologic and clinical analysis. *Dermatol Surg.* 2007;33(12):1470–6.
6. Goldberg DJ. Nonablative laser surgery for pigmented skin. *Dermatol Surg.* 2005;31(10):1263–7.
7. Friedman PM, Jih MH, Skover GR, Payonk GS, Kimyai-Asadi A, Geronemus RG. Treatment of facial atrophic scars with the 1064 nm Q-switched Nd:YAG laser-six month follow up study. *Arch Dermatol.* 2004;140(11):1337–41.
8. Brauer JA, Kazlouskava V, Alabdulrazzaq H, Bae YS, Bernstein LJ, Anolik R, Heller P, Geronemus RG. Use of a picosecond duration laser with specialized optic for treatment of facial acne scarring. *JAMA Dermatol.* 2015;151(3):278–84.
9. Bernstein EF, Schomacker KT, Basilavecchio LD, Plugis JM, Bhawalkar JD. Treatment of acne scarring with a novel fractionated dual wavelength picosecond domain laser incorporating a novel holographic beam splitter. *Lasers Surg Med.* 2017;49(9):796–802.
10. Yaghmai D, Garden JM, Bakus AD, Massa MC. Comparison of a 1064 nm laser and a 1320 nm laser for the nonablative treatment of acne scars. *Dermatol Surg.* 2005;31(8 Pt 1):903–9.
11. Chua SH, Ang P, Khoo LS, Goh CL. Nonablative 1450 nm diode laser in the treatment of facial atrophic scars in type IV to V Asian skin: A prospective clinical study. *Dermatol Surg.* 2004;30(10):1287–91.
12. Narurkar V. Skin rejuvenation with microthermal fractional photothermolysis. *Dermatol Ther.* 2007;20(Suppl 1):S10–3.
13. Chrastil B, Glaich AS, Goldberg LH, Friedman PM. Second generation 1550 nm fractional photothermolysis for the treatment of acne scars. *Dermatol Surg.* 2008;34(10):1327–32.
14. Taub AF. Fractionated delivery systems for difficult to treat clinical applications: Acne scarring, melasma, atrophic scarring, striae distensae and deep rhytides. *J Drugs Dermatol.* 2007;6(11):1120–8.
15. Geronemus RG. Fractional photothermolysis: Current and future applications. *Lasers Surg Med.* 2006;38(3):169–76.
16. Byalekere S, Siriam R, Mysore R, Bhaskar S, Shetty A. Evaluation of microneedling fractional radiofrequency device for treatment of scars. *J Cutan Aesthet Surg.* 2014;7(2):93–7.
17. Chapas AM, Brightman L, Sukal S, Hale E, Daniel D, Bernstein LJ, Geronemus RG. Successful treatment of acneiform scarring with CO_2 ablative fractional resurfacing. *Lasers Surg Med.* 2008;40(6):381–6.
18. Jeong JT, Kye YC. Resurfacing of pitted facial acne scars with a long pulsed Er:YAG laser. *Dermatol Surg.* 2001;27(2):107–10.
19. Walia S, Alster TS. Prolonged clinical and histologic effects from CO_2 laser resurfacing of atrophic acne scars. *Dermatol Surg.* 1999;25(12):926–30.

12

Surgical Techniques: Subcision, Grafting, Excision, and Punch Techniques

Rohit Kakar, Farhaad Riyaz, Megan Pirigyi, and Murad Alam

KEY FEATURES

- Treatment approaches for acne scarring should be individualized and primarily determined by the morphological features of each patient's scars.
- The surgical interventions described in this chapter are indispensable in the revision of deep and fibrotic acne scars.
- Subcision is a simple, well-tolerated procedure capable of producing long-term improvement of rolling acne scars.
- Dermal grafts are autologous implants that may provide permanent augmentation of depressed acne scars.
- Excision and punch techniques remain the treatments of choice for deep, sharply punched-out acne scars.
- All the procedures that are described in this chapter may be incorporated into multistep treatment plans tailored to address patients' individual needs.

Introduction

Anecdotal experience and medical investigation have shown that most cases of acne scarring cannot be solved by a single "best" treatment. Acne scars come in a variety of structures and depths, and each of the currently available treatments is ideally suited to address a subset of this spectrum. While resurfacing procedures are useful in resolving texture and pigment irregularities caused by shallow-to-medium-depth acne scars, fillers are more effective at augmenting depressed, distensible scars. The surgical interventions described in this chapter, including subcision, dermal grafting, excision and punch techniques, are often the best options for improving the deepest and most fibrotic forms of acne scarring in addition to correcting superficial scars.

Both subcision and dermal grafting are aimed at achieving long-term augmentation of depressed acne scars with indistinct borders. Subcision, or subdermal undermining, is designed to treat rolling acne scars that result from abnormal fibrous tethering of scar surfaces to deeper structures. Due to their underlying physiology, these scars are not amenable to correction by fillers alone but may be improved when subcision is used to disrupt the fibrous bands below their surfaces. Dermal grafting involves implantation of an autologous strip or plug of dermis into a subcised recipient pocket and may achieve long-term augmentation of deeper depressed scars caused by dermal loss.

Excision and punch techniques are used to replace deep, sharply delineated scars, such as ice pick and deep boxcar scars, with less conspicuous secondary defects. In elliptical and punch excision, this is accomplished by surgical removal of a scar and careful closure of the resultant defect to create a flat, linear scar that lies along a relaxed skin tension line. Punch grafting entails replacing an excised scar

TABLE 12.1

Patient Characteristics that are Possible Contraindications for Surgical Scar Treatment

Characteristic	Reason for Contraindication
History of poor wound healing or tendency toward keloid formation/hypertrophic scarring	Risk of unacceptable secondary defect
Unreasonable expectations for improvement	Complete elimination of a scar is highly unlikely. Optimal results may require a combination of treatment modalities over the course of several months
Active or recently resolved acne lesions	Disruption of pilosebaceous units during surgical procedures may lead to the formation of acneiform cysts

with a full-thickness, autologous punch graft, and punch elevation involves preserving an excised scar base and allowing it to rise to the level of the surrounding skin.

For all of the surgical techniques described in this chapter, careful patient selection and ongoing communication are paramount. While these procedures have the potential to improve the appearance of even the most severe forms of acne scarring, patients must have realistic expectations and should be counseled regarding the degree of improvement they are likely to achieve. Although irregularities in contour, texture and pigmentation may be ameliorated, complete erasure of a scar is highly unlikely. Since many patients have a variety of different acne scar types and because some of these treatments involve the creation of secondary defects, a combination of different procedures over the course of many months is often required to produce optimal results. In addition, when designing a treatment strategy, the clinician should carefully consider a patient's willingness to accept downtime. Before recommending any scar revision procedure it is crucial to obtain a thorough medical and surgical history. Patients with increased risk of keloid and hypertrophic scarring and those with active or recently active acne are not good candidates for surgical scar revision [1] (Table 12.1).

Subcision

History

In 1995, Orentreich and Orentreich introduced the technique of subcision as a stand-alone treatment for depressed scars and wrinkles [2]. Subdermal undermining of scars, however, was used as early as 1957 when it was described as a method to prepare sites for fibrin foam injection [3]. Since that time, undermining has been used frequently in conjunction with fibrel implantation [4,5], microlipoinjection, [6] and dermal grafting [7] procedures.

Structure and Function

Subcision is designed to address the underlying pathophysiology of rolling acne scars. These scars appear as broad, undulating depressions on the surface of the skin and lack the sharply delineated edges seen in boxcar and ice pick scars. Despite their superficial appearance, rolling scars result from deep fibrous attachments tethering the epidermis to the subcutis. Subcision is designed to sever these fibrous bands while causing minimal damage to the overlying skin. Typically, this technique results in elevation of the depressed scar to the level of the surrounding skin. The originators of this technique, David and Norman Orentreich, propose that the augmenting effect seen after subcision is the result of two distinct processes [2]. An immediate, partial elevation results from the scar base being cut free from the downward pull of its tethers [2,8]. In the weeks following subcision, additional augmentation of the depressed defect is typically observed. This subsequent elevation is thought to result from trauma caused during the procedure, which initiates a wound-healing response culminating in the deposition of new connective tissue beneath the scar surface [2,9].

Technology

Indication

Subcision is best used to treat rolling acne scars with normal-appearing overlying skin and a lack of sharply delineated borders [2]. It is contraindicated for areas of active infection and in patients with bleeding diathesis or a tendency toward keloid formation [2]. Other cutaneous depressions, such as rhytids, depressed skin grafts, surgical wounds and cellulite dimples are also considered valid indications for subcision [2,10].

Advantages/Disadvantages

The main advantage of subcision is that it has the potential to produce long-term improvement in the appearance of rolling acne scars while causing minimal injury to overlying skin. The procedure is easy to perform and is generally safe and well tolerated. Although it may cause some bruising and swelling, the recovery time is brief. Furthermore the required materials are both inexpensive and widely available.

One disadvantage of subcision is that a single treatment is not guaranteed to produce substantial improvement. Since the final result of the procedure depends on the unique wound-healing response of the individual, it is often difficult to predict the outcome of an initial treatment [2]. In order to achieve optimal results, some patients require several treatment sessions or adjunct procedures such as resurfacing or filler injection [2].

Complications

Erythema, bruising, edema and tenderness are expected sequelae and may persist at the subcision site for 1–2 weeks [2,11]. Another potential complication is the formation of cystic acneiform lesions, which are thought to result from disruption of acne sinus tracts or pilosebaceous units [2,11].

While partial improvement of a depressed scar is common, an excessive or hypertrophic response may also occur in 5%–10% of cases [2,11]. An excessive response usually results in a small, palpable induration at the treated site [12]. Such areas of firmness may not be visible and may typically flatten over time. Patients may be informed that palpable but invisible bumps may be desirable to the extent that they tend to improve the smoothness of the final skin contour.

Combination Possibilities

Subcision may be readily combined with other treatments such as filler injection, laser resurfacing, needling or cryorolling, microneedling with radiofrequency, trichloroacetic acid peeling or chemical reconstruction [13–19]. In many instances a combined treatment protocol will produce superior results, especially when rolling scars are interspersed with other forms of acne scars.

Practical Advice for the Clinician

Some bleeding and ecchymosis during the procedure is considered normal and beneficial, as the collection of blood beneath the defect may instigate new collagen formation [11] (Figure 12.1).

Prior to treatment it is important for patients to understand that complete improvement after a single treatment with subcision is unlikely and several sessions may be required to achieve maximal correction.

Technical Procedure

Before beginning the procedure, the skin is cleansed and the depressed scars are carefully outlined using a surgical marking pen. The sites are then infiltrated with a solution of 1% lidocaine with 1:100,000 epinephrine. The anesthetized area should extend far enough beyond the borders of each scar to allow for painless needle insertion. Once adequate anesthesia and vasoconstriction has been obtained, a tri-bevelled

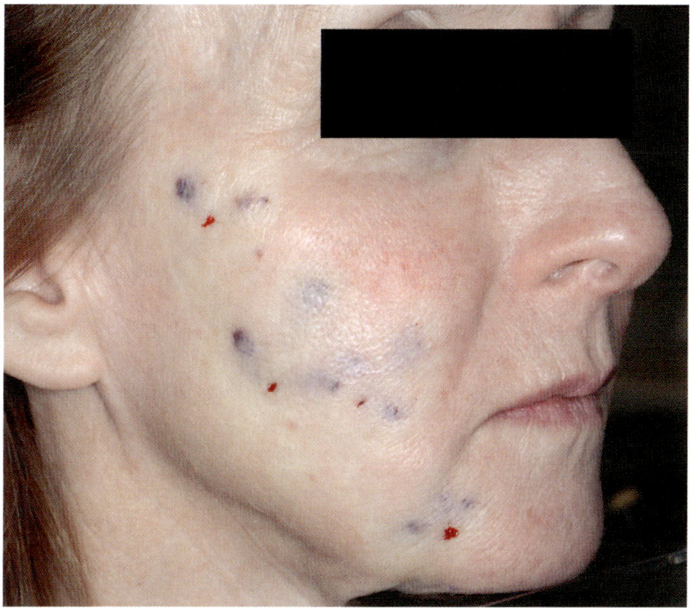

FIGURE 12.1 Immediately following subcision there may be bleeding and ecchymosis at the treated sites. This is expected and may be beneficial in promoting the formation of new collagen beneath the depressed scars.

hypodermic needle [2] or Nokor needle [11,12] (Becton Dickinson, Franklin Lakes, NJ, USA) is inserted into the skin adjacent to the depression and advanced until it lies directly beneath the scar (Figure 12.2). The depth of needle insertion will depend upon the severity of each scar, with more superficial scars being subcised at the level of the mid-dermis and more deeply depressed scars being undermined in the deep dermis or subcutis [11].

The subcision needle is initially moved forwards and backwards in a tunneling motion to pierce through the fibrotic scar tissue (Figure 12.2). Once the fibrous mass is sufficiently fragmented, the needle is swiped side-to-side in a direction parallel to the skin surface to free the scar from its tethers (Figure 12.2). For densely fibrous scars it may be useful to use multiple needle insertion sites to undermine the defect from different angles [1]. Upon severing the final tethers, the skin may visibly elevate. Following the procedure, antibiotic ointment and a compression bandage may be applied [1].

Modifications to this procedure have been suggested. Altering the instrument has been the primary focus of technique advancement: bending the subcision needle at a 90° angle to prevent penetration of and/or damage to the skin [20]; using a needle holder for the Nokor needle to create horizontal orientation and avoid withdrawing [21]; using an 18- or 21-gauge metal spinal needle cannula (Hakko Co., Chikuma, Japan) that demonstrated a high cure rate [22]; using a 20-gauge cataract blade due to its increased sharpness, increased control of depth and precision, longer cutting distance, and easier grasp of the handle [23]; and injecting a tumescent solution followed by the use of a blunt blade in order to avoid needlestick injury [24]. All of these modifications have demonstrated improvement of acne scars.

A recent device innovation has been the Taylor Liberator, a long metal apparatus with a handle, a shaft and a fork-like tip. Inserted through a nick into the superficial subcutis at the preauricular area, this is advanced from that ipsilateral single point to the area under acne scars in the mid-cheek and the perioral area. Benefits include the need for fewer entry points and less epidermal trauma. The instrument must be kept superficial throughout its course to avoid excess trauma and transient paresthesia.

An additional suggested enhancement involves attempting to physically lift the treatment area. Patients who underwent suctioning with a microdermabrasion device on the third day after subcision and continued every other day for at least 2 weeks had a significant improvement [25]. Similarly, although not studied for use with acne scars, the creation of a looping suture at the center of an atrophic scar that is pulled vertically upward to create a virtual plane via retraction during subcision improved scars [26]. The authors

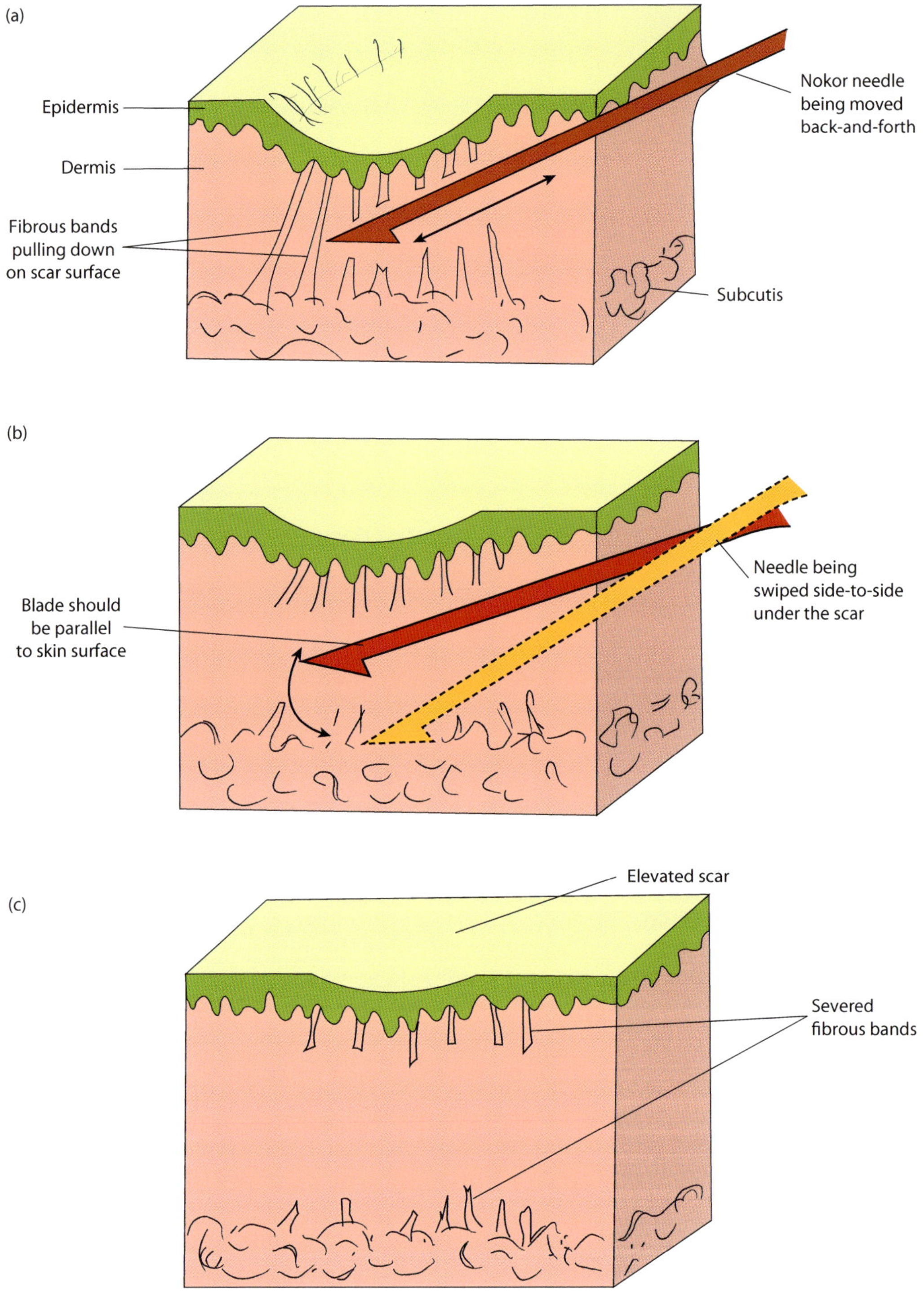

FIGURE 12.2 Subcision. (a) A Nokor needle (Becton Dickinson, Franklin Lakes, NJ, USA) is inserted at an angle into the skin adjacent to the scar so that its blade lies directly beneath the depressed area and is parallel to the skin surface. The needle is first advanced in a back-and-forth tunneling motion to pierce through the fibrous tissue. (b) Next, the needle is swept from side-to-side beneath the scar to ensure that all tethers are cut. (c) After healing the scar is no longer bound down to the subcutis and its surface has elevated.

contend that lifting allows for the release of retracted bands located at a deeper plane, which may be of utility with deeper, more tethered acne scars and requires further research [26].

Management of Complications

If a cyst forms at a subcision site, it may be treated with intralesional steroid injection and oral antibiotics. Induration caused by a hypertrophic response usually disappears without intervention, but resolution may be accelerated by daily firm fingertip massage of the sites [12] or low-dose intralesional corticosteroid injections [1,2,11].

Dermal Grafting

History

Dermal grafts and dermal fat grafts have been used since the 1930s [27] but were initially employed primarily for the correction of defects in organs other than the skin [11,28,29]. For many decades the use of dermal grafts in the skin was limited due to their tendency toward cyst formation and inconsistent results [28,29]. Recent improvements in harvesting and graft placement techniques have allowed dermal grafting to gain acceptance as an option for permanent augmentation of cutaneous depressions [29].

Structure and Function

In the dermal grafting procedure, a depressed recipient site is undermined immediately prior to implantation of the graft. This step is intended to create a recipient pocket lined with highly vascular granulation tissue that can accept the graft and promote anastomosis of capillaries [28]. It is thought that this encourages rapid restoration of circulation to the graft and is consequently responsible for the high success rate of the procedure [28].

Technology

Indication

Dermal grafting is indicated for the correction of broad (3 mm to 2 cm in diameter) and linear scars that are soft and distensible [28,30]. Like subcision, dermal grafting can augment depressed scars while leaving the overlying epidermis largely intact, so it is best suited to treat scars with normal overlying skin and a lack of sharp walls. Dermal grafting has also been used to augment wider, deep rhytids such as nasolabial folds and glabellar creases [28] and to correct deep nasal and alar rim defects resulting from Mohs surgery [31].

Advantages and Disadvantages

Dermal grafting is a useful technique for correcting deep contour defects and the grafts have several advantages over other augmenting agents. They are readily available, inexpensive, nonallergenic implants that are autologous and not susceptible to rejection [7,29]. They also have the potential to provide long-term or permanent correction [29]. They also can be precisely created to match the size and shape of nearly any depressed area [7]. Dermal grafting spares a scar's surface from injury and typically results in only mild bruising and swelling, similar to subcision.

The primary disadvantage of dermal grafting is the requirement of a donor site, and patients and physicians may be reluctant to create a new defect for this purpose. In addition, although dermal grafts have some advantages over other fillers, the process of harvesting and implanting the grafts is considerably more time consuming and challenging than alternative augmenting procedures. The recent increased availability of numerous safe and relatively long-acting prepackaged injectable soft-tissue augmentation materials has resulted in a reduced interest in dermal grafting.

Complications

Following dermal grafting, some bruising, edema and crusting at the insertion sites are expected [7]. The most frequent complication is cyst formation, which has an incidence of approximately 10% [31]. The best way to avoid this outcome is to take meticulous care to completely remove the epidermis and appendageal structures from the donor sites before harvesting grafts [29].

Combination Possibilities

Multiple dermal grafts taken from a single donor site may be implanted at different sites during the same procedure. Patients may also undergo resurfacing via dermabrasion, chemical peeling or laser therapy at the time of graft placement or following healing [29,32]. Although no formal studies have been conducted with dermal grafts, platelet-rich plasma may potentially serve to enhance results, as shown with autologous fat grafts with and without laser resurfacing for various scar types [33,34].

Practical Advice for the Clinician

Although dermal grafting is recommended for the treatment of distensible scars, one or two sessions of subcision can make some fibrotic scars soft enough to accept dermal grafting [29].

When selecting punches to harvest round dermal grafts, it should be noted that while epidermal punch grafts are normally designed to be slightly larger than their recipient sites to allow for graft shrinkage, a dermal punch graft should exactly match the size and shape of the recipient defect [29].

Technical Procedure

There is some difference of opinion concerning the optimal preparation for dermal grafting. While Swinehart recommends undermining a scar 10–14 days prior to graft placement and then again at the time of the procedure [28], others prefer to subcise the scar only at the time of dermal grafting [29]. Regardless of whether this additional step is taken, scars should be examined carefully with overhead and tangential light immediately prior to dermal grafting and both the scars and donor site should be carefully outlined with a marker pen. Photographs should be taken before and after marking, and postmarking photographs should be available as a reference during the procedure.

Next, both sites are typically injected with 1%–2% lidocaine with 1:100,000 epinephrine for local anesthesia and hemostasis. The donor site, usually the postauricular crease, is then de-epithelialized to a level below the papillary dermis using either dermabrasion [7] or a resurfacing laser [30]. Care should be taken to remove all appendageal structures, especially sebaceous glands that may lead to cyst formation if left behind [29]. The method of graft harvesting is then determined based upon the size and shape of the defect to be corrected. A scalpel or laser may be used to collect linear strips of dermis, while appropriately sized punches are ideal for producing grafts destined for small, round scars. The grafts should be placed in chilled sterile saline and, if necessary, should be precisely trimmed to fit the recipient scar sites [28].

The scar should then be freshly undermined to create a pocket underneath its depressed surface. For small, round scars, grafts may be inserted into their recipient pockets through the opening made by the subcision needle and manipulated into place with diamond-tipped Jewelers forceps [28] (Figure 12.3).

For the correction of large linear scars, Goodman suggests using an intravenous cannula to undermine the scar and provide a means of guiding the graft into place [29]. The cannula is inserted into one end of the linear defect, passed forward and backward several times to create the recipient pocket, and then passed out via the distal end of the scar [29]. The plastic sleeve surrounding the instrument is left within the wound as the introducer is removed so that the sleeve protrudes from both ends of the recipient pocket [30]. This sleeve acts as a tunnel into which one can pull a dermal graft attached with a polydioxanone suture to a straight needle [16]. The needle is passed through one end of the tunnel until the graft is about to enter the sleeve, then the trailing end of the graft is grasped with Jewelers forceps so that it can be more easily manipulated into its final position [29]. With the graft still held by the Jewelers forceps, the sleeve and graft are pulled through the recipient tunnel as a unit so that the

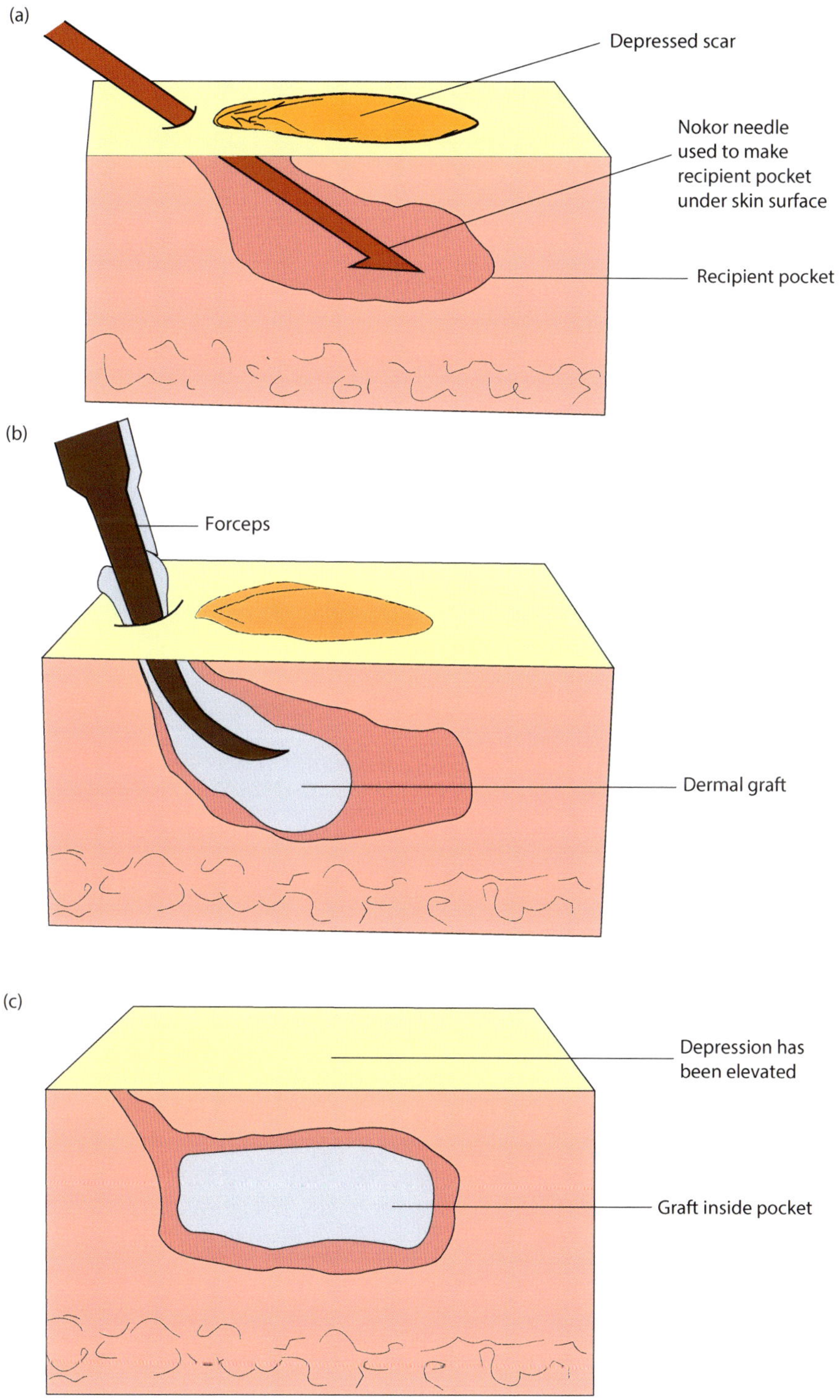

FIGURE 12.3 Dermal grafting. (a) The depressed scar is first subcised to create a recipient pocket for the graft. (b) Using Jewelers forceps, a freshly harvested dermal graft is inserted into the recipient pocket through the incision made by the subcision needle. (c) Upon completion of the procedure, the depressed area is augmented to the level of the surrounding skin.

plastic sleeve is removed, and only the sutured graft remains in the tunnel [29]. Once the graft is in a satisfactory position, the Jewelers forceps are removed and the suture is cut proximally [29]. Removal of the suture from the graft is not required. If necessary, the ends of the graft may be secured in place with highly degradable sutures and the ends of the recipient tunnel may be closed with Steri-Strips (3M Corp, St. Paul, MN, USA) or fine degradable sutures [28]. Finally, the donor site should be closed using a running horizontal mattress suture [29].

Following the procedure, the patient should be advised to immobilize the graft site as much as possible for 1–2 days in order to maximize graft survival [29]. Immediate results of dermal grafting are typically very good, with complete or nearly complete correction of the defect evident upon dressing removal [28]. Unfortunately these impressive initial results may not be permanent as grafts often lose volume over time. Nonetheless, in Goodman's 1997 study involving 11 patients with 32 dermal grafts, 84% of the grafts provided substantial improvement or complete correction of defects at follow-up periods from 3 to 30 months [30].

A modified technique describes mincing grafts with a #15 surgical blade or curved iris scissors to form smashed dermal grafts, moldable to any shape and suitable for boxcar, rolling, linear or irregular geometrical scars [36]. The smashed dermal grafts are aspirated into 1 mL tuberculin syringes with 18-gauge needles and inserted with graft-holding forceps. This may be followed by external manipulation until maximum correction is achieved [36].

Management of Complications

In the event of cyst formation, intralesional corticosteroid injections may be used. Alternatively, cysts may be drained or excised [28].

Excision, Punch Elevation and Punch Grafting

History

Excision and punch techniques have been used for several decades in the treatment of deep, atrophic acne scars [8,36–41]. These techniques remain indispensable for the correction of acne scars whose depth precludes correction by resurfacing and whose irregular scar bases and sharply defined walls make them unsuitable candidates for filler correction.

Technology

Indication

Elliptical or punch excision should be used when one's aesthetic goal is to replace a prominent scar with a less conspicuous linear, superficial scar. Punch excision is indicated for the treatment of ice pick and deep boxcar scars that are <3.5 mm in diameter [1]. Scars larger than 3.5 mm should be removed with elliptical excision so that the resultant wound can be repaired more effectively without the risk of standing cone formation. Excision is also often the best option for the treatment of acne scars with cutaneous bridges or persistent cysts and tunnels [42]. It may also be an option for certain hypertrophic or keloidal acne scars [35] (Table 12.2).

For some patients with ice pick and deep boxcar scars, punch grafting may produce better cosmetic results than excision, particularly if the scars are in regions of the face where linear defects are not easily hidden in relaxed skin tension lines. Punch grafting is only feasible, however, if the patient has a suitable donor site with skin that matches the scar site in color and texture. Punch grafting is most successful in less mobile areas of the face such as the forehead and upper cheeks [35] (Table 12.2).

Punch elevation has a very narrow indication for deep boxcar scars with bases that are smoothly textured, normal in pigmentation, and not fibrotic. The scar must also have vertical walls, as a scar that tapers along its depth does not have a large enough base to fill its surface opening (Table 12.2).

TABLE 12.2

Indications for Excision and Punch Techniques

Technique	Indicated Scar Types
Punch excision	Ice pick scars; deep boxcar scars <3.5 mm in diameter
Elliptical excision	Ice pick scars; deep boxcar scars ≥ 3.5 mm in diameter; scars with bridges, cysts or tunnels
Punch grafting	Ice pick scars; deep boxcar scars
Punch elevation	Deep boxcar scars with vertical walls and scar bases that match surrounding skin in texture and pigmentation

Advantages and Disadvantages

Excision and punch techniques have a distinct advantage over nonsurgical scar revision techniques in their capacity to substantially improve the appearance of ice pick and deep boxcar scarring. Until the development of the focal trichloroacetic acid chemical reconstruction of skin scars technique for the treatment of narrow ice pick scars [43], cold-steel surgical techniques were the only effective treatments for deep, sharply punched-out acne scars and scars with irregular atrophic bases.

The primary disadvantage of all excision and punch techniques is that they necessitate the creation of secondary defects. The concept of replacing old scars with fresh ones may be unappealing to some patients and physicians. In addition, these procedures are unlikely to produce optimal results in patients with tendencies toward poor wound healing. It should be noted that some patients develop severe acne scars due to a propensity toward abnormal healing, and these particular patients would be poor candidates for these interventions. Even when performed in well-selected candidates, excision and punch techniques carry the risk of leaving behind conspicuously elevated or depressed scars. Punch grafting has the added disadvantages of requiring a donor site and involving the risks of graft extrusion or visual mismatch between the graft and recipient skin.

Complications

Following elliptical excision, depression and widening of scars may occur, particularly in regions of high sebaceous gland activity [44,45]. This outcome is best prevented by careful patient selection and meticulous technique. Care should be taken while excising the defect to preserve as much subcutaneous tissue as possible to act as an anchoring foundation for the healing wound [44]. A precise suturing technique [46] and the use of Steri-Strips (3M Corp., St. Paul, MN, USA) for up to 10 days following the procedure [47] can prevent scar spread. When planning to treat more substantial areas of scarring, large excisions should be avoided in favor of a series of small excisions performed at 4–6-week intervals [46].

Some complications of punch transplantation include poor graft take, graft extrusion, depressed grooves around the margins of the grafts, depressed or elevated grafts, and color or texture mismatch between grafts and surrounding skin. To prevent these outcomes, the donor site should be carefully selected prior to the procedure. The risk of depressed borders around the grafts or depression or elevation of the grafts themselves can be minimized by ensuring that the graft is slightly larger in diameter than the recipient site and using Steri-Strips to hold the grafts in place for a minimum of 5 days [48]. To decrease the chance of graft extrusion, patients should be advised not to touch or press on their graft sites and to minimize their facial movements for the 3 days following the surgery [48]. In addition, grafts are less likely to succeed in the lower cheeks and perioral area due to mouth and jaw movement. If grafts are placed in these areas, extra care should be taken to secure them in place and patients should be strongly advised to limit talking and chewing for several days following the procedure [48].

In punch elevation, the most frequent complication is persistent elevation of a plug above the level of the surrounding skin [48].

Combination Possibilities

Excision and punch techniques are frequently combined with resurfacing procedures in order to improve the appearance of secondary defects. Traditionally, dermabrasion is performed 4–8 weeks after excision or punch grafting [38]; a newer alternative is to perform a single combined procedure of excision or punch grafting and laser resurfacing [49,50]. A split-face randomized study comparing punch elevation followed by two treatments of fractional carbon dioxide (CO_2) laser separated by a 1-month interval to fractional CO_2 laser alone for atrophic acne scars found the combination to be more efficacious [51].

Practical Advice for the Clinician

Since excision and punch procedures involve the creation of secondary defects, it is essential that patients have realistic expectations prior to undergoing these treatments. Patients should be well informed about the potential outcomes and should be willing to accept the possibility that subsequent procedures, such as laser resurfacing, may be necessary to produce an optimal result.

With all of these techniques it is possible to treat multiple areas simultaneously. If two or more scars are to be excised, they should be at least 4–5 mm apart to prevent excess traction during healing [1]. If multiple punch transplants of different sizes are to be performed in a single procedure, it is helpful to devise a way of organizing and labeling the grafts before starting.

In punch grafting, careful donor-site selection is crucial. The postauricular area is most frequently used, but if it is not a good match with the recipient site or if it has active acne lesions, other sites including the preauricular area, supraclavicular area, posterior arms and hairline may be considered [48].

Technical Procedure

Prior to an excision or punch procedure, scars are examined and marked, the treatment area is cleansed and the tissue is infiltrated with 1% lidocaine plus epinephrine (1:100,000). For all punch techniques, a variety of disposable punch biopsy instruments are available with diameters ranging in 0.25 mm increments from 1.5 to 3.5 mm (Goodman GJ, unpublished work). The walls of the punches are seamless and straight.

For punch excision, a punch instrument is selected that is just large enough to encompass the scar and its walls [1]. The first finger and thumb are placed on either side of the scar and used to create outward traction perpendicular to a resting skin tension line [35]. This creates an elongated wound that will be camouflaged along a natural facial line. The punch is inserted at a 90° angle and inserted to the level of the subcutaneous fat; the scar will easily lift out unless the base is overly fibrotic. Forceps and iris scissors can be used to gently release the scar from any fibrous attachments if necessary [1]. If smaller than 2 mm, a wound may be left to heal by second intention [28] or may be closed with one or two simple interrupted sutures [1]. Punch sites larger than 2.5 mm may heal better when closed with a single buried deep suture [1]. Any epidermal sutures are removed within 7 days to prevent track-mark formation [1].

Elliptical excision is preferable to punch excision for acne scars larger than 3.5 mm. A scalpel blade is used to excise a longitudinally oriented ellipse along a resting skin tension line. The scar is encompassed at the center of the ellipse and the wound angles are 30 degrees or less to allow for aesthetic closure [35]. Undermining may be used to mobilize the wound edges for tension-free wound closure [47]. Small excisions may be closed with buried dermal sutures [46] while larger excisions may be closed with several simple, interrupted sutures [1] or buried vertical mattress [35] sutures.

To perform punch elevation, a punch instrument is chosen that exactly matches the diameter of the scar base (Figure 12.4). The punch is inserted down to the level of subcutaneous fat so that the tissue may be manipulated [48]. Next, forceps are used to gently elevate the scar base until it sits slightly higher than the surrounding surface, and the tissue is held in place for 1 or 2 minutes until a coagulum forms beneath it [48] (Figure 12.4). The plug is then secured in place using sutures, Dermabond (2-octyl cyanoacrylate, Ethicon, Inc., Somerville, NJ, USA), or Steri-Strips [19]. The area is covered with a topical antibiotic and

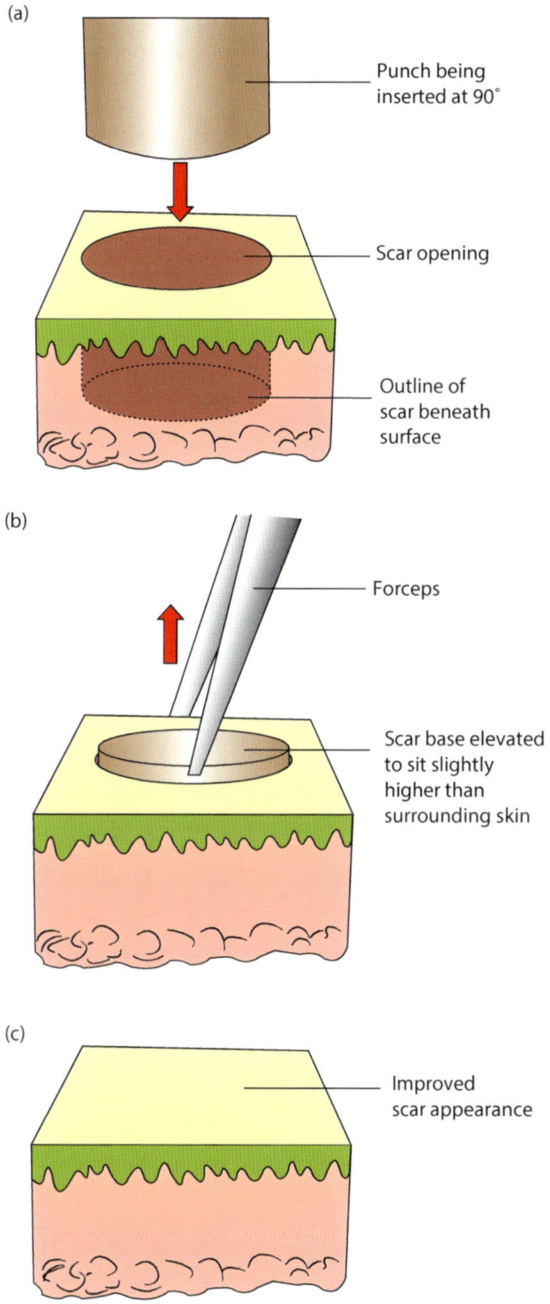

FIGURE 12.4 Punch elevation of a deep boxcar scar. (a) A punch is selected that matches the diameter of the scar base and is inserted at a 90° angle down to the level of the subcutaneous tissue. (b) Forceps are then used to gently elevate the scar base so that it sits slightly higher than the surrounding skin. (c) The elevated plug should flatten on its own during healing.

dressed with gauze, and the patient is instructed to gently wash the area and reapply a topical antibiotic twice a day [1].

Prior to punch grafting, an appropriate donor site is prepared and anesthetized in the same manner as the recipient site. First, the entire scar, including its walls, is excised (Figure 12.5). The punch should be inserted at a 90° angle to the skin surface with a twisting motion. In contrast with the punch excision

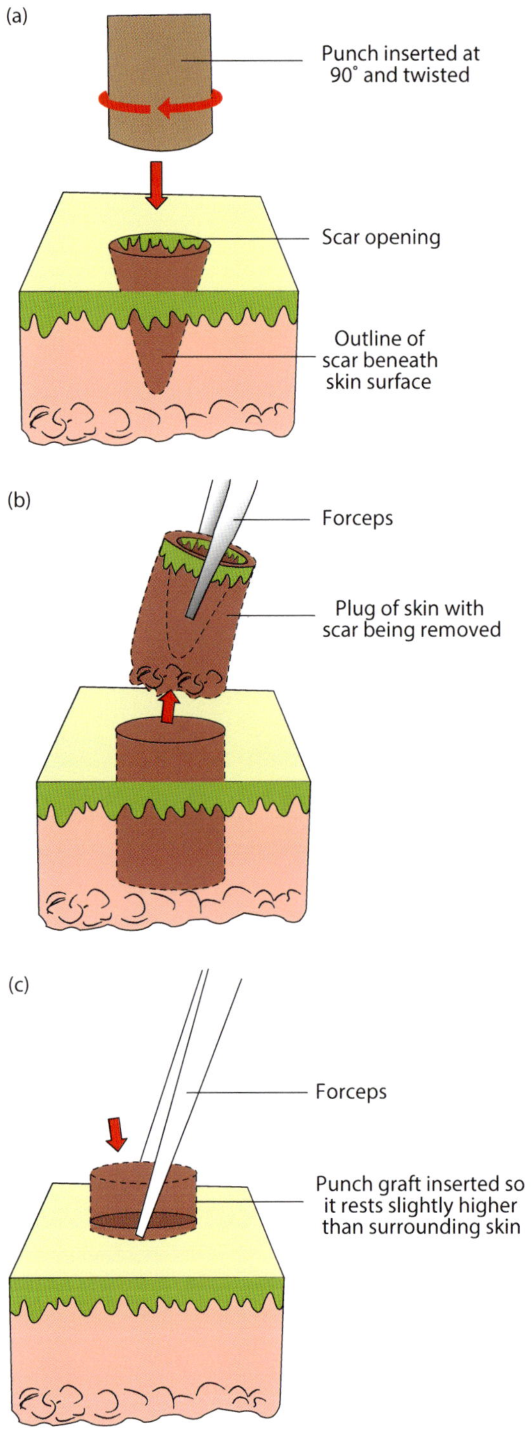

FIGURE 12.5 Punch grafting of an ice pick scar. (a) A punch is selected that will fully encompass the scar and its walls and is inserted at a 90° angle with a twisting motion down to the level of the subcutis. (b) Next, forceps are used to remove the scar from the recipient hole. (c) A full-thickness graft that is slightly larger than the recipient hole is inserted using forceps. Its surface should rest slightly higher than the surrounding skin.

procedure described before, care should be taken to avoid lateral stretching of the skin so that the resulting recipient hole will be perfectly round [42]. The excised scars are removed and discarded. A graft is then harvested using a punch 0.25–0.5 mm larger in diameter using the same procedure to create a full-thickness, cylindrical graft. Use of a slightly larger graft is recommended because grafts have a tendency to contract while the recipient wounds may expand, and it is important for the graft to maintain contact with the margins of the recipient hole [38,42]. The graft is gently inserted and manipulated into the recipient site using forceps so that its surface rests slightly higher than the surrounding skin (Figure 12.5). The graft is either sutured or glued in place and secured with Steri-Strips and the donor site is sutured closed. Patients should be advised to limit their facial movements and to avoid touching graft sites for the first several days.

Management of Complications

As described above, the risk of complications from excision and punch procedures may be minimized through careful technique. With larger punch excisions and elliptical excisions, meticulous suturing is necessary to produce the least conspicuous secondary defects. In punch grafting, careful donor site selection, precise harvesting techniques and painstaking graft placement are all integral to the achievement of a good result.

When secondary defects are not aesthetically acceptable their appearance can often be improved with subsequent procedures. An elevated graft, plug or excision scar is often adequately managed by laser resurfacing that is performed approximately 4–8 weeks after the original procedure [40]. In the event of punch graft extrusion or the development of a depressed scar, the original procedure should be repeated [38,42].

In punch elevation, plugs that are initially elevated above the level of the surrounding skin usually flatten without intervention, but persistently elevated plugs may be planed with resurfacing performed 4–8 weeks after the original procedure (Goodman GJ, unpublished work).

Additional Modalities and Future Developments

Although many of the surgical treatments for acne scarring have been in use for decades, there has been a limited amount of research evaluating the long-term response to these treatments and comparing outcomes from different modalities. While some treatments, such as dermabrasion, have fallen out of favor, novel treatments, newer protocols and more comparative studies continue to be reported. Further work on the aforementioned modalities in this chapter along with the discovery of new treatments may refine and/or enhance future outcomes.

Dermabrasion is the use of a motorized device with an abrasive material, such as a high-speed brush, diamond cylinder, fraise or silicon carbide sandpaper for removal of the epidermis and/or a portion of the dermis and for collagen formation [52–54]. It is purported to allow for the clinician to etch scar edges with increased accuracy, but without thermal injury [54]. Dermabrasion appears best suited for rolling scars and superficial boxcar scars, but less useful for deeper acne scars such as ice pick or deep boxcar scars [54–56]. Previous studies have demonstrated efficacy similar to that of fractional lasers [57]. However, the procedure typically involves significant pain, erythema, edema, long recovery times, a risk of scarring, dyschromia and milia formation [55,57].

Recent work in stem cell biology and regenerative medicine suggests that novel approaches to scar revision may be available in the future. Great strides have been made in elucidating the differences between the process of fibrotic wound healing that leads to scarring and the pathways that produce perfect regeneration of injured tissues, a phenomenon that can be observed in human fetuses and other organisms [58]. Skin progenitor cells have already been identified in mammals, and it is expected that by grafting such cells into injured skin and providing the right microenvironmental conditions, healing by regeneration may be induced [58]. Thus, it may eventually become possible to excise a fibrotic scar and manipulate the resultant wound in such a way that it will be replaced by normal, healthy skin. A recently described therapeutic intervention study involves the use of stem cells for the rejuvenation and visual improvement of scars. Stem cells are found in the bone marrow, adipose tissue and blood where they function as undifferentiated cells that can differentiate into specialized cells [59]. Ibrahim et al. found a significant qualitative and quantitative improvement in 14 patients where acne scars were directly injected with autologous bone marrow stem cells [60]. Similarly, Zhou and colleagues evaluated the use of topical adipose-derived stem cells at baseline, 1 week after the first treatment and 1 month after each treatment with fractional CO_2 laser for facial atrophic acne scars and skin rejuvenation [61]. Both groups saw an increase in subject satisfaction, elasticity and skin hydration, and decreased transepidermal water loss, roughness and melanin index. Histologic analysis from one patient showed an increase in dermal collagen and elastin densities [61]. Consequently, the use of stem cells may be considered as a sole treatment or in conjunction with surgical management for potentially improved outcomes. Recently, outpatient clinic-based stem cell treatments for various clinical indications have come under United States Food and Drug Association scrutiny and clinics have been sanctioned for unsafe practices and making untested claims.

Autologous fat transplantation, or fat grafting, is a treatment option that has been more recently explored for its use in acne scarring. Although originally described by Neuber in 1893, Coleman in 2006 demonstrated an improvement of acne scars in a patient who underwent fat grafting [62,63]. Efficacy of the fat graft is thought to be related to adipose-derived stem cells that have the potential to differentiate, synthesize collagen and stimulate angiogenesis [64]. The fat graft is harvested and small parcels of fat are injected into multiple tunnels for maximal access to blood supply [59]. Results are best appreciated approximately 3 months following the procedure [59].

Seidel and Moy evaluated the use of twice-daily synthetic epidermal growth factor serum for acne scars. Following 12 weeks of treatment in eight patients, 25% had an excellent result and 37% had a good result [65]. A multitude of additional topical serums with stem cell additives are on the market that may be utilized to improve efficacy when combined with surgical treatments [59].

An additional potential adjunctive treatment that has undergone investigation is the use of low-level light therapy (LLLT). Barolet and Boucher reported three patients with hypertrophic scars or keloids due to acne or surgery who underwent CO_2 laser ablation and had one of two scars treated with a non-thermal, non-ablative near-infrared light-emitting diode 805 nm at 30 mW/cm^2 for 30 days [66]. Following treatment, all three patients, including one patient with hypertrophic acne scars on the chest, showed improvement of visual impression, severity and skin surface topography compared with the untreated side. Although additional research is necessary, LLLT is thought to possibly decrease interleukin-6 and modulate transforming growth factor-β, which are associated with abnormal wound healing [67].

Alternatively, hair transplantation has been used to camouflage boxcar and rolling acne scars in the beard region of a patient with Fitzpatrick V skin type [68]. The authors describe the use of follicular unit extraction with donor supply taken from the submandibular and submental regions and placed in and around individual scars [68]. The acne scars were noted to be less visible and aesthetically acceptable [68].

Summary for the Clinician

Revision of acne scarring is a complex task in which treatment protocols are designed on a case-by-case basis following critical evaluation of scar type, overall patient characteristics and thorough consideration of patients' preferences, goals and budget [59]. Each scar revision technique is best suited to address a subset of scars and being equipped to treat the full range of acne scarring requires familiarizing oneself with a variety of surgical, non-surgical and resurfacing procedures. The surgical techniques described in this chapter are essential components of such a repertoire and are among the few procedures capable of improving deep and fibrotic acne scars (Figure 12.6). The clinician should consider combining these surgical modalities with non-surgical and resurfacing procedures, which potentially function synergistically for a superior result [59]. Since severe acne scars are frequently the source of profound social and emotional distress for patients, learning these techniques is essential for the cosmetic dermatologist.

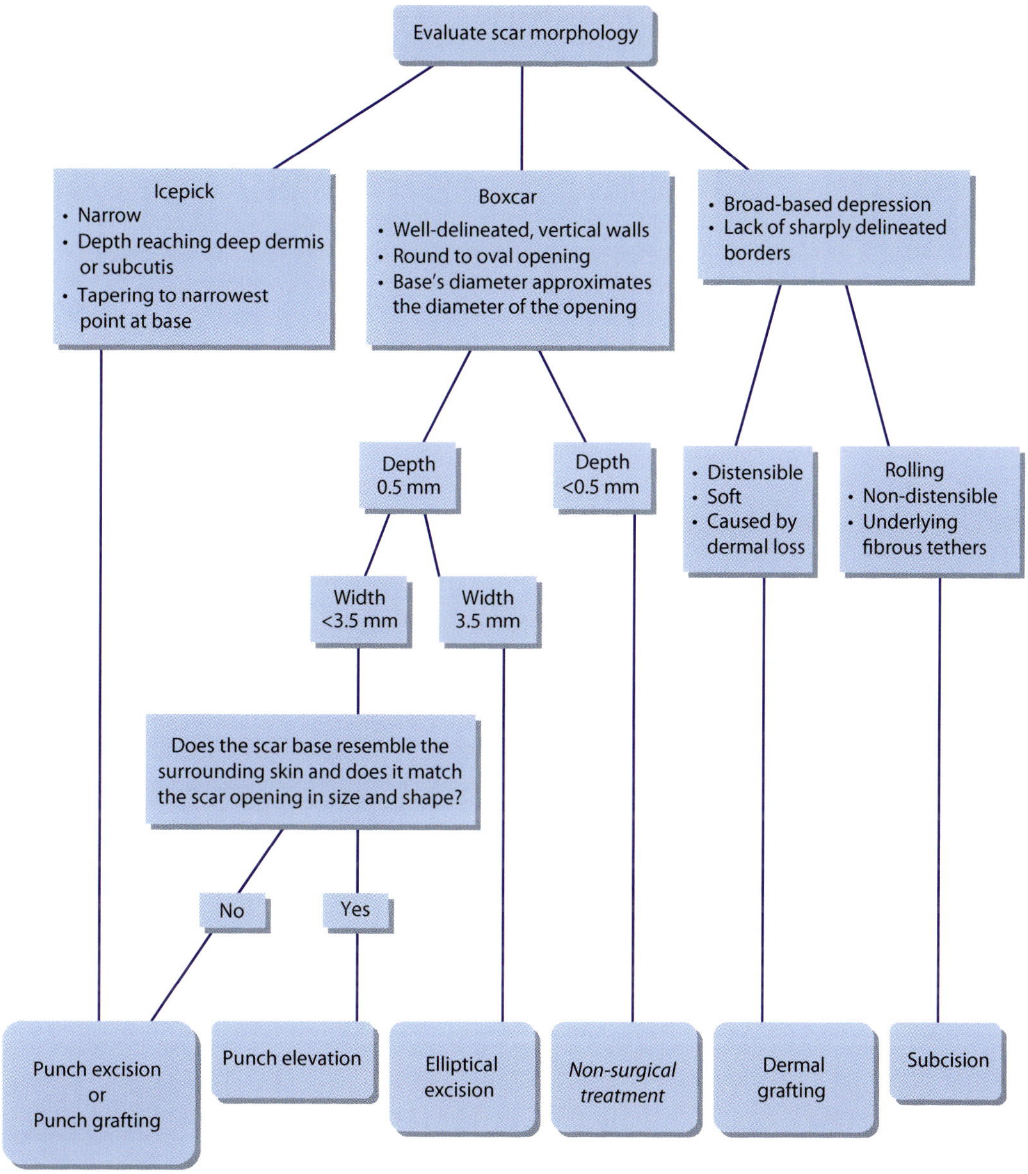

FIGURE 12.6 Flowchart linking different acne scar types to appropriate surgical procedures. With the exception of superficial boxcar scars <0.5 mm in depth, each scar type may be improved by surgical revision. Punch excision and punch grafting are suitable for treating ice pick and deep boxcar scars, punch elevation may be used to correct deep boxcar scars with regular bases, subcision is ideal for treating rolling scars and dermal grafting is an option for improving distensible depressed scars.

REFERENCES

1. Jacob CI, Dover JS, Kaminer MS. Acne scarring: A classification system and review of treatment options. *J Am Acad Dermatol*. 2001;45:109–17.
2. Orentreich DS, Orentreich N. Subcutaneous incisionless (subcision) surgery for the correction of depressed scars and wrinkles. *Dermatol Surg*. 1995;21:543–9.
3. Spangler AS. New treatment for pitted scars; preliminary report. *AMA Arch Derm*. 1957;76:708–11.
4. Millikan L, Rosen T, Monheit G. Treatment of depressed cutaneous scars with gelatin matrix implant: A multicenter study. *J Am Acad Dermatol*. 1987;16:1155–62.

5. Cohen I. Fibrel®. *Semin Dermatol.* 1987;6:228–37.
6. Hambley RM, Carruthers JA. Microlipoinjection for the elevation of depressed full-thickness skin grafts on the nose. *J Dermatol Surg Oncol.* 1992;18:963–8.
7. Swinehart J. Pocket grafting with dermal grafts: Autologous collagen implants for permanent correction of cutaneous depressions. *Amer J Cosm Surg.* 1995;12:321–31.
8. Orentreich D, Orentreich N. Acne scar revision update. *Dermatol Clin.* 1987;5:359–68.
9. Goodman GJ. Post-acne scarring: A short review of its pathophysiology. *Australas J Dermatol.* 2001;42:84–90.
10. Hexsel DM, Mazzuco R. Subcision: A treatment for cellulite. *Int J Dermatol.* 2000;39:539–44.
11. Goodman GJ. Therapeutic undermining of scars (subcision). *Australas J Dermatol.* 2001;42:114–7.
12. Alam M, Omura N, Kaminer MS. Subcision for acne scarring: Technique and outcomes in 40 patients. *Dermatol Surg.* 2005;31:310–7.
13. Balighi K, Robati RM, Moslehi H, Robati AM. Subcision in acne scar with and without subdermal implant: A clinical trial. *J Eur Acad Dermatol Venereol.* 2008;22:707–11.
14. Fulchiero GJ Jr., Parham-Vetter PC, Obagi S. Subcision and 1320 nm Nd:YAG nonablative laser resurfacing for the treatment of acne scars: A simultaneous split-face single patient trial. *Dermatol Surg.* 2004;30:1356–9.
15. Branson DF. Dermal undermining (scarification) of active rhytids and scars: Enhancing the results of CO_2 laser skin resurfacing. *Aesthet Surg J.* 1998;18:36–7.
16. Gadkari R, Nayak C. A split-face comparative study to evaluate efficacy of combined subcision and dermaroller against combined subcision and cryoroller in treatment of acne scars. *J Cosmet Dermatol.* 2014;13(1):38–43.
17. Faghihi G, Poostiyaan N, Asilian A, Abtahi-Naeini B, Shahbazi M, Iraji F, Fatemi Naeini F, Nilforoushzadeh MA. Efficacy of fractionated microneedle radiofrequency with and without adding subcision for the treatment of atrophic facial acne scars: A randomized split-face clincal study. *J Cosmet Dermatol.* 2017;16(2):223–9.
18. Taylor MB, Zaleski-Larsen L, McGraw TA. Single session treatment of rolling acne scars using tumescent anesthesia, 20% trichloroacetic acid, extensive subcision, and fractional CO_2 laser. *Dermatol Surg.* 2017;43(Suppl 1):S70–4.
19. Kaur J, Kalsy J. Subcision plus 50% trichloracetic acid chemical reconstruction of skin scars in the management of atrophacne scars: A cost-effective therapy. *Indian Dermatol Online J.* 2014;5(1):95–7.
20. AlGhamdi KM. A better way to hold a Nokor needle during subcision. *Dermatol Surg.* 2008;34:378–9.
21. Khunger NKM. Subcision for depressed facial scars made easy using a simple modification. *Dermatol Surg.* 2011;37:514–7.
22. Nilforoushzadeh M, Lotfi E, Nickkholgh E, Salehi B, Shokrani M. Can subcision with the cannula be an acceptable alternative method in treatment of acne scars? *Medical Archives.* 2015;69(6):384–6.
23. Ayeni O, Carey W, Muhn C. Acne scara treatment with subcision using a 20-G cataract blade. *Dermatol Surg.* 2011;37(6):846–7.
24. Barikbin B, Akbari Z, Youseif M, Dowlati Y. Blunt blade subcision: An evolution in the treatment of atrophic acne scars. *Dermatol Surg.* 2017;43(Suppl 1):S57–63.
25. Aalami Harandi S, Balighi K, Lajevardi V, Akbari E. Subcision-suction method; a new successful combination therapy in treatment of atrophic acne scars and other depressed scars. *J Eur Acad Dermatol Venerol.* 2011;25(1):92–9.
26. Pereira O, Bins-Ely J, Paulo EM, Lee KH. Treatment of skin depression with combined upward suture traction and percutaneous subcision. *Plast Reconstr Surg Glob Open.* 2015;3:e534.
27. Peer LA, Paddock R. Histologic studies on the fate of deeply implanted dermal grafts: Observations on sections of implants buried from one week to one year. *Arch Surg.* 1937;34:268.
28. Swinehart JM. Dermal grafting. *Dermatol Clin.* 2001;19:509–22.
29. Goodman GJ. Autologous fat and dermal grafting for the correction of facial scars. In: *Surgical Techniques for Cutaneous Scar Revision.* Harahap M, ed. New York: Marcel Dekker, 2000, 311–48.
30. Goodman G. Laser-assisted dermal grafting for the correction of cutaneous contour defects. *Dermatol Surg.* 1997;23:95–9.
31. Meyers S, Rohrer T, Grande D. Use of dermal grafts in reconstructing deep nasal defects and shaping the ala nasi. *Dermatol Surg.* 2001;27:300–5.

32. Shilpa K, Sacchidanand S, Leelavathy B, Shilpashree P, Divya G, Ranjitha R, Lakshmi DV. Outcome of dermal grafting in the management of atrophic facial scars. *J Cutan Aesthetic Surg*. 2016;9:244–8.
33. Nita AC, Orzan OA, Filipescu M, JIanu D. Fat graft, laser CO_2, and platelet-rich plasma synergy in scars treatment. *J Med Life*. 2013;6(4):430–3.
34. Tenna S, Cogliandro A, Barone M, Panasiti V, Tirindelli M, Nobile C, Persichetti P. Comparative study using autologous fat grafts plus platelet-rich plasma with or without fractional CO_2 laser resurfacing in treatment of acne scars: Analysis of outcomes and satisfaction with FACE-Q. *Aesthetic Plast Surg*. 2017;41(3):661–6.
35. Choi JM, Rohrer TE, Kaminer MS, Batra RS. Surgical approaches to patients with scarring. In: *Scar Revision*. Arndt KA, ed. Philadelphia: Elsevier Saunders, 2006, 45–66.
36. Nagaraju U, Chikkaiah MK, Raju BP, Agarwal P. Autologous smashed dermal graft with epidermal re-closure: Modified technique for acne scars. *J Cutan Aesthet Surg*. 2016;9(4):258–62.
37. Solotoff SA. Treatment for pitted acne scarring–postauricular punch grafts followed by dermabrasion. *J Dermatol Surg Oncol*. 1986;12:1079–84.
38. Johnson WC. Treatment of pitted scars: Punch transplant technique. *J Dermatol Surg Oncol*. 1986;12:260–5.
39. Stal S, Hamilton S, Spira M. Surgical treatment of acne scars. *Clin Plast Surg*. 1987;14:261–76.
40. Dzubow LM. Scar revision by punch-graft transplants. *J Dermatol Surg Oncol*. 1985;11:1200–2.
41. Eiseman G. Reconstruction of the acne-scarred face. *J Dermatol Surg Oncol*. 1977;3:332–8.
42. Stegman SJ. *Cosmetic Dermatologic Surgery*. 2nd ed. Chicago: Year Book Medical Publishers, Inc., 1990.
43. Lee JB, Chung WG, Kwahck H, Lee KH. Focal treatment of acne scars with trichloroacetic acid: Chemical reconstruction of skin scars method. *Dermatol Surg*. 2002;28:1017–21.
44. Tsao SS, Dover JS, Arndt KA, Kaminer MS. Scar management: Keloid, hypertrophic, atrophic, and acne scars. *Semin Cutan Med Surg*. 2002;21:46–75.
45. Koranda FC. Treatment and modalities in facial acne scars. In: *Facial Scars: Incision, Revision, and Camouflage*. Thomas JR, Holt GR, eds. St. Louis: The C.V. Mosby Company, 1989, 278–89.
46. Haneke E. Fusiform excision and serial excisions. In: *Surgical Techniques for Cutaneous Scar Revision*. Harahap M, ed. New York: Marcel Dekker, 2000, 359–80.
47. Usatine R. Elliptical excision. In: *Skin Surgery: A Practical Guide*. Usatine RP, Moy RL, eds. St. Louis: Mosby, 1998, 120–36.
48. Griffin E. Punch transplant technique for pitted scars. In: *Surgical Techniques for Cutaneous Scar Revision*. Harahap M, ed. New York: Marcel Dekker, 2000, 259–74.
49. Grevelink JM, White VR. Concurrent use of laser skin resurfacing and punch excision in the treatment of facial acne scarring. *Dermatol Surg*. 1998;24:527–30.
50. Goodman GJ. The limitations of skin resurfacing techniques. The necessity to combine procedures. *Dermatol Surg*. 1998;24:687–8.
51. Faghihi G, Nouraei S, Asilian A et al. Efficacy of punch elevation combined with fractional carbon dioxide laser resurfacing in facial atrophic acne scarring: A randomized split-face clinical study. *Indian J Dermatol*. 2015;60(5):473–8.
52. Lanoue J, Goldenberg G. Acne scarring: A review of cosmetic therapies. *Cutis*. 2015;95(5):276–81.
53. Frank W. Therapeutic dermabrasion back to the future. *Arch Dermatol*. 1994;130:1187–9.
54. Abdel Hay R, Shalaby K, Zaher H, Hafez V, Chi CC, Dimitri S, Nabhan AF, Layton AM. Interventions for acne scars. *Cochraine Database Sys Rev*. 2016;4:CD011946.
55. Goodman GJ. Treatment of acne scarring. In: *Pathogenesis and Treatment of Acne and Rosacea*. Zouboulis Christos C, Katsambas Andreas D, Kligman Albert M, eds. Heidelberg: Springer Berlin, 2014, 527–36.
56. Hession MT, Graber EM. Atrophic acne scarring: A review of treatment options. *J Clin Aesthet Dermatol*. 2015;8:50–8.
57. Christophel JJ, Elm C, Endrizzi BT et al. A randomized controlled trial of fractional laser therapy and dermabrasion for scar resurfacing. *Dermatol Surg*. 2012;38:595–602.
58. Gurtner GC, Werner S, Barrandon Y, Longaker MT. Wound repair and regeneration. *Nature*. 2008;453:314–21.
59. Zaleski-Larsen LA, Fabi SG, McGraw T, Taylor M. Acne scar treatment: A multimodality approach tailored to scar type. *Dermatol Surg*. 2016;43(Supply 2):S139–49.

60. Ibrahim ZA, Eltatawy RA, Ghaly NR, Abd El-Naby NM, Abou El Fetouh HM, Abd Elateef AE, Abdou S, Tahaa A, El Afandy M. Autologous bone marrow stem cells in atrophic acne scars: A pilot study. *J Dermatol Treat.* 2015;26(30):260–5.
61. Zhou BR, Zhang T, Bin Jameel AA, Xu Y, Xu Y, Guo SL, Wang Y, Permatasari F, Luo D. The efficacy of conditioned media of adipose-derived stem cell combined with ablative carbon dioxide fractional resurfacing for atrophic acne scars and skin rejuvenation. *J Cosmet Laser Ther.* 2016;18(3):138–48.
62. Neuber F. Fetttranspalntation. *Zentrabl Chir.* 1893;22:66.
63. Coleman SR. Structural fat grafting: More than a permanent filler. *Plast Reconstr Surg.* 2006;118(Suppl 3):108S–120S.
64. Zuk PA, Zhu M, Mizuno H et al. Multilineage cells from human adipose tissue: Implications for cellbased therapies. *Tissue Eng.* 2001;7(2):211–28.
65. Seidel R, Moy RL. Improvement in atrophic acne scars using topical synthetic epidermal growth factor (EGF) serum: A pilot study. *J Drug Dermatol.* 2015;14(9):1005–10.
66. Barolet D, Boucher A. Prophylactic low-level light therapy for the treatment of hypertrophic scars and keloids: A case series. *Lasers Surg Med.* 2010;42(6):597–601.
67. Avci P, Gupta A, Sadasivam M, Vecchio D, Pam Z, Pam N, Hamblin MR. Low-lever laser (light) therapy (LLLT) in skin: Stimulating, healing, restoring. *Semin Cutan Med Surg.* 2013;32(1):41–52.
68. Sarangal R, Yadav S, Dogra S. Hair transplant for acne scars: An innovative approach. *J Cosmet Dermatol.* 2012;11(2):158–61.

13

Clinical Importance of Corrective Cover Cosmetic (Camouflage) and Quality-of-Life Outcome in the Management of Patients with Acne Scarring and/or Post-Inflammatory Hyperpigmentation

Aurora Tedeschi and Giorgia Giuffrida

KEY FEATURES

- Camouflage or corrective maquillage is based on the use of particular and tested cover products.
- It is a non-invasive technique that allows an immediate coverage of several skin conditions, including post-inflammatory acne hyperpigmentation and superficial acne scars.
- It does not interfere with the ongoing pharmacological therapies of cosmetics procedures.

Introduction

Acne is one of the most common dermatologic disorders that can be very distressing to patients. Facial lesions may cause depression, loss of self-esteem, quality-of-life deterioration, sexual dysfunction and increased prevalence of emotional distress compared with the general population [1,2]. Moreover, inflammatory acne if not promptly and appropriately managed, may result in scarring with varying degrees of cosmetic disfigurement. This may cause, or worsen, psychological problems, with the result of impairing the quality of life (QoL) [1].

Acne scars represent a difficult issue to manage: long-term therapy with topical retinoids may provide minimal improvement in mild cases [3] while surgical and medical procedural approaches, such as punch or handled elliptical excision, punch elevation, chemical peeling, dermabrasion and needling, may provide effective treatment only if managed by experienced practitioners. However, different types of scar may be present at the same time in the same patient, so the choice of the best treatment option may be troublesome and different techniques may be required in order to achieve satisfactory results [1,3].

Finally, the physician should carefully choose the procedures that are best able to treat the different types of scars successfully.

Camouflage, or corrective cover cosmetic (CCC), may be used as an alternative to medications, procedures, and surgery and is notably used as a temporary post-procedure cover for erythema resulting from dermabrasion, needling or chemical peel [1] (see Figures 13.1–13.5). In addition, CCC may also be used as an adjuvant to dermatologic therapy in order to enhance the outcome more than that achieved by therapy alone [4]. Finally, CCC is reported to improve mental well-being, self-esteem, and social acceptance [5–14].

Many dermatologists are reluctant on the use of makeup products in acne patients, since they are afraid of "acne cosmetica." This is a particular variety of acne, described around the 1970s and caused or worsened by the use of inappropriate comedogenic cosmetics, an event that with appropriate patient

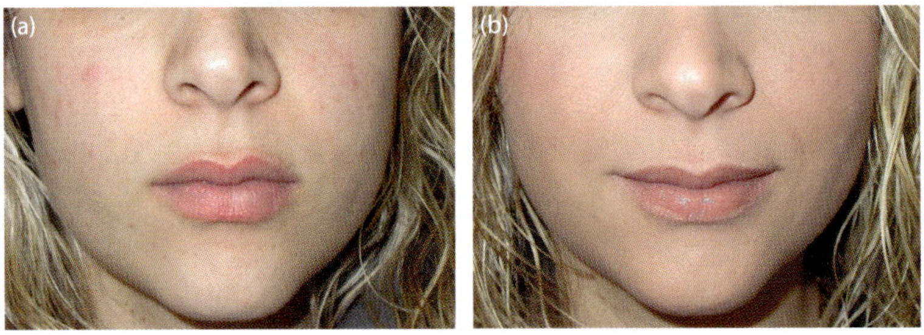

FIGURE 13.1 Papules and post-inflammatory erythematous lesions (a) before and (b) after camouflage.

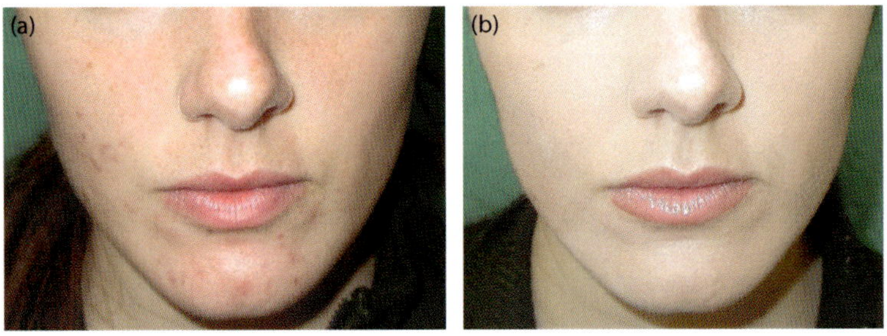

FIGURE 13.2 Post-inflammatory erythematous lesions and scars (a) before and (b) after camouflage.

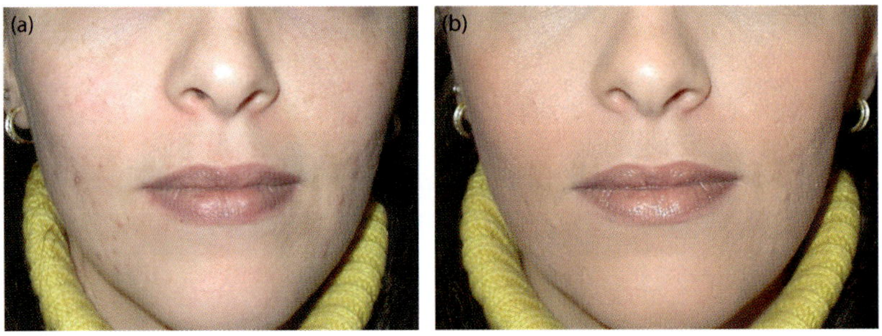

FIGURE 13.3 Papules, post-inflammatory erythematous lesions and scars (a) before and (b) after camouflage.

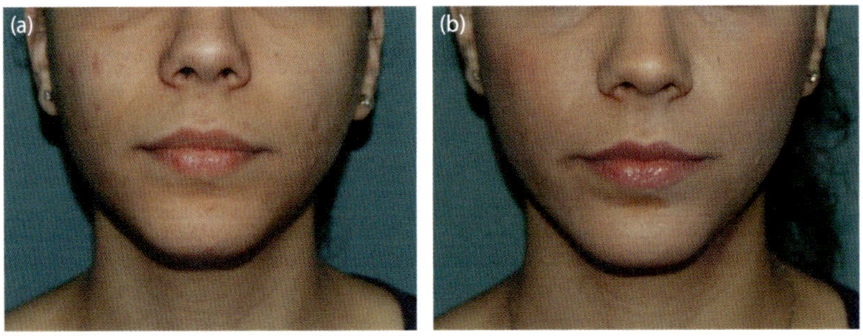

FIGURE 13.4 Papules, pustules and post-inflammatory erythematous lesions (a) before and (b) after camouflage.

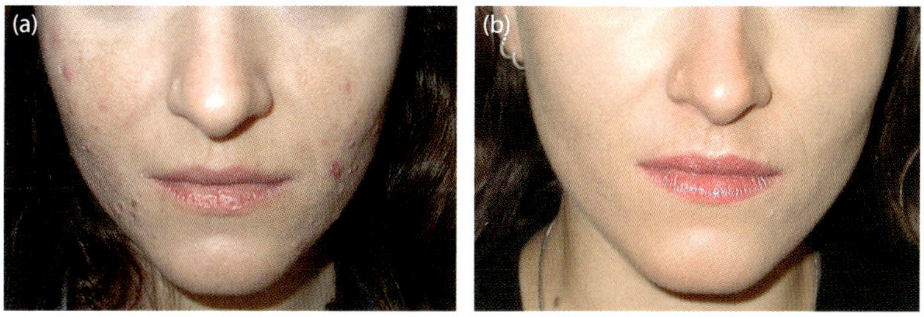

FIGURE 13.5 Papules, pustles and post-inflammatory erythematous lesions (a) before and (b) after camouflage.

counseling, can be easily avoided [12]. In addition, the modern concept of health—intended, nowadays, not only as the "absence of illness" but also as "psycho-physical well-being"—point toward the use of CCC as an adjunct to the standard pharmacological therapies [6–14].

CCC is a corrective makeup used in the United States since the late 1960s based on the use of water-resistant and concealing cover products that are able to correct and minimize skin defects that have resulted from various dermatological disorders.

Table 13.1 [6–14] reports the most common dermatologic disorders that can have beneficial effects from CCC.

In our department, a CCC unit has been active from 2001 and different dermatoses, including post-inflammatory acne hyperpigmentation and acne scars have been successfully treated [6–14].

CCC procedure generally consists of two steps. The first regards a preliminary examination aimed to evaluate the need, expectations and likely outcome for CCC on patient lifestyle, and to provide more detailed information about the products. During this step, a QoL questionnaire is provided in order to investigate the relation between acne scarring and psychological discomfort [1].

After this preliminary consultation, CCC-eligible patients routinely undergo skin cleansing and hydrating procedures with nonallergenic and noncomedogenic/nonacnegenic products. The most

TABLE 13.1

Selected Dermatoses Manageable with Corrective Cover Cosmetic
Acne
Acne scars
Achanthosis nigricans
Allergic contact dermatitis
Becker nevus
Blue nevus
Burn scars
Chloasma/melasma
Guttate idiopathic hypomelanosis
Lentigo
Lichen verrucosus
Melanocytic nevus
Nevus of Ota
Palpebral hyperpigmentation
Post-inflammatory pigmentations of immunobullous disorders (i.e., pemphigus)
Psoriasis
Rosacea
Surgery scars
Telangiectasias
Xeroderma pigmentosum
Vitiligo

appropriate foundation is applied, from a color selection of light to very opaque, water-resistant or waterproof, noncomedogenic/nonacnegenic and/or hypoallergenic products, and fixed with a powder application.

Pigmentary changes are corrected through the application of green and/or yellow undercover, in order to respectively neutralize reddish and gray/brownish or blue defects; for post-inflammatory hyperpigmentation from facial acne, green undercover is commonly used as a masking technique [1]. During the corrective cover makeup procedure patients are carefully instructed on how to correctly apply the products at home.

Patients are invited to return to the CCC clinic 2 weeks later in order to check the quality of their CCC technique and also to obtain follow-up on their QoL.

In our experience, despite an average CCC outcome, patients with acne scars and/or post-inflammatory hyperpigmentation reported a higher degree of satisfaction with CCC compared with other patients affected by other dermatoses [1]. CCC products provided an immediate result in terms of coverage and with no recrudescence of acne observed [12].

Discussion

After its introduction in the late 1960s, the use of CCC has become popular worldwide from the 1980s [15–18]. It represents a non-invasive technique that allows an immediate coverage of some skin dermatoses, including post-inflammatory acne hyperpigmentation and acne scars. Dermatologists should be aware of this simple and safe procedure and should be able to suggest the best cover products to meet every specific demand as well to educate patients to their correct use [12].

Importantly, CCC products are not conventional "glamour" or "fashion" makeup products. Advanced noncomedogenic and nonacnegenic formulations developed by trusted companies known in the dermatologic community are developed containing a high percentage of pigments and a wide range of colors in order to cover different types of dermatoses in different skin phototypes [12,19].

Unfortunately, CCC products remain somewhat less successful in covering acne scars than for other other dermatologic disorders, and this is primarily due to the difficulty in "filling" hypotrophic scars, while the shadows from such scars (i.e., acne pitting) remain visible [1].

REFERENCES

1. Tedeschi A, West L. Camouflage: Clinical importance of corrective cover cosmetic (camouflage) and quality-of-life outcome in the management of patients with acne scarring and/or post-inflammatory hyperpigmentation. In: *Acne Scars*. Tosti A, De Padova MP, Beer KR, eds. UK: Informa Healthcare Ltd, 2009.
2. Matsuoka Y, Yoneda K, Sadahira C et al. Effects of skin care and makeup under instructions from dermatologists on the quality of life of female patients with acne vulgaris. *J Dermatol*. 2006;33:745–52.
3. Rivera AE. Acne scarring: A review and current treatment modalities. *J Am Acad Dermatol*. 2008;59: 659–76.
4. Hayashi N, Imori M, Yanagisawa M et al. Make-up improves the quality of life of acne patients without aggravating acne eruptions during treatments. *Eur J Dermatol*. 2005;15:284–7.
5. Boehncke WH, Ochsendorf F, Paeslack I et al. Decorative cosmetics improve the quality of life in patients with disfiguring skin diseases. *Eur J Dermatol*. 2002;12:577–80.
6. Tedeschi A, Dall'Oglio F, Micali G et al. Our experience in the corrective camouflage in dermatology practice. *Proceedings XI Congress of the European Academy of Dermatology and Venereology*; Prague, October 2–6, 2002, 75–8.
7. Tedeschi A, Pappalardo S. Camouflage dell'acne. In: *Principi di dermocosmetologia dell'acne*. Barbareschi M, Bettoli V, Fabbrocini G et al. eds. Salerno: Momento Medico Editore, 2011, 115–9.
8. Tedeschi A, Dall'Oglio R, Micali G, Schwartz RA, Janniger CK. Corrective camouflage in dermatology practice. *Aesthetic Dermatology*. 2003;5:273–5.

9. Tedeschi A, Dall'Oglio F, Micali G, Schwartz RA, Janniger CK. Corrective camouflage in pediatric dermatology. *Cutis.* 2007;79:110–2.
10. Dall'Oglio F, Tedeschi A, Puglisi G, Carbone C. Principi di cosmetologia. In: *Le basi della dermatologia.* Micali G, Innocenzi D, Fabbrocini G et al. eds. Italia: Spinger-Verlag, 2011, 258–9.
11. Tedeschi A, Guzzardi L, Dall'Oglio F. Camouflage nell'acne. In: *Dermocosmetologia dell'acne.* Mediprint, 2013, 160–5.
12. Tedeschi A, Dall'Oglio F, Micali G. Camouflage. *J Medical Books.* 2017;219–28.
13. Tedeschi A, Dall'Oglio F, Micali G. Terapia topica dell'acne lieve e moderata. I dermocosmetici. In: *Linee guida e raccomandazioni SIDeMAST.* Pisa: Pacini Editore, 2016.
14. Tedeschi A, Dall'Oglio F, Micali G. Terapia topica dell'acne grave. I dermocosmetici. In: *Linee guida e raccomandazioni SIDeMAST.* Pisa: Pacini Editore, 2016.
15. Caputo R, Barbareschi M, Baggini G, Bovo D. The corrective make-up lab: The Italian experience. *Poster, 60th Meeting of the American Academy of Dermatology*, New Orleans (LA), February 22nd–27th, 2002.
16. Roberts NC. Corrective cosmetics—Need, evaluation, and use. *Cutis.* 1988;41:439–41.
17. Westmore MG. Camouflage and makeup preparations. *Clin Dermatol.* 2001;19:406–12.
18. Holme SA, Beattie PE, Fleming CJ. Cosmetic camouflage advice improves quality of life. *Br J Dermatol.* 2002;147:946–9.
19. Grimes PE. Skin and hair cosmetic issues in women of color. *Dermatol Clin.* 2000;18:659–65.

14

Acne Scarring and Asian Patients

Evangeline B. Handog, Maria Juliet E. Macarayo, and Chee Leok Goh

KEY FEATURES

- Acne vulgaris remains as the leading cause of dermatological consults in Asia.
- Acne scarring is a common sequela of untreated acne vulgaris, even among Asians.
- Early management of all types of acne vulgaris help prevent scarring.
- Several modalities to treat acne scars are available for Asian patients, with variable results.

Introduction

Asians, categorically belonging to the brown race [1] and identified as a skin of color [2], are more of a heterogeneous group, considering several factors as migration and intermarriages [1]. Generally classified as having Fitzpatrick skin type IV–V and Lancer Ethnicity Scale IV [1,3], Asian skin now encompasses skin phototypes II–V with skin tone varying from the lightest to the darkest shade of brown [4].

Acne vulgaris and its sequelae, post-inflammatory hyperpigmentation (PIH) and scarring are not uncommon among Asians. Attempts to treat the acne, at any of its stages, is a common practice. With the Asian population having different cultural practices and beliefs, delays in treatment have been noted. However, from the time we originally wrote this chapter 7 years ago, there has been a notable rise in the consciousness of the Asian populace as to the menace acne can bring if left unattended. Hence, there has been an increase in acne consultations in most of the hospitals and clinics around Asia.

Management practices are evolving, yet acne scarring remains a problem. With the introduction of newer laser and light devices, doors have been opened to many possibilities for acne scar treatment. Many Asian dermatologists, with access to these devices, have created their own study trials and have shaped experiences to fit the Asian skin.

Acne Vulgaris among Asians: What Recent Studies Say

There are many skin diseases unique to each race [2] but acne vulgaris is one condition common to all, including Asians. It is considered one of the top reasons for patient consultation in dermatological clinics [2,4–6].

From 2011 to 2016, there were 475,967 consults in the 11 training institutions of the Philippine Dermatological Society; of these, there were 45,085 (9.47%) Filipino patients seen and treated for acne, with new cases accounting for 32,948 (6.9%). Two thirds were females and only a third were males, with an age range from less than a year to 67 years old [7]. A high percentage of Filipino dermatologists see at least 10 acne patients a week of varying types and degrees in their clinics, making it one of the most common reasons a patient would seek a consultation (Handog EB, unpublished data).

Similarly, in Singapore-based studies, acne has always been among the top ten conditions for which patients seek treatment [8–10]. In a ten-year (2004–2013) epidemiological study on adolescent (<25 years) and post-adolescent (≥25 years) acne conducted in Singapore by Han *et al.* [11], an increasing number and proportion of acne cases with a consistently higher number among females than males, was shown. Subgroup analysis, however, showed more male patients among the adolescent acne group (61.3% males vs 38.8% females). Post-adolescent acne comprised 30% of all the cases seen, with more females than males (69.0% females vs 31.0% males). As to acne types, comedonal acne was noted to be more prevalent among adolescents and cystic acne among the post-adolescent group. Interestingly, 40.5% of the post-adolescent acne subjects reported acne from adolescence persisting into adulthood. Among the adult persistent acne and adult onset acne groups, truncal acne occurred more often with the former, and pustular lesions frequented the latter. Singapore is a good example of a country with an intermix of Asian races (i.e., Chinese, Malay, Indians). Although the study recorded an increase in the number of acne cases in all races, the Chinese had the highest number and proportion of acne vulgaris seen.

A recently published profile study of acne vulgaris in Nepal [12] showed a low acne frequency of 1.068%. Patient age varied from 13 to 45 years with more patients in the 16–20 year group (mean age 19.78 years). Although a male-to-female ratio of 1.25:1 was noted, acne in the older age groups showed a higher number among females and the degree of acne was more severe. Duration of acne ranged from 1 month to 25 years, with a mean of 45.55 months. Similar to other studies, Nepalese patients with a longer duration of acne had a more severe type. Facial acne predominated but the back, chest, and neck were likewise involved. Comedonal acne was observed in all patients and the ratio of non-inflammatory to inflammatory lesions was 8.55:1.

A multicenter epidemiological study of acne in Korea involving 1,236 participants [13] revealed a significant male-to-female ratio of 1:1.6 with more females in the older age group (19–35 years old) and carrying a longer acne duration (mean 7.7 years). Facial acne affected both sexes but the perioral area showed a female preponderance. Acne on the nose, neck, chest and back were more common among males. A more recent 10-year (2004–2013) multicenter study on 180,782 acne patients completed by the Korean Society for Acne Research [14] revealed a similar higher number among females. Adult acne (>18 years old) still accounted for the majority of cases (83.8%) with 14.4% belonging to the adolescent acne group (13–18 years). Childhood acne (<13 years old) at a proportion of 1.8%, had a male-to-female ratio of 4:6. There was a 60% increase in the total number of acne patients within the 10-year study and the authors attributed this significant rise to the increased awareness of Koreans about acne and its complications.

It is interesting to note that among the studies done on acne in Asian patients, different acne severity assessment grading systems were used [12,15–17]. As such, there exists no uniformity, even among experts, on how acne severity must be evaluated. Although each one has a sound basis, confusion may arise when different grades and terms are implemented.

The psychosocial effects of acne can never be underrated [6,15,17–20]. Among 429 Singaporeans, 17–35 years of age, more than half expressed embarrassment and self-consciousness with their acne condition, with a third considering it an interference in their social or leisure activities [6]. Even the perception of the severity of one's acne varied greatly with the actual physician's objective assessment, affecting the patient's treatment-seeking behavior [6,15].

Etiopathogenesis of acne vulgaris has been known to be multifactorial and this is true for all races and ethnicities [4,6]. All forms and degrees of acne may be experienced by Asians but the severe nodulocystic form occurs to a lesser degree [21] and PIH, on the other end, is almost always a notable sequela [4,5,12, 15,16,21–23].

Acne Scarring among Asians: What the Data Shows

Scarring is a dreaded outcome of acne vulgaris and can occur in all levels of acne severity [24]. If acne vulgaris affects the quality of life of its sufferers, more so does scarring [25]. Inflammatory acne, if left untreated or incurred a delay in treatment, is likely to result in scarring (Figures 14.1 and 14.2). Moreover, studies have shown that this dreaded endpoint can even occur in non-inflammatory acne or in acne classified to be mild [24–27].

In the past three decades, several acne scar classification systems have been proposed and used [28]. As with the assessment of acne severity, different acne scar studies utilized different modes of evaluating

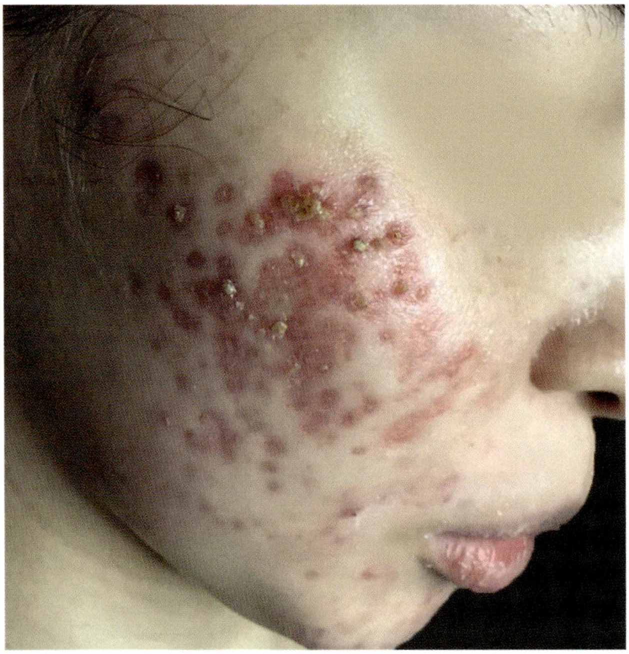

FIGURE 14.1 Severe acne leading to scarring.

their acne scar patients. In simpler terms, true acne scarring may result from either a loss or excess in tissue formation [1]. The latter is seen as hypertrophic or keloidal scarring and has been noted to have a higher incidence among Asians, compared with Caucasians [29] (Figures 14.3 and 14.4). Atrophic scars, represented by ice pick, rolling, and boxcar scars, are the most common type of acne scarring seen in many races and ethnicities, including Asians (Figure 14.5).

Post-acne scarring was observed in 39.5% of the Nepalese patients in Jha's study, with the cheeks involved in all the cases. Ice pick scars were the most common type. A longer disease duration of more than 3 years were noted to be a factor in the tendency for acne scarring [12]. Among adolescent acne patients in Hong Kong, scarring and pigmentation, considered as a reflection of acne severity, were noted to be higher than the western population and were more commonly seen in females [20]. Hazarika and

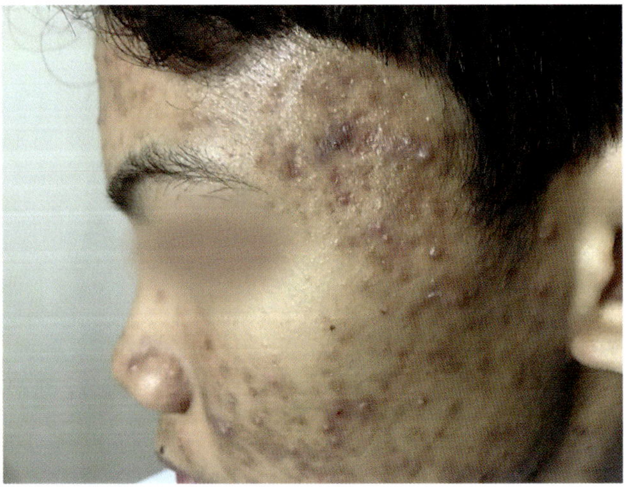

FIGURE 14.2 Papulopustular acne.

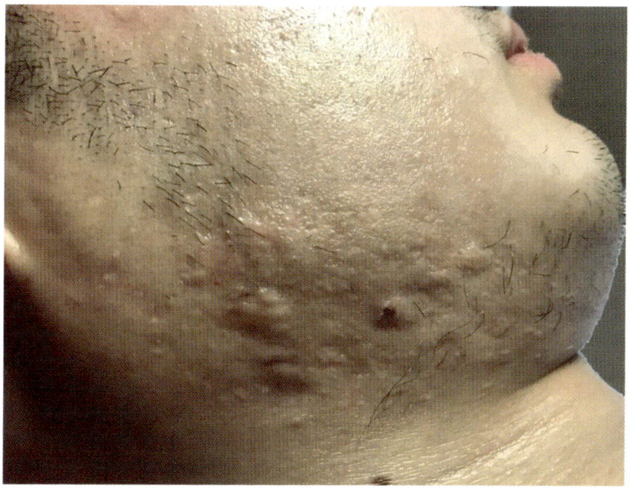

FIGURE 14.3 Hypertrophic scars.

Rajaprabha, however, in a study conducted in a suburban Indian population, noted that scarring affected the male gender more than females (86 vs 38%) [30].

Acne scars are commonly observed along with the acne lesions of many Filipino patients. All types of acne scars were seen by Filipino dermatologists, with a predominance of the atrophic scar type, managed mostly using lasers and light, chemical exfoliation and microneedling. Hypertrophic scars, on the other hand, were managed mostly by intralesional corticosteroid injection with or without the aid of laser and light devices, and topical silicon application. Post-acne hyperpigmentary changes were predominantly seen compared with hypopigmentation. Chemical peeling using trichloroacetic acid (TCA), glycolic or salicylic acid , was a common choice for dealing with acne scars. This procedure was performed once or twice monthly by the majority with a notable 50% improvement (Handog EB, unpublished data).

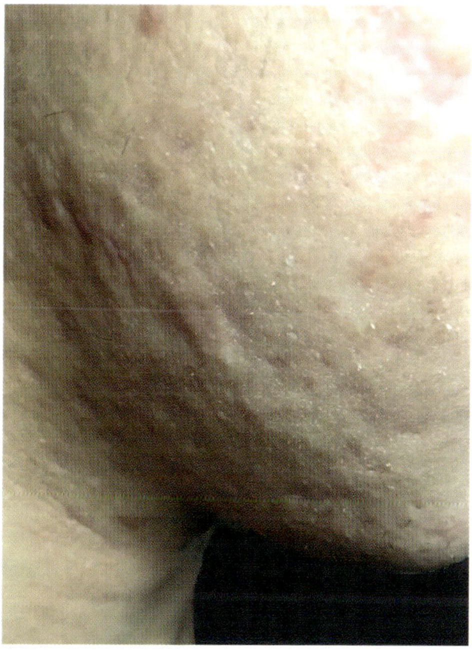

FIGURE 14.4 Keloidal scars.

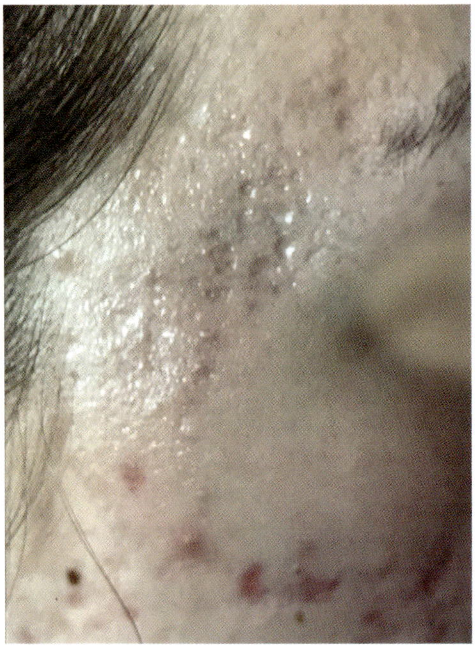

FIGURE 14.5 Atrophic scars.

Papular acne scars of the nose and chin have been proposed as a distinct entity, different from elastolytic scars predominantly seen on the chest and trunk [31,32]. This entity is not uncommon among Asian patients. Management with CO_2 laser ablation or cauterization may, however, lead to hypopigmentation. Lee, et al [33] presented two Korean females, aged 34 and 20 years, treated with the pinhole method using an erbium:yttrium–aluminum garnet (Er:YAG) laser with a hydrocolloid dressing applied for a week after treatment. The first case had a good aesthetic result after a single treatment with no sign of relapse even after a year post laser. The second case had two sessions with a 1-month interval with a significant cosmetic result.

Recently, Chaudhary and associates [34] compared the treatment outcome of different chemical peels and surgical procedures in the management of acne scars among 80 Indian patients. They found a male-to-female ratio of 1.2:1 with 62% belonging to the adolescent age group and a duration of acne scars of 2–5 years. Boxcar scars were the most common type, followed by rolling and ice pick scars. Four groups of 20 patients each were designated either to (A) glycolic acid with serial increase in concentration from 35 to 70% fortnightly for a minimum of 10 sessions, (B) 95% TCA chemical reconstruction of skin scars (CROSS) every month for a minimum of four sessions, (C) microneedling/dermaroller every 6 weeks for a minimum of three sittings, and (D) subcision every month for a minimum of four sittings. Microneedling showed the highest percentage reduction in acne scar score, followed by TCA CROSS, subcision, and glycolic peel. Improvement of acne scars with surgical management over chemical exfoliation was statistically significant. Only seven out of the 80 patients reported adverse events. Common were prolonged erythema and hematoma for the surgical treatment and pigmentary changes with chemical peels.

Dealing with Acne Scars among the Asian Population

Once scarring develops, it is very difficult to treat. It is not possible to restore the skin back to normal. At present, all modalities intended to treat acne scars do not eliminate them completely.

The majority of patients are concerned with PIH and post-inflammatory erythema (PIE) (Figures 14.6 and 14.7). Topical management with skin lightening agents together with daily sunscreen, a practice among Asian dermatologists, usually suffice. In fact, the PIH can fade in time.

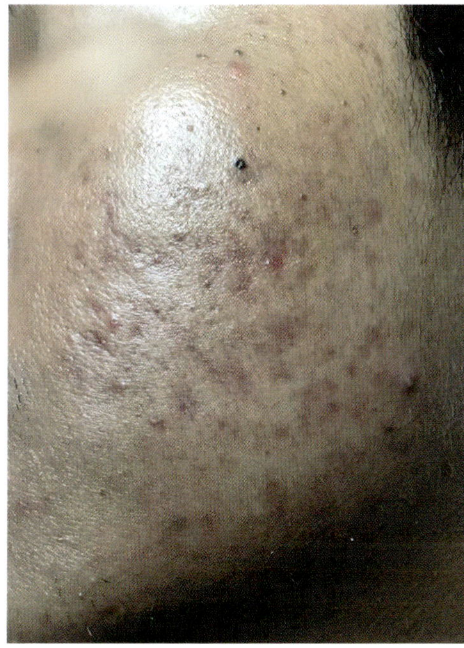

FIGURE 14.6 Post-inflammatory hyperpigmentation.

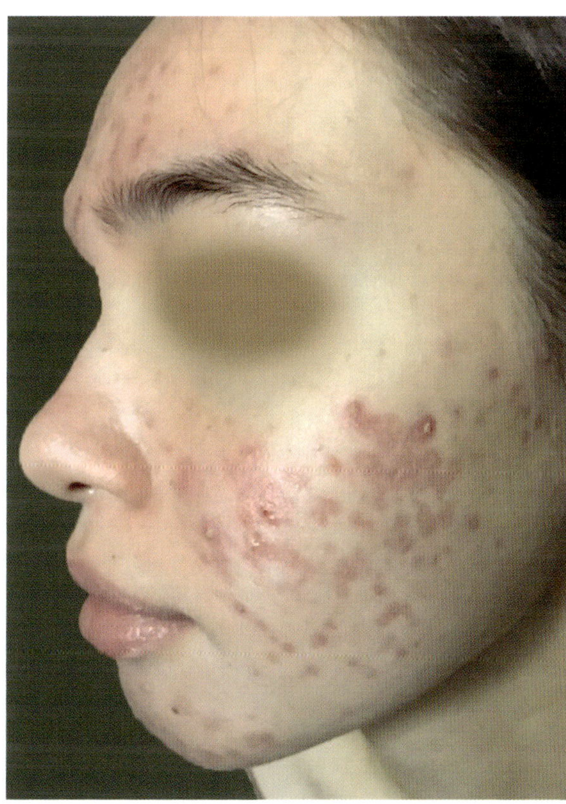

FIGURE 14.7 Post-inflammatory erythema.

Chemical peeling is still a favorite modality for treating PIH, PIE, and acne scars among many dermatologists, especially in Asia. This may be due to the lower cost of this procedure. However, its effectivity is influenced by many factors such as the kind of existing acne scars and the patient's age and skin type.

When treating post-acne scars, it is essential to differentiate scars (atrophic and hypertrophic) from macular marks (PIH and PIE). The latter are self-limiting and clear with time, but atrophic, hypertrophic, and keloidal scars tend to persist without treatment. Management options include technologies which are either energy or non-energy based [35]. Energy-based devices include ablative and non-ablative lasers, fractional radiofrequency, intense pulsed light and plasma skin regeneration. Non-energy-based technologies are the subcutaneous incisionless surgery or subcision, dermabrasion and microdermabrasion, microneedling, dermal fillers and chemical peels. Various surgical modalities, lasers, and energy-based devices have been used to treat post-acne scars in Asians [36].

The improvement achieved with acne scar treatments among Asians is variable and may range from 10 to 50%. Complications are not uncommon. Asian patients can develop hypertrophic and keloidal scars, especially those with a darker skin type. PIH, however, is the most common complication from procedural treatments of acne scars [37,38]. More than 40% of Asian patients who undergo aggressive laser treatment for acne scars will experience some degree of PIH. Although various measures have been tried to reduce PIH following laser treatment, pre- and post-laser application of skin whitening agents (e.g., hydroquinone) has been contentious [39,40]. Sun avoidance and sunscreens, however, have been shown to be effective.

Hypertrophic and Keloidal Scars

Hypertrophic scars tend to resolve spontaneously over time but keloidal scars are best treated with intralesional triamcinolone injections. Surgery tends to provoke aggravation of keloidal scars.

Pulsed-dye lasers, set at the lowest fluence to produce mild purpura, have been used to decrease the volume of hypertrophic scars. Skin texture and pliability were noted to improve together with reduction in the degree of erythema [41]. This device has been tried by Asian dermatologists, with variable rates of success for hypertrophic scars.

Atrophic Scars

Surgical Techniques

Ice pick, boxcar, and rolling scars often occur simultaneously [36] (Figures 14.8 and 14.9). Surgical techniques often employed for atrophic scars include subcision, punch or elliptical excision, and punch elevation.

The subcision technique aims to free the fibrous bands within the scar and is used mainly for rolling scars. Insertion of a Norkor needle or an 18-gauge needle horizontally in the deep dermis with a sweeping motion releases the fibrous bands and enables the skin to become distensible again. Bruising and hematoma are common complications.

Punch or elliptical excision is used for ice pick scars and boxcar scars <3 mm diameter. Removal of the whole scar up to the subcutaneous fat is done with a punch biopsy instrument under local anaesthesia. The gap is then sutured using 6–0 suture with avoidance of excessive traction. Complications include scarring and infection.

Punch elevation is done for boxcar scars >4 mm diameter. The procedure consists of a punch excision around the walls of the scar down to subcutaneous fat. The floating punched specimen is then fixed at a slightly elevated level to the surrounding skin by sutures or Steri-Strips. Complications include scarring and infection.

Dermal Fillers

Dermal fillers can be used to correct mild distensible atrophic acne scars [42]. Suitable dermal fillers include temporary (e.g., hyaluronic acid) and longer-lasting fillers (e.g., poly-L-lactic acid and calcium hydroxylapatite). Autologous fat transplant is another option. The duration of effect varies according to the type of filler used. Hyaluronic acid is a safer option among the dermal fillers but it is short lasting.

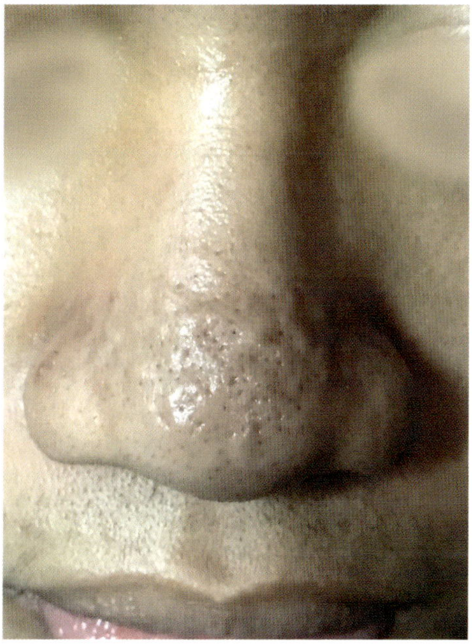

FIGURE 14.8 Pitted scars.

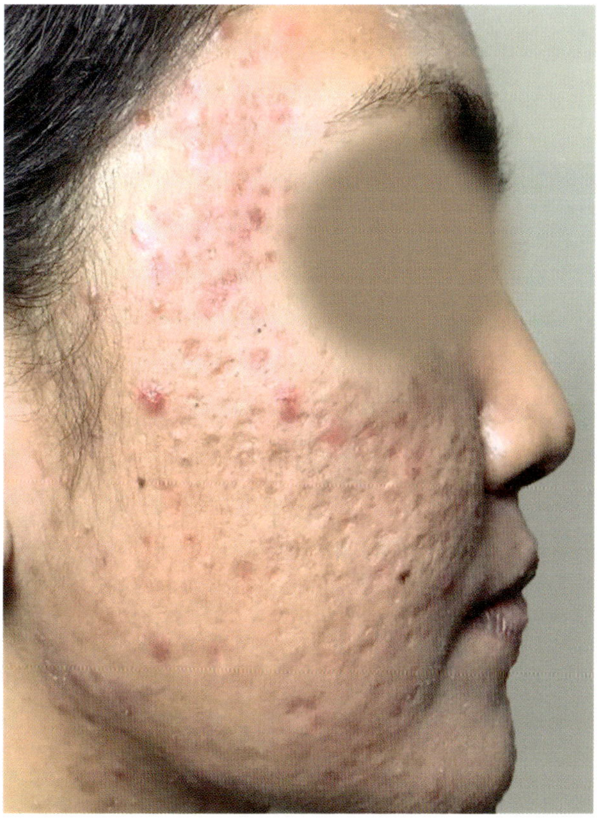

FIGURE 14.9 Depressed scars.

Laser, Light, and Energy-Based Devices

Lasers and energy-based devices have been the gold standard for treating acne scars, with many devices introduced over the last two decades. Unfortunately, none has been shown to eliminate acne scars completely. Improvements of acne scars post-treatment ranged from very minimum to around 50% in Asian patients. A high incidence of post-procedural PIH was noted among Asians and, although various preventive measures have been tried including the use of pre- and post-treatment with skin whiteners [43,44], this was met with varying degrees of success.

Ablative Skin-Resurfacing Lasers

Ablative skin laser resurfacing with a scanner was the first laser procedure introduced to treat acne scars. It served as the gold standard, providing the best outcome of 50%–60% improvement of scars [45]. At present, it is rarely used due to its prolonged downtime and associated complications. Two to three weeks post-resurfacing, erythema and oozing are still evident, carrying a high risk of secondary bacterial and herpes simplex virus (HSV) infection. Even after 3–6 months post-treatment, erythema persists. More than 40% of Asian patients tend to develop PIH post- procedure [46]. In addition, overtreatment can lead to further scarring and delayed skin hypopigmentation. Most commonly used ablative lasers for this purpose were the CO_2 laser (10600 nm) and the Er:YAG laser (2940 nm). Ablation of the full thickness of the epidermis and upper papillary dermis leads to the regeneration ofa healthier skin with improved skin texture. A single treatment is usually enough. Patients with the desire to further improve their scars may have more treatments, 12 months or more later.

Complications from this procedure include prolonged erythema (up to 12 months), protracted visible healing, dyspigmentation (PIH and delayed hypopigmentation), milia, acneiform eruption, infection, telangiectases and scarring. Those with history of HSV infection on the face should receive prophylaxis antivirals.

Non-ablative Lasers

To minimize downtime and complications from ablative laser resurfacing, a number of non-ablative lasers were introduced. These consist of diode lasers, neodymium-doped:YAG laser and other lasers that do not cause any epidermal injury. Heat is delivered into the dermis with water as the target chromophore, damaging the collagen in the dermis. This will stimulate the production of new collagen and improve acne scars. In this procedure, the epidermis is protected from thermal injury with epidermal cooling. Examples of such lasers include the Smoothbeam (1450 nm) and Cooltouch (1320 nm). Unfortunately, the treatment outcome was poor [47] such that these lasers end up seldom used. Complications (e.g., redness and PIH) are uncommon.

Fractional Photothermolysis Lasers

Fractional photothermolysis is now the preferred and gold standard for the treatment of acne scars. It provides middle-ground effects between ablative laser resurfacing and non-ablative laser for acne scars. Fractional photothermolysis provides a controlled and effective skin injury with reduced downtime compared with ablative laser resurfacing, but with more significant improvements of the acne scars than non-ablative laser. However, as expected, the improvements in treatment outcome from fractional photothermolysis are inferior to that of ablative laser resurfacing.

Fractional lasers create columns of microthermal treatment zones with surrounding spared tissue called fractional photothermolysis. The result is faster wound healing, shorter downtime and less risk of complications, especially PIH. The skin (epidermis and dermis) tissue is ablated to a much greater depth (up to the deep dermis), in columns several hundred microns in diameter, sparing untreated epidermis and dermis in between to act as a reservoir of normal tissue to enhance wound healing. The procedure stimulates dermal collagen remodeling and neocollagenesis in a columnar fashion.

Fractional photothermolysis devices can either be ablative or non-ablative. The non-ablative type causes fractional photothermolysis of the skin without much thermal injury to the epidermis and dermis. Coagulation necrosis may be observed in both skin layers but the epidermis remains intact. Such injuries are adequate to partially damage the dermal collagen, stimulating neocollagenesis with relatively little downtime and complications. There is minimal crusting and erythema. A short downtime allows patients to return to work 3–4 days post-treatment [48]. The erbium- (1550 nm) and thulium-doped fiber lasers (1927 nm) are some of the non-ablative fractional laser resurfacing devices. Patients usually need a series of three to four treatments at monthly intervals to achieve an optimal outcome.

The ablative fractional resurfacing devices (e.g., CO_2 fractional resurfacing lasers 10,600 nm) were introduced shortly after the first non-ablative-fractional resurfacing devices. It is believed that more thermal injury to the dermis will stimulate more neocollagenesis and produce better treatment outcomes for acne scars. In ablative fractional resurfacing, thermal injury with breakdown in the epidermis and dermis is more intense with obvious tissue necrosis and columnar damage to both skin layers. This is associated with more downtime and complications. Crusting is seen 1–2 days after laser resurfacing and erythema lasts longer. The patient can only return to work after 5–7 days.

The treatment outcomes comparing non-ablative and ablative fractional laser resurfacing are variable. Some reports indicated that both produced similar efficaciousness while others reported that the ablative fractional laser resurfacing confer better treatment outcome [49]. The reported improvement from fractional laser resurfacing ranges from 20 to 30% after three treatment sessions.

Fractional laser resurfacing causes much less PIH than ablative laser resurfacing, even in Asian skin. PIH is also less severe and short lived. Hence fractional laser resurfacing can be safely carried out in the darker skin type. The prevalence of PIH from fractional laser has been reported to range from 5 to 90% among Asians.

Fractional Radiofrequency Devices

Radiofrequency (RF) consists of electromagnetic wave frequencies ranging from 3 kHz to 300 GHz. The fractional bipolar RF devices deliver energy to produce sublative fractional heating of the dermis, creating microzones of treated and untreated tissue via tiny electrodes that come into contact with the skin. The RF wavelength generates heat beneath the epidermis in the upper dermis, heating the collagen in this area. This stimulates dermal collagen generation and remodeling with minimal epidermal disruption and injury. Examples of fractional RF resurfacing devices include eMatrix and eTwo. To enhance the effects and delivery of RF energy into the dermis, microneedles are attached to the hand piece of such devices so that RF energy can be delivered into the dermis directly. ePrime and Infiny are two such devices (Figures 14.10 and 14.11).

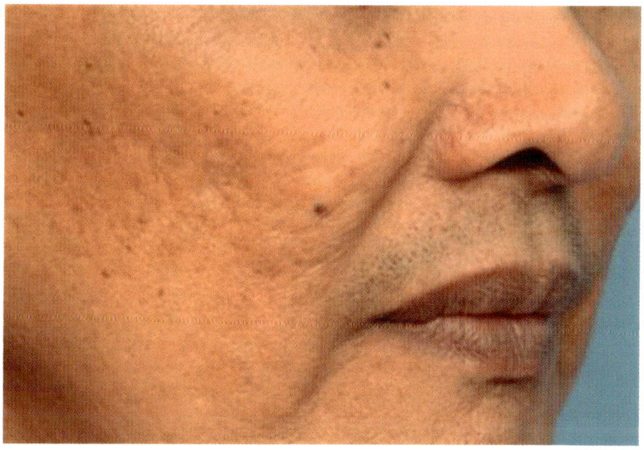

FIGURE 14.10 Before treatment with bipolar fractional RF (eTwo device) 80 mJpin, 64 pin tip, three passes at monthly intervals (skin type 5).

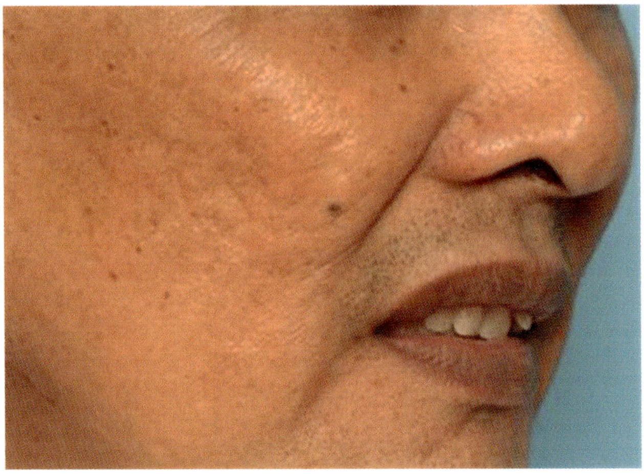

FIGURE 14.11 After treatment with bipolar fractional RF.

The treatment outcome of fractional RF devices is comparable with the fractional photothermolysis laser treatment, with 20%–35% improvements after three treatments [50]. The advantages include minimal complications and downtime. As the epidermis is not damaged, post-treatment erythema is minimal. The patient is often able to return to work the next day. The risk of PIH is very low. It is thus suitable especially for darker skin type, especially Asian patients [50]. The devices, however, should not be used in patients with heart implant/pacemaker as the wavelength may interfere with the implants.

Pearls to Live by

It is apt to close this chapter with words of wisdom we have learned to live by in our practice as Asian dermatologists.

- Prevention is the best policy.
  - Acne scars, to be prevented, must start with aggressive but proper acne treatment.
- Each patient is unique, no matter what skin color one bears.
  - Once an acne patient comes into one's clinic, evaluation right from history taking through the physical examination must be thorough.
  - Treatment of acne, no matter how mild, must ensue.
  - Treatment, to be successful, must consider the patient's preference, but with the physician's final decision as to what is best for one's condition.
- Not a single person should be scarred for life.
  - Realistic goals must be set at the very beginning.
  - What cannot be attained must not be falsely claimed.
  - What can be attained must be explained thoroughly, setting an approximate time frame for expected results.
  - Possible adverse reactions must never be missed.
  - Adherence to the management can thus be attained by the patient, once all the cards are laid properly.
- Science is ever evolving.
  - There will always be new kids on the block.
  - Use what you deem is best for each patient, by your experience and by what medical evidence is presenting.

REFERENCES

1. Handog EB, Macarayo MJE, Gabriel MTG. Acne scars in Asian patients. In: *Acne Scars Classification and Treatment.* Tosti A, De Padova MP, Beer KR, eds. London: Informa UK Ltd, 2010, 90–7.
2. Taylor SC, Kyel A. Defining skin of color. In: *Taylor and Kelly's Dermatology for Skin of Color 2E.* Taylor SC, Paul Kelly A, Lim HW, Serrano AMA, eds. New York: McGraw Hill Education, 2016, 9–14.
3. Enriquez-Macarayo MJ, Handog EB. The concept of brown skin. In: *Melasma and Vitiligo in Brown Skin.* Handog EB, Enriquez-Macarayo MJ, eds. India: Springer, 2017, 4.
4. Handog EB, Macarayo, MJE, Datuin MSL. Maritime Southeast Asia. In: *Taylor and Kelly's Dermatology for Skin of Color 2E.* Taylor SC, Paul Kelly A, Lim HW, Serrano AMA, eds. New York: McGraw Hill Education, 2016, 650–1.
5. Lim JTE, Choon SE. Mainland Southeast Asia. In: *Taylor and Kelly's Dermatology for Skin of Color 2E.* Taylor SC, Paul Kelly A, Lim HW, Serrano AMA, eds. New York: McGraw Hill Education, 2016, 642–3.
6. Su P, Chen Wee Aw D, Lee SH, Han Sim Toh MP. Beliefs, perceptions and psychosocial impact of acne amongst Singaporean students in tertiary institutions. *J Dtsch Dermatol Ges.* 2015; 13(3):227–33.
7. Philippine Dermatological Society Health Information System Registry. Accessed June 2017.
8. Yeung CK, Teo LHY, Xiang LH, Chan HHL. A community-based epidemiological study of acne vulgaris in Hong Kong adolescents. *Acta Derm Venereol (Stockh).* 2002;82:104–7.
9. Chau-Ty G, Goh CL, Koh SL. Pattern of skin diseases at the National Skin Centre (Singapore) from 1989–1990. *Int J Dermatol.* 1992;31:555–9.
10. Goh CL, Akarapanth R. Epidemiology of skin disease among children in a referral skin clinic in Singapore. *Pediatr Dermatol.* 1994;11:125–8.
11. Han XD, Oon HH, Goh CL. Epidemiology of post-adolescence acne and adolescence acne in Singapore: A 10-year retrospective and comparative study. *J Eur Acad Dermatol Venereol.* 2016;30(10):1790–3.
12. Jha BN. To study the profile of acne vulgaris, its seasonal variation, relationship with smoking and possible correlation between acne vulgaris and markers of androgenecity in females. *Adv Res J Life Sci.* 2016;2(3):1–6.
13. Suh DH, Kim BY, Min SK et al. A multicenter epidemiological study of acne vulgaris in Korea. *Int J Dermatol.* 2011;50:673–81.
14. Park MY, Kim KH, Kang H et al. Analysis of Korean acne patients according to age groups based on two multicenter studies. *J Dermatol.* 2017;44(2):186–8.
15. Zari S, Turkistani A. Acne Vulgaris in Jeddah Medical students: Prevalence, severity, self-report, and treatment practices. *J Cosm Dermatol Sci Applic.* 2017;7:67–76.
16. Abad-Casintahan F, Chow SKW, Goh CL et al. Frequency and characteristics of acne-related post-inflammatory hyperpigmentation. *J Dermatol.* 2016;43:826–8.
17. Tan HH, Tan AWH, Barkham T et al. Community-based study of acne vulgaris in adolescents in Singapore. *Br J Dermatol.* 2007;157:547–51.
18. Tan JKL. Psychosocial impact of acne vulgaris: Evaluating the evidence. *Skin Therapy Lett.* 2004;9(7):1–3.
19. Suh DH, Kim BY, Min SK et al. A multicenter epidemiological study of acne vulgaris in Korea. *Int J Dermatol.* 2011;50:673–81.
20. Yeung CK, Teo LHY, Xiang LH, Chan HHL. A community-based epidemiological study of acne vulgaris in Hong Kong adolescents. *Acta Derm Venereol (Stockh).* 2002;82:104–7.
21. Kim IH. Salicyclic acid peel (acne peel). *Hong Kong J Dermatol Venereol.* 2005;13:83–5.
22. Dainichi T, Ueda S, Imayama S et al. Excellent clinical results with a new preparation for chemical peeling in acne: 20% salicylic acid in polyethylene glycol vehicle. *Dermatol Surg.* 2008;34:891–9.
23. Sarkar R, Gokhale N, Sharma S. South Asia. In: *Taylor and Kelly's Dermatology for Skin of Color 2E.* Taylor SC, Paul Kelly A, Lim HW, Serrano AMA, eds. New York: McGraw Hill Education, 2016, 664–5.
24. Tan J, Kang S, Leyden J. Prevalence and risk factors of acne scarring among patients consulting dermatologists in the United States. *J Drugs Dermatol.* 2017;16(2):97–102.
25. Layton A, Dreno B, Finlay AY et al. New patient-oriented tools for assessing atrophic acne scarring. *Dermatol Ther (Heidelb).* 2016;6(2):219–33.
26. Perkins AC, Cheng CE, Hillebrand GG et al. Comparison of the epidemiology of acne vulgaris among Caucasian, Asian, Continental Indian and African American women. *J Eur Acad Dermatol Venereol.* 2011;25:1054–60.

27. Tan JK, Tang J, Fung K et al. Development and validation of a Scale for Acne Scar Severity (SCAR-S) of the face and trunk. *J Cutan Med Surg.* 2010;14:156–60.
28. Micali G, Francesconi L, Nardone B, Lacarrubba F. Classification of acne scars: a review with clinical and ultrasound correlation. In: *Acne Scars Classification and Treatment.* Tosti A, De Padova MP, Beer KR, eds. London: Informa UK Ltd 2010, 1–7.
29. Rivera A. Acne scarring: A review and current treatment modalities. *J Am Acad Dermatol.* 2008;59:659–76.
30. Hazarika N, Rajaprabha RK. Assessment of Life Quality Index among patients with acne vulgaris in a suburban population. *Indian J Dermatol.* 2016;61:163–8.
31. Ali FR, Kirk M, Madan V. Papular acne scars of the nose and chin: An under- recognised variant of acne scarring. *J Cutan Aesthet Surg.* 2016;9:241–3.
32. Gan SD, Graber EM. Papular scars: An addition to the acne scar classification scheme. *J Clin Aesthet Dermatol.* 2015;8:19–20.
33. Lee SJ, Kim JM, Kim YK, Seo SJ, Park KY. The pinhole method using an erbium: YAG laser for the treatment of papular acne scars. *Dermatologic Therapy.* 2017;e12512. https://doi.org/10.1111/dth.12512
34. Chaudhary RG, Pitroda HS, Modi KR, Chauhan AP. Comparative outcome study of various chemical peels and surgical procedures in the management of acne scarring. *Int J Med Sci Pub Health.* 2016;5:1128–33.
35. Kravvas G, Al-Niaimi F. A systematic review of treatments for acne scarring. Part 1: Non-energy-based techniques. *Scars, Burns & Healing.* 2017;3:1–17.
36. Zaleski-Larsen LA, Fabi SG, McGraw T, Taylor M. Acne scar treatment: A multimodality approach tailored to scar type. *Dermatol Surg.* 2016;42(S2):S139–49.
37. Wat H, Wu DC, Chan HH. Fractional resurfacing in the Asian patient: Current state of the art. *Lasers Surg Med.* 2017;49(1):45–59.
38. Dai R, Xie H, Hua W et al. The efficacy and safety of the fractional radiofrequency technique for the treatment of atrophic acne scar in Asians: A meta-analysis. *J Cosmet Laser Ther.* 2017;7:1–8.
39. Duke D, Grevelink JM. Care before and after laser skin resurfacing. A survey and review of literature. *Dermatol Surg.* 1998;24(2):201–6.
40. Wanitphakdeedecha R, Phuardchantuk R, Manuskiatti W. The use of sunscreen starting on the first day after ablative fractional skin resurfacing. *J Eur Acad Dermatol Venereol.* 2014;28(11):1522–8.
41. Philip Werschler W, Herdener RS, Victor Ross E, Zimmerman E. Treating acne scars: What's new? *J Clin Aesthet Dermatol.* 2015;8(S8):S2–8.
42. Wollina U, Goldman A. Fillers for the improvement in acne scars. *Clin Cosmet Investig Dermatol.* 2015 8:493–9.
43. Goldman MP. The use of hydroquinone with facial laser resurfacing. *J Cutan Laser Ther.* 2000;2(20):73–7.
44. West TB, Alster TS. Effect of pretreatment on the incidence of hyperpigmentation following cutaneous CO2 laser resurfacing. *Dermatol Surg.* 1999;25(1):15–17.
45. Goh CL, Khoo L. Laser skin resurfacing treatment outcome of facial scars and wrinkles in Asians with skin type III/IV with the Unipulse CO2 laser system. *Sing Med J.* 2002;43(1):28–32.
46. Kim YJ, Lee HS, Son SW et al. Analysis of hyperpigmentation and hypopigmentation after Er:YAG laser skin resurfacing. *Lasers Surg Med.* 2005;36(1):47–51.
47. Chua SH, Ang P, Khoo LS, Goh CL. Nonablative 1450-nm diode laser in the treatment of facial atrophic acne scars in type IV to V Asian skin: A prospective clinical study. *Dermatol Surg.* 2004;30(10):1287–91.
48. Alexis AF, Coley MK, Nijhawan RI et al. Nonablative Fractional Laser Resurfacing for acne scarring in patients with Fitzpatrick skin phototypes IV-VI. *Dermatolo Surg.* 2016;42(3):392–402.
49. Abdel Hay R, Shalaby K, Zaher H et al. Interventions for acne scars. *Cochrane Database Syst Rev.* 2016;4:CD011946.
50. Qin X, Li H, Jian X, Yu B. Evaluation of the efficacy and safety of fractional bipolar radiofrequency with high-energy strategy for treatment of acne scars in Chinese. *J Cosmet Laser Ther.* 2015;17(5):237–45.

15

Acne Scarring and Patients of African Descent

Aldo D. Galvez and Amy J. McMichael

KEY FEATURES

- Acne is a frequent problem among all races and ethnicities. Darker-skinned individuals are at increased risk of post-inflammatory hyperpigmentation and hypertrophic scarring such as keloids.
- Regarding how to decrease these risks in patients of African descent, it is important to consider prevention and prompt treatment of inflammatory acne without inducing skin.
- Medical management of post-inflammatory hyperpigmentation is usually performed with retinoids, lightening creams and chemical peels.
- Types of scarring: atrophic (ice pick, rolling, and boxcar) and hypertrophic (hypertrophic scar and keloid).
- Management of hypertrophic scars in patients of African descent include injectable steroids and cytotoxic agents, silicone dressings, and laser therapies with pulsed-dye laser.
- Management of ice pick scars has the limited options of punch excision and the chemical reconstruction of skin scars technique.
- Management of rolling and boxcar scars in patients of African descent has more therapeutic options. These include: chemical peels, microneedling, subcision (only for rolling scars), dermal fillers, and laser therapies with fractional non-ablative and ablative lasers.

Introduction

Acne is a common disorder affecting up to 45 million people in the United States [1] with a prevalence of 80% in people between 11 and 30 years of age and occurring in 5% of older adults [2,3]. It is the skin disease most commonly treated by physicians [3] and occurs in people of all ethnicities and races. Currently it is accepted that the pathophysiology, presentation, and treatment of acne are similar in all skin phenotypes. However, acne in pigmented skin is distinguished by the higher incidence of post-inflammatory hyperpigmentation (PIH) and scarring. This chapter will focus on these two major acne sequelae occurring primarily in individuals of African descent.

Acne scarring and PIH can have significant psychosocial impact on patients. Scarring can lead to emotional debilitation, embarrassment, poor self-esteem, social isolation, depression, and many other effects [4]. Although these effects cannot be easily quantified in patient terms, healthcare affect or social expense, scarring is a significant issue that requires attention especially in darker-skinned individuals, as the incidence rates for hypertrophic scarring are higher in this population [5,6] (Figure 15.1).

Epidemiology

As the population of the world becomes increasingly diverse, understanding ethnic and racial differences in dermatologic disease is becoming increasingly important. Genetic, environmental, socioeconomic,

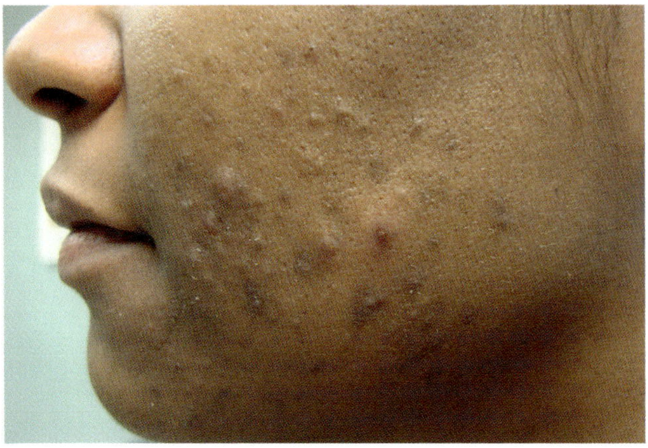

FIGURE 15.1 Inflammatory acne lesions (papules and nodules) and PIH. Both lesions motivated the patient's consult.

and cultural factors are likely to contribute to these differences [7]. Currently, there is still a paucity of reliable studies investigating racial and ethnic differences in the epidemiology of dermatologic disease [6]. Most of the data we have is based on practice surveys and individual clinical experience [7,8]. Most surveys show that this skin disorder consistently ranks as the top dermatologic diagnosis in populations of all skin types [6–8] and suggests that ethnicity might have an influence in disease presentation [9].

Dermatological visits in the African-American population were related to acne in 22.1% according to the National Ambulatory Medical Care Survey Database Study between 1993 and 2009 [1]. Based on a retrospective chart review conducted between August 2004 and July 2005, the six most common diagnoses observed in Black patients were acne, dyschromia, contact dermatitis and other eczema, alopecia, seborrheic dermatitis, and lesion of unspecified behavior. This study also found that dermatologic visits for acne were the most common in both Black (28.4%) and White (21.0%) patients [7].

Ethnicity might influence acne prevalence and some of its features. A survey study published by Perkins et al. in 2011, performed in four cities (in the United States, England, Japan, and Italy) with a sample of 2895 women ranging from 10 to 70 years, of whom 385 (13.3%) were Black showed interesting data. Other populations included were classified as Caucasian, Hispanic, Asian, and Continental Indian. This study estimated a prevalence of 37% of acne in the African-American population, which was the highest of the included groups. Hyperpigmentation, hypertrophic, and atrophic scarring were more common in African-American woman than in other groups [9].

The quality of life and treatment expectations in Caucasian and non-Caucasian (including the African-American population and others) were also investigated by Callender and colleagues in a study published in 2014. They did not find any statistically significant differences in quality of life between these groups. Nevertheless, they did find that non-Caucasian patients were more worried about PIH and two out of three patients in this group wanted acne treatment to be designed to their specific skin needs [10] (Figure 15.2).

As previously reviewed, PIH is a major acne sequelae in skin of color. In a survey of 2,000 Black patients seen by dermatologists, PIH was the third most common dermatosis, seen in 9% of patients (acne 28% and eczema 20%) versus 2% of White patients [8,11]. A high rate of PIH was also documented in a 2002 survey of African-American, Hispanic, and Asian patients. Acne and hyperpigmented macules were found in 65, 53 and 47%, of these populations, respectively [12]. It is clear that even though the incidence of acne is fairly equivalent among different skin phototypes, the PIH of acne is a much larger concern for patients of color than for White patients [6,13].

Hypertrophic and keloidal scarring is not as common in the general population as PIH and atrophic scarring; however, it is more frequent in skin of color and can be more permanent and disfiguring [9]. In general, keloidal overgrowths of scar tissue are seen between five and 16 times more frequently in patients of color [14]. These lesions can be very persistent and are equal in incidence among both sexes. They are less common in the very young or old. Familial and genetic influences with both autosomal dominant and recessive traits are associated with these lesions [5,14].

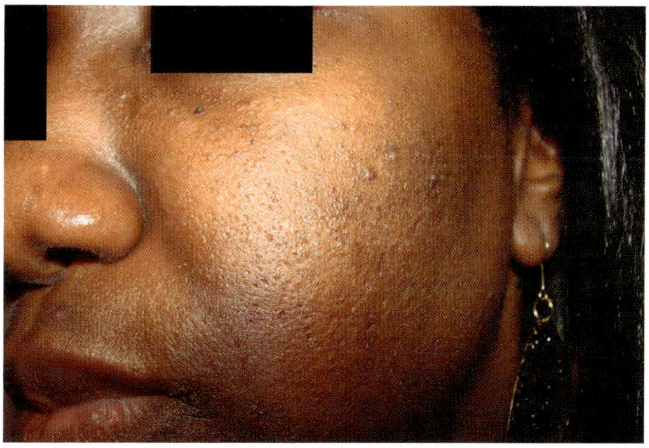

FIGURE 15.2 A patient consulting for PIH and acne scars. Although the findings in the physical exam are mild, they cause distress for the patient and decrease her quality of life.

The morbidity of acne is due to the lesions themselves, which may be painful and tender, as well as from residual scarring and PIH after the nodules and cysts resolve. Morbidity may be generated by adverse effects of treatments as well. There can be a huge impact on quality of life, especially in terms of psychological morbidity. An estimated $100 million per year is spent on over-the-counter remedies by consumers for acne. When the loss of productivity and unemployment are included the direct cost of acne may exceed $1 billion per year in the United States [1].

It is therefore important to keep in mind not only the lesions themselves (inflammatory and non-inflammatory) but also their consequences (PIH and scarring), and their combined morbidity in the quality of life of patients. Greater understanding of acne in people with skin of color can lead to more tailored treatment and more favorable outcomes [15].

History

PIH and scarring are the two most disfiguring sequelae of inflammatory acne [6]. The use of topical applications of substances to treat dyspigmentation has existed for centuries. The ancient Egyptians applied animal oils, salt, alabaster, and sour milk to the skin for aesthetic improvement [16]. Dermatologists have continued to advance on these earlier treatments. It was dermatologists who pioneered skin peeling for therapeutic benefit. As early as 1871, Fox, a dermatologist, was treating pigmentary changes using phenol for the treatment of freckles [17].

Over the years, there have been many attempts to improve acne scarring as well. Ablative techniques such as deep chemical peels, dermabrasion, and, more recently, laser-driven skin-resurfacing procedures with carbon dioxide (CO_2) and/or erbium:yttrium–aluminum garnet (Er:YAG) as well as fractionated lasers have been used [18]. Ablative procedures such as laser treatment have been attempted for scar revision since the 1990s [19,20].

Post-inflammatory Hyperpigmentation

PIH represents the skin's response to any type of trauma or cutaneous injury and is often the major sequela of acne. It is visibly more pronounced in darker-skinned individuals. PIH can be either epidermal or dermal. Acne typically results in the epidermal form of hyperpigmentation in which there is an increase in melanin production and/or transfer to keratinocytes. Various inflammatory mediators such as prostaglandins E2 and D2 have been shown to enhance pigment production in animal models and may have a similar role in humans [21].

The development of PIH in the setting of acne may be multifactorial. The lesions of acne itself, including comedones, papules, pustules, and nodules induce hyperpigmentation, but physical manipulation of lesions by the patient or over-aggressive, irritating acne treatment regimens can trigger this unwanted skin reaction.

In general, comedonal acne in White skin is characterized as non-inflammatory. In biopsies of comedonal acne in Black skin, comedonal lesions exhibit marked inflammation with infiltrates of polymorphonuclear leucocytes [22]. This disparity in histological inflammation between Black skin and White skin helps explain the propensity for darker-skinned individuals to develop PIH (Figure 15.3).

Clinical Features

For many dark-skinned patients, PIH is more aesthetically unacceptable than the original acne lesions. Subsequently macular hyperpigmentation of the face is often the chief complaint of the acne patient with dark skin when presenting to the dermatologist.

PIH presents as asymptomatic tan-to-dark-brown patches or macules corresponding to the areas of injury. The discoloration typically outlasts the acne lesions themselves and can persist for months to years and consequently poses a lingering problem for the patient. In a survey of 239 African Americans with acne, 27.2% tried using over-the-counter 1%–2% hydroquinone preparations prior to presentation to the dermatologist [23]. Another report states 80% of African patients with acne use skin-lightening agents [24]. Agents commonly employed by patients for the purpose of skin lightening include various over-the-counter acne washes, vinegar, cocoa butter and hydroquinone; clearly PIH is a major sequela mandating treatment (Figure 15.4).

Treatment

It is essential to understand that it is more convenient to prevent PIH rather than to treat it. An aggressive approach to treat acne will be convenient and products used for that purpose (retinoids and antibiotics) are similar for all Fitzpatrick skin types.

Nevertheless, it is important to avoid irritation of the skin, since it can worsen PIH. Recognition of the patient's skin type, that is, dry/sensitive skin prone to irritation, normal skin with minimal propensity for irritation, oily skin or combination skin, can aid in choosing an appropriate regimen with the least amount of irritation [23]. In addition, many patients consider their skin "sensitive." It is important to determine what "sensitive" means and if there are true allergies, irritant reactions or simply dryness in response to treatment.

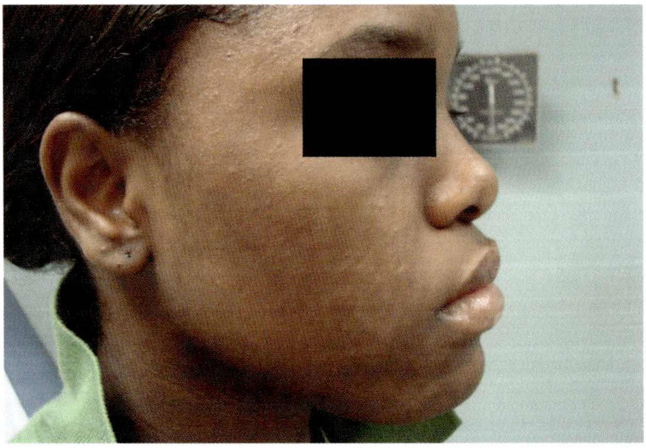

FIGURE 15.3 Patient with PIH secondary to acne lesions that had resolved by the time of the consult.

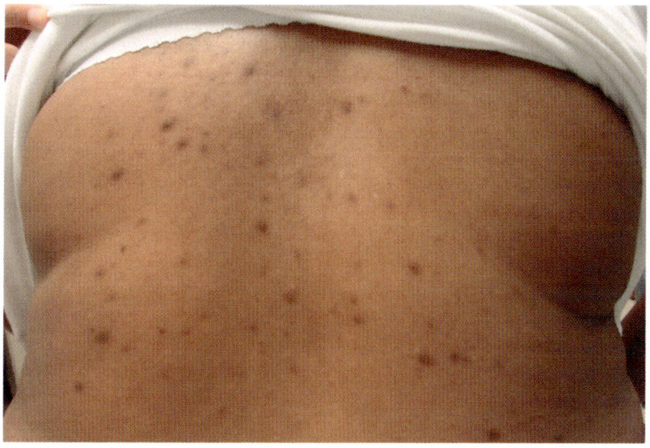

FIGURE 15.4 Papular and nodular acne in the back of a patient with subsequent postinflammatory hyperpigmentation.

Topical Agents

Topical agents used for treating PIH are summarized in Table 15.1. In using these agents, the dermatologist must set expectations for the patient. Advising the patient prior to commencing treatment that it will take 3 months or more to improve PIH will help the patient remain compliant with treatment. Additionally, the patient must understand that photoprotection is especially important, including avoiding sun exposure, using an adequate hat with a wide brim, and sunscreen if prescribed by their physician.

Irritation is a well-documented adverse effect with these medications in all skin types. In pigmented skin, minimizing this predictable adverse effect rests on choosing the right vehicle, starting with lower concentrations, considering alternate day dosing, proper patient education on use, and selecting a tolerable formulation. The treatment of hyperpigmentation can be a long, arduous process even with treatment, requiring patience and compliance. Realistic goals must be discussed with the patient.

The retinoids, such as tretinoin, adapalene, and tazarotene, represent a class of topicals that not only treat acne but also hyperpigmentation and, therefore, should be initiated early in treatment and remain as maintenance therapy. It is beneficial to explain to the patient the dual role of retinoids in treatment of

TABLE 15.1

Therapeutic Agents for Hyperpigmentation According to Severity

Mild
Hydroquinone 2, 3 and 4%
Azelaic acid 20%
Kojic acid 2%–4%
Glycolic acid
Tretinoin and other retinoids
Moderate
Hydroquinone 4%–10%
Kojic acid
Azelaic acid/tretinoin
Hydroquinone/tretinoin
Hydroquinone/glycolic acid
Combination therapies
Chemical peels: salicylic acid 20%–30%, salicylic/mandelic acid
Severe
Combination therapies
Chemical peels: salicylic acid 20%–30%, salicylic/mandelic acid

acne and hyperpigmentation to foster improved adherence. Retinoids are not only well known for their effect on non-inflammatory and inflammatory acne but they can also directly affect PIH in dark-skinned individuals [25–27].

Azelaic acid, a dicarboxylic acid obtained from *Pityrosporum ovale*, is another topical that acts on acne lesions and hyperpigmentation. It inhibits melanin synthesis by interfering with tyrosinase and has direct cytotoxic effects on melanocytes. It has no effect on normally pigmented skin and is considered to have a low irritancy profile, so may be useful in those with sensitive skin and a history of PIH. It can be used in combination with retinoids.

Some individuals, especially those with prominent PIH, will also require skin-lightening agents in addition to the traditional acne regimen to combat hyperpigmentation. Hydroquinone, a hydroxylphenol, has been the gold standard for treatment of hyperpigmentation for over 50 years [28]. There are numerous other skin-lightening agents available and may be used as alternatives to hydroquinone. A few of these agents will be briefly mentioned.

Hydroquinone reduces the production of melanin by inhibiting tyrosinase, which is responsible for converting L-3,4-dihydroxyphenylalanine (DOPA) to melanin. Other mechanisms of action, including destruction of melanocytes, degradation of melanosomes, and inhibition of deoxyribose nucleic acid and ribonucleic acid synthesis, have been attributed to hydroquinone. It is available in over-the-counter concentrations of 1%–2%, with a prescription strength of 3%–4% and compounded at 5%–10%. It is recommended to begin treatment after the acne is under control, or even after 2–4 weeks of acne treatment and should be applied after application of topical acne medication. Treatment can be used as spot treatment or diffusely once to twice a day. Results may be noticed within 8–12 weeks [6]. Adverse effects include irritant and allergic dermatitis, temporary hypopigmentation of surrounding normal skin, giving a halo appearance, and the much-debated exogenous ochronosis with prolonged use. Instruction on how to apply the hydroquinone product over an entire cosmetic unit will help to avoid the localized halo side effect. Various formulations are available; some with additives such as glycolic acid, tretinoin, vitamin C, steroids, sunscreens, and microsponges enhance delivery and efficacy of hydroquinone [29].

Mequinol, also known as 4-hydroxyanisole, methoxyphenol, hydroquinone monomethyl ether, and p-hydroxyanisole, is approved in the United States and Europe and is the primary prescription alternative to hydroquinone [29]. The exact mechanism of action is unknown. It does not damage melanocytes, unlike hydroquinone. Kojic acid, a naturally occurring fungal derivative, is used increasingly in Japan, for treatment of hyperpigmentation. It is available over the counter. It also inhibits tyrosinase by binding to copper, with a reported efficacy similar to over-the-counter hydroquinone [28].

Arbutin, available over the counter, is a derivative of hydroquinone used in PIH. Obtained from the leaves of the bearberry plant, it decreases tyrosinase activity and inhibits melanosome maturation. Aleosin is a glycoprotein derived from *Aloe vera* that inhibits tyrosinase without cytotoxicity. It has limited ability to penetrate the skin due to its hydrophilic property. It is commonly used with Arbutin. Licorice extract is considered the safest pigment-lightening agent [29]. Its mechanism of action is similar to kojic acid. The main component is glabridin.

A number of cosmeceutical pigment-lightening agents are available with varying effects and these include N-acetylglucosamine, soybean trypsin inhibitor and ascorbic acid. Other botanically derived topicals have been included in cosmeceuticals for the treatment of hyperpigmentation including: resveratrol, niacinamide, extracts of coffeeberry, soy, green tea, orchids, and grape seed.

Chemical Peels

Chemical peels can also be used for treating this condition, but it is important to choose the acids that have the lowest profile for inducing PIH. This strategy is to treat the epidermal rather than dermal component. Salicylic acid is a β-hydroxy acid that can treat both inflammatory acne and PIH, or PIH alone [30]. One study compared chemical peels with glycolic acid 35% versus salicylic acid 20%–mandelic acid 10% (SM) solution for the treatment of acne, scars and PIH; they found that SM solution was more effective for acne lesions, PIH and had lower adverse effects [31]. Some authors also suggest the use of 25% trichloroacetic acid (TCA) and Jessner's solution [32], but caution is best when treating darker Fitzpatrick skin types with these strong peeling agent. Do no harm should be a guide to choosing treatment of PIH.

Hypertrophic and Atrophic Scarring

Acne scars can be divided into atrophic and hypertrophic scars, the latter include hypertrophic and keloid scars [33]. The literature reports a 3:1 ratio between atrophic and hypertrophic scars [34]. Nevertheless, in patients of African descent this ratio might be lower because keloid scars are considered to be more common in this population [35].

Keloids are unique to humans and can be described as a disproportionate formation and excess deposition of collagen outside the margins of the original injury [5]. Common locations include the chest, back, shoulders and ears. Clinically, there may be pain, itching, burning or a limited range of motion [35] (Figure 15.5).

Histology shows a normal-appearing dermis with relaxed, randomly aligned collagen. Both hypertrophic scars and keloids demonstrate thicker, more abundant collagen that is stretched and aligned in the same plane as the epidermis. Islands of dermal collagen fibers, small vasculature, and fibroblasts can be seen throughout hypertrophic scars [36]. Their pathogenesis is related to an excess of collagen deposition and decreased collagenase activity [34].

On the other hand, atrophic acne scars are classified by Jacob in three different types: ice pick, rolling, and boxcar. Ice pick scars are the most common atrophic scars found in patients with acne [37]. Sometimes a patient can present with facial scars that are difficult to classify, even for experts. For all of these scar types, their pathogenesis is related to an increase of collagenase activity and lack of collagen deposition [34].

Treating acne scars can be one of the most difficult cosmetic surgery procedures that exists [38]. The difficulty in achieving total correction of damage caused by severe inflammatory acne is that the epidermis, dermis, and underlying fat are often involved. The goal of treatment should be to obtain as much improvement as possible rather than perfection [39]. Medical, surgical, and procedural options will be discussed for the management of scarring. These are summarized in Table 15.2.

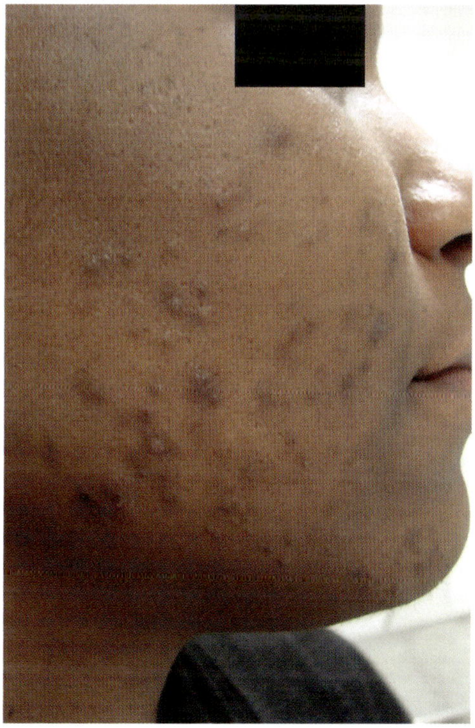

FIGURE 15.5 Late stage acne scars with fibrous change.

TABLE 15.2

Classification of Acne Scars with Suggested Treatment in Patients with Dark Skin

Hypertrophic scarring	
Hypertrophic scars Keloid scars	Topical and intralesional steroids, intralesional steroids with 5-FU, silicone dressing, pulsed-dye laser
Atrophic scarring	
Ice pick scars	CROSS technique, punch excision
Boxcar scars Rolling scars	Punch elevation or grafting (small boxcar), subcision (rolling), microneedling, chemical peels, dermal fillers, ablasive and nonablasive fractional lasers

Management of Hypertrophic Scarring

Topical and Intralesional Steroid

Steroids are one of the more popular choices for medical therapy for hypertrophic scars and keloids [40]. Clinical responses can be varied as steroids can be used topically with and without occlusion. Possible side effects of topical steroids are well known and include telangiectasias, bruising, atrophy, pain or pigmentary change [41]. Intralesional steroid injections are another route; this remained as first-line treatment for hypertrophic scars and keloids for many years [40].

To flatten keloids, a concentration of triamcinolone acetonide (TAC) between 10 and 20 mg/cc should be used. Repeat injections can be given every 2–4 weeks [6]. With intralesional injections, often multiple injections spaced one or several months apart are required to determine the final result and prevent excess atrophy [5].

Intralesional steroids can also be used to create atrophy in an area where there has been an overcorrection with permanent filler for augmentation. Other side effects of injected steroids include intolerance, necrosis, allergy, bruising, hyperpigmentation or hypopigmentation, injection pain, and telangiectasias. Of these side effects hypopigmentation can be a major concern for patients of color. Minimizing the amount of steroid injected, selecting a few lesions for trial, and spacing injections by at least 4 weeks can help prevent hypopigmentation. Choosing lesions that are located in inconspicuous areas for the first treatment may also give an idea of how the skin will respond to a given concentration of injected steroid.

Intralesional 5-Fluorouracil with Steroids

Updated evidence reviews support the use of intralesional 5-fluorouracil (5-FU) in combination with corticoids in order to get an effective treatment and reduce steroids side effects formerly mentioned [40]. This treatment strategy had enhanced therapeutic efficacy when compared with pulsed-dye laser (PDL) [42] and surgical excision + intralesional steroids [43]. Concentration used for this purpose can be achieved with TAC 4 mg (0.1 mL of 40 mg/mL TAC) mixed with 5-FU 45 mg (0.9 mL of 50 mg/mL 5-FU) [44]. This treatment can also be used after surgery to prevent the development of keloid scars [40].

Silicone Dressings

Silicone dressings are another treatment option for hypertrophic scars and to a lesser extent for keloids. These are completely safe to use in darker skin types, although there are variable results with this treatment modality. The results are likely attributable to occlusion or hydration. Pressure, temperature, increased oxygen tension, electrostatic properties and immunologic effects have all been other rationales for the use of silicone dressings. There are conflicting reports as to its efficacy [5].

In one randomized control trial, an improvement in pruritus, pain, and pliability was reported, but no improvement in pigmentation, average elevation or minimum elevation of scars was found [45]. Another review of effects, efficacy, and safety determined that side effects rarely occur but can include pruritus, contact dermatitis, maceration, skin breakdown, xerosis, and odor [5].

In terms of ease of use, silicone dressings do not suit facial scars well since they would be visible to others if worn in public. Thus, these dressings may best serve large areas on the chest or back that can easily be camouflaged with clothing. Another worry with these dressings is that most studies support their use in early forming scars as opposed to late scars [5].

Pulsed-Dye Laser

Treatment of hypertrophic scars with PDL was previously demonstrated in patients with lighter skin tones. Technological advances in laser devices (refinements in laser technology and epidermal cooling) and protocols for darker skin patients allow it to be attempted as treatment cautiously in recalcitrant patients. Relatively low PDL energy densities (4.5–5.0 J/cm^2, 10 mmspot) are typically applied to hypertrophic scars and keloids at 2-month time intervals [46]. Transient PIH is the most common adverse effect of PDL treatment of vascular lesions and scars in pigmented skin [47] (Figure 15.6).

Management of Atrophic Ice pick Scars

Chemical Reconstruction of Skin Scars Technique

Chemical reconstruction of skin scars (CROSS) consists of the focal application of 100% TCA using a sharpened wooden applicator in ice pick scars. The treatment is done until achieving focal frosting (usually within 10 seconds) every 1–3 months. It is a technique that does not require much equipment and achieves good results [48].

Khunger and colleagues performed a study in 2011 proving its safety in 30 patients with a Fitzpatrick's phototypes IV and V, where priming was done previous to the procedure using a cream with 4% hydroquinone in the morning and 0.025% tretinoin at night. The procedure was repeated every 2 weeks for a total of four sessions. Excellent results were achieved in more than 70% of patients; transient hypopigmentation was seen in two patients and hyperpigmentation in one [49].

Punch Excision

This represents a way to surgically remove an ice pick scar, exchanging it for a less noticeable scar. This latter scar can be treated with a resurfacing laser in order to improve its cosmetic appearance [50]. We

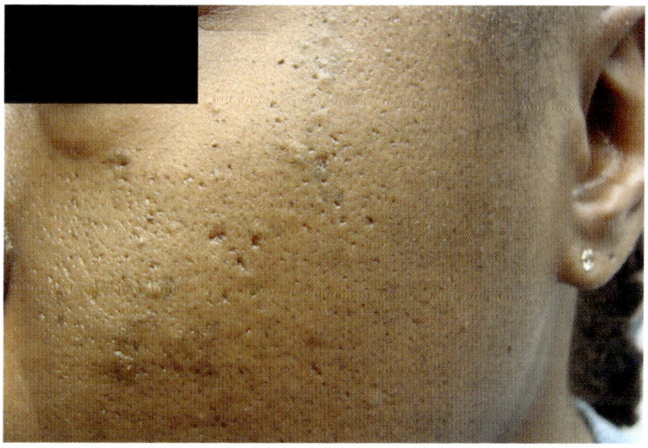

FIGURE 15.6 Patient with ice pick scars.

need to keep in mind that patients of African descent are prone to keloid scars, so the physician needs an adequate follow-up. Strategies for treatment of hypertrophic scars, previously reviewed, need to be kept in mind.

Management of Other Atrophic Scars

Punch Grafting and Elevation (for Small Boxcar Scars)

Punch grafting represents a modification for the punch excision technique. The graft is usually provided from the post-auricular area. This technique is highly dependent on the surgeon's skills. Punch elevation represents the intermediate technique between punch excision and grafting. The scar is punched and the skin is elevated and fixed into place at a plane even to the surface of the skin [50]. As with all invasive techniques, possible further scarring can occur and should be discussed with the patient before such a procedure (Figure 15.7).

Subcision (for Rolling Scars)

Rolling scars usually present fibrous attachments from the dermis to the subcutis. Subcision is a technique that uses a needle to manipulate and release those attachments and requires a clot formation in place to release the scar tissue. Multiple treatments may be needed to achieve the desired result. Complications include bruising, bleeding and infection; this technique should be done when the patient's acne is no longer active to avoid its reactivation. Some authors suggest the use of a dermal filler to raise the dermis without clot formation [50].

Chemical Peels

Differently to what was discussed on PIH, to treat atrophic acne scars, the dermal component must be addressed. This puts the patient with dark skin in an increased risk of PIH. Priming with a hydroquinone cream some weeks before is useful to avoid PIH due to the procedure. Combination of 70% glycolic acid gel is suggested with focal application of 25% TCA over the gel into the atrophic scars. Frosting will be noted but the physician should not let it finish, just keeping the solution in action for 2–4 minutes before the face is neutralized with 1% sodium bicarbonate solution [30].

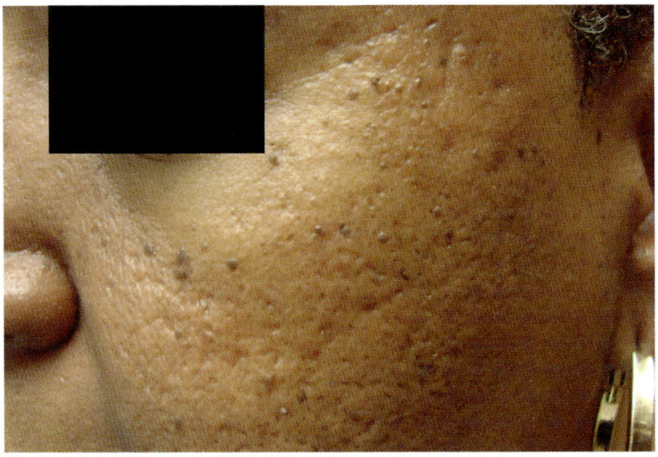

FIGURE 15.7 Patient with boxcar and ice pick acne scars.

Microneedling

Microneedling is a technique that allows the physician to make many rapid healing punctures, allowing the formation of collagen and elastin as a wound-healing response. Side effects, such as infection or PIH, are minimal as it keeps the epidermis partially intact [51]. Microneedling is usually done with a device called the Dermaroller, with most protocols suggesting rolling the device in four to six different directions in the targeted area. These procedures are usually done every 6 weeks and its safe in patients with dark skin [52]. Some protocols in patients with phototype VI and V combine microneedling treatment with chemical peels as high as 35% which are performed every 6 weeks in between the resting period for microneedling, achieving better results than with microneedling alone and without a significant risk for PIH [53].

Dermal Fillers

For patients with few scars, augmentation is another alternative for the management of acne scarring. The past decade has seen the advent of a multitude of injectable fillers including human collagen, polylactic acid and hyaluronic acid among the short-term agents and many agents of a longer-term nature with the reintroduction of silicone and variations of polyacrylamides for longer correction. Agents may be xenografts, autografts, homografts or synthetics [54]. For those with few scars, simple dermal augmentation with hyaluronic acid containing fillers would be most appropriate. In patients with limited acne scarring overcorrection should be avoided.

There are few to no studies that specifically examine the use of filler agents in skin of color. The safety and use of Restylane (Galderma Laboratories), a hyaluronic acid, have been studied off-label in patients with Fitzpatrick skin types IV to VI in isolated cases. There were no transient or permanent adverse outcomes among the type IV to VI subjects in those cases. If proper injection techniques are used, patients with Fitzpatrick skin types IV to VI can benefit from this kind of treatment [55].

Nonablasive and Ablasive Fractionated Lasers

When using light and lasers in the treatment of acne scarring, there is a higher risk of side effects in darker-skinned patients due to the nonspecific energy absorption by the relatively large quantities of melanin in the basal layer of the epidermis. These side effects include permanent depigmentation, textural changes, focal atrophy and scarring. Epidermal melanin can also compete for absorption of energy and decrease the total amount of energy reaching deeper dermal lesions.

It is imperative to consider power level as well as the wavelength of the laser when treating darker skin. Power setting should be conservative, using the minimal threshold fluences necessary to produce the desired tissue effect in a given individual. Test spots should be performed whenever possible. In treating darker skin, it is always best to err on the side of caution rather than risk excessive thermal injury. All of this makes it more difficult to achieve the desired clinical result [56,57]. The absorption coefficient of melanin decreases exponentially as wavelengths increase [58]. Therefore, to produce a safer laser system, it needs to generate wavelengths that are less efficiently absorbed by endogenous melanin but can still achieve the desired results [59].

Cutaneous laser resurfacing can be an effective approach for improving the appearance of atrophic scarring in patients with darker skin phototypes. Several reports document the long-term safety of the high-energy, pulsed, and scanned CO_2, and short- and long-pulsed Er:YAG lasers for the treatment of more darkly pigmented patients [60]. Fractionated lasers are preferred over traditional non-fractionated lasers in patients with darker-skin phototypes because the remaining intact epidermis allows a faster recovery time and minimizes side effects [33].

Skin resurfacing with the CO_2 laser remains the gold-standard technology for production of the most dramatic clinical and histologic improvement in scarred facial skin. Use of the CO_2 laser for skin resurfacing yields an additional benefit of collagen tightening through heating of dermal collagen. To minimize the risk of adverse events, it is best to avoid overlapping or stacking of laser scans or pulses. If patients have scarring on their neck or chest, it is best to avoid resurfacing in these areas due to the scarcity of pilosebaceous units in these regions with resultant slow re-epithelialization and potential for scarring [60]. The wavelength of the CO_2 laser is 10,600 nm and the target chromophore is extracellular and intracellular water. Hyperpigmentation is observed in all skin phototypes following CO_2 laser irradiation, however, at a higher incidence in darker skin tones [61].

The Er:YAG laser attempts to duplicate the results of the CO_2 laser while minimizing the side effects. The wavelength emitted is designed to be absorbed more efficiently and superficially, and the short pulses limit the amount on thermal necrosis. Thus, the Er:YAG is able to provide shorter recovery times, reduced post-treatment erythema, and a decreased risk of dyspigmentation [62,63]. The most common side effect post-laser skin resurfacing is transient hyperpigmentation and it affects approximately one third of all patients. It is important to note that the incidence rises to 68%–100% among patients with the darkest skin phototypes [64].

A study from Korea was performed in exclusively dark-skinned patients (Fitzpatrick skin phototypes III–V) to evaluate the clinical and histologic effects of long-pulsed Er:YAG laser resurfacing for pitted facial acne scars. In this study, 35 patients with pitted facial acne scars were treated with a long-pulsed Er:YAG. The results of long-pulsed Er:YAG laser resurfacing for pitted facial acne scars were excellent in ten patients (36%), good in 16 patients (57%), and fair in two patients (7%). Erythema occurred in all patients after laser treatment and lasted longer than 3 months in 15 patients (54%). PIH occurred in eight patients (29%). However, the pigmentation faded or disappeared within 3 months. No scarring, infection or contact dermatitis was observed. This study showed that resurfacing with a long-pulsed Er:YAG laser can be safe and effective treatment for pitted facial acne scars in moderately dark skin phototypes III–V [65]. Since there are no data on patients of African descent with this laser treatment, more studies are warranted before it can be considered a viable option for a dark-complexioned patients.

Of particular importance is strict avoidance of excessive sun exposure and the use of a full-spectrum sunblock consistently before and after laser treatment [66]. Some pre-surgical topical treatments may enhance the eventual post-operative results by decreasing the risk of PIH. There are conflicting opinions regarding pre-treatment with hydroquinone, tretinoin or glycolic acid to decrease the incidence of hyperpigmentation after ablative laser resurfacing in any skin phototype [67]. However, topical tretinoin, hydroquinone, and mild topical steroids are thought to be important post-laser procedure, especially in patients with darker skin [65]. Retinoic acid topically appears to speed re-epithelialization rates, and it can reduce rates of melanin production after the initial stage of healing is completed and the skin can tolerate the retinoic acid [68]. Critical in darker-skinned patients, even if retinoic acid does not decrease the actual incidence of post-treatment PIH, it may reduce its severity and duration.

Another approach is the newer non-ablative laser technology that may provide both greater efficacy and safety in patients with darker skin. They have a lower risk of pigmentary alterations when compared with ablative technologies adding to their appeal for use in darker skin types. These modalities are less aggressive, side effects are minimized (PIH, downtime) but it is not as effective as ablative devices and requires more treatments [64]. Typically, patients will receive several treatments monthly. These treatments create a controlled thermal injury in the dermis, leading to inflammation, cytokine upregulation, and fibroblast proliferation for improvement of scars.

Fractional photothermolysis, a more current concept was first introduced and discussed in 2004 [69]. It is one of the latest technologies introduced for laser skin resurfacing and treatment of atrophic scars without a significant risk of side effects [64]. It creates minute columns of thermal injury in the dermis called microscopic treatment zones (MTZ) that contain areas of localized epidermal necrosis and collagen denaturation. Rapid healing occurs from the viable epidermal and dermal cells residing in the intact tissue surrounding each MTZ. Since there is selective sparing of skin rather than total ablation, there tend to be fewer problems overall when compared with the CO_2 laser [70].

A study of 53 patients (Fitzpatrick I–V) using a 1550-nm erbium-doped fractional laser on facial skin with mild-to-moderate atrophic acne were treated with several sessions. Blinded assessments of photographs revealed 91% to have 25%–50% improvement after a single treatment, whereas 87% of patients undergoing three treatments had 51%–75% improvement. Age, sex, and skin type (I–V) did not alter the outcome with maintained results at 6-month follow-up [71].

Alajlan and Alsuwaidan published a retrospective study in South Arabia in year 2011, in which they compared 45 patients treated with non-ablative fractional (NAF) erbium fiber 1550 nm versus 37 patients treated with ablasive fractional (AF) CO_2 laser for atrophic acne scars. All patients had a Fitzpatrick skin phototype between III and V, treatment with NAF was performed monthly (mean number of treatments: five) and with AF every 2 months (mean number of treatments: 2.5), a hydroquinone-based bleaching cream was started at the middle of the treatment. Usually, patients with deeper scars were more likely found to be treated with AF rather than NAF. Evaluators compared photographic improvement, patient satisfaction, and adverse effects. The grade of improvement and patient satisfaction score were similar in both groups, hydroquinone cream significantly decreased the magnitude of PIH, and only one patient with AF treatment had transient PIH, which resolved within 3 months [72]. Again, with no data in skin of patients of African descent, this is not recommended for scar treatment in this population (Figure 15.8).

Unique Acne Considerations in Pigmented Skin

Nodulocystic acne appears to be less common in people of African descent than in Caucasians and Hispanics. This has been reported in various surveys [1,12,73]. Studies have also found that isotretinoin is prescribed less often for African Americans than for Caucasians [74]. There were 35 million visits to physicians for the treatment of acne between 1990 and 1997, and isotretinoin was prescribed at 5.8 million (17%) of these visits. Per capita visit rates for acne among Whites were 2.3 times that of Blacks, and Whites were 1.8 times more likely to receive isotretinoin at acne visits [75].

Nodulocystic acne has implications for the patient as it is more likely to lead to scarring. A systemic retinoid such as isotretinoin is the treatment of choice for nodulocystic acne in patients with ethnic skin [6]. Still, studies have shown that there is a relatively low usage of isotretinoin among patients of color [74]. Early treatment with isotretinoin in patients of color with moderate or mild acne may be justified in some cases as a way to subvert development of PIH and keloidal scarring [76]. Skin dryness, a common side effect of isotretinoin, is of particular importance to patients of color as it can result in PIH. Emollients and topical corticosteroids can be used to minimize this side effect [6].

As previously discussed, early and aggressive treatment of acne in patients with dark skin reduces the possibility of PIH and scarring. The objective is to perform this in a safe way, without irritating the patient's skin. There are some strategies that can be performed in patients with dark skin (Table 15.3).

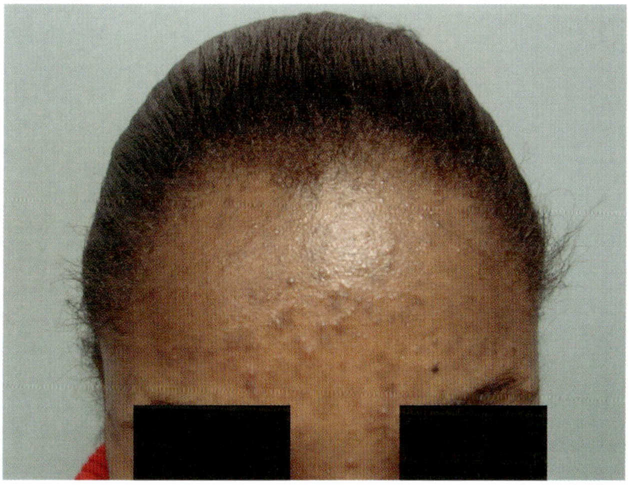

FIGURE 15.8 Pomade acne on forehead. Without addressing the habits that worsen active acne lesions, the efficacy of treating its consequences is reduced.

TABLE 15.3

Treatment Goals in Patients with Acne and Dark Skin

1.	Aggressively manage current acne signs and symptoms
2.	Minimize emergence of new acne lesions
3.	Reduce the risk of PIH and keloidal scarring
4.	Maximize tolerability
5.	Manage patient expectations regarding time-to-treatment benefits
6.	Identify and avoid cosmetic practices related to acne (pomade acne)

Summary

In treating acne scarring in patients of African descent, prevention of the acne is key. While the deeper pigmentation plays a large role in the PIH observed in this population, all the factors that contribute to scarring in patients of African descent are not known, but are likely further reaching than simple pigmentation. These patients are at increased risk for PIH, atrophic scarring, hypertrophic scarring and keloids.

Treatment of PIH and true scars resulting from acne must reflect several considerations by the physician: cost, severity of lesions, physician goals, patient expectations, side-effect profiles, and psychological or emotional effect to the patient. Side-effect profiles must be carefully weighed against benefits, particularly in darker-skinned individuals who may be more prone to adverse reactions to common treatments for acne scarring. Close follow-up, an emphasis on compliance and counseling regarding the use of noncomedogenic and nonirritating skin and hair care products will aid in yielding better outcomes.

Most importantly, the physician and the patient must agree on realistic treatment goals. As acne scarring is one of the most difficult conditions to treat, especially in darker-skinned individuals, often the goal is improvement, not perfection of acne scarring.

REFERENCES

1. Centers for Disease Control and Prevention. National Center for Health Statistics. National ambulatory medical care survey. http://www.cdc.gov/nchs/about/major/ahcd/ Plnamcsdes.htm (Accessed June 25, 2018).
2. Jacob CI, Dover JS, Kaminer MS. Acne scarring: A classification system and review of treatment options. *J Am Acad Derma*. 2001;45:109–17.
3. Pochi PE. The pathogenesis and treatment of acne. *Annu Rev Med*. 1990;41:187–98.
4. Koo J. The psychosocial impact of acne: Patients' perceptions. *J Am Acad Dermatol*. 1995;32(Suppl): S26–30.
5. Rivera A. Acne scarring: A review and current treatment modalities. *J Am Acad Dermatol*. 2008;59(4):659–76.
6. Callender, VD. Considerations for treating acne in ethnic skin. *Cutis*. 2005;76(2 Suppl):19–23.
7. Alexis AF, Sergay AB. Taylor SC. Common dermatologic disorders in skin of color: A comparative practice survey. *Cutis*. 2007;80(5):387–94.
8. Taylor SC. Epidemiology of skin disease in ethnic populations. *Dermatol Clin*. 2003;21:601–7.
9. Perkins AC, Cheng CE, Hillebrand GG et al. Comparison of the epidemiology of acne vulgaris among Caucasian, Asian, Continental Indian and African American women. *J Eur Acad Dermatol Venereol*. 2011;25(9):1054–60.
10. Callender VD, Alexis AF, Daniels SR. Racial differences in clinical characteristics, perceptions and behaviors, and psychosocial impact of adult female acne. *J Clin Aesthet Dermatol*. 2014;7(7):19–31.
11. Halder RM, Grimes PE, McLaurin CI, Kress MA, Kenney JA. Incidence of common dermatoses in a predominantly black dermatologic practice. *Cutis*. 1983;32:388–90.
12. Taylor SC, Cook-Bolden F, Rahman Z, Strachan D. Acne vulgaris in skin of color. *J Am Acad Dermatol*. 2002;46(Suppl):S98–106.
13. McMichael AJ. Diagnosis and treatment of acne vulgaris. *Monthly Prescribing Reference*. 2004 ed.

14. Shaffer JJ, Taylor SC, Cook-Bolden F. Keloidal scars: A review with a critical look at therapeutic options. *J Am Acad Dermatol.* 2002:46(Suppl):S63–S97.
15. Shah SK, Alexis AF. Acne in skin of color: Practical approaches to treatment. *J Dermatolog Treat.* 2010;21(3):206–11.
16. Brody HJ, Monheit GD, Resnik SS, Alt TH. A history of chemical peeling. *Dermatol Surg.* 2001;26(5):405–9.
17. Brody HJ. Variations and comparisons in medium-depth chemical peeling. *J Dermatol Surg Oncol.* 1989;15:953–63.
18. Kwon HH, Park HY, Choi SC, Bae Y, Kang C, Jung JY, Park GH. Combined fractional treatment of acne scars involving non-ablative 1,550-nm erbium-glass laser and micro-needling radiofrequency: A 16-week prospective, randomized split-face study. *Acta Derm Venereol.* 2017;97(8):947–51.
19. West TB. Laser resurfacing of atrophic scars. *Dermatol Clin.* 1997;15(3):449–57.
20. Sawcer D, Lee HR, Lowe NJ. Lasers and adjunctive treatments for facial scars: A review. *J Cutan Laser Ther.* 1999;1(2):77–85.
21. Chang MW. Disorders of hyperpigmentation. In: *Dermatology.* Bolognia JL, Jorizzo JL, Rapini RP, eds. New York: Mosby, 2008, 947.
22. Halder RM, Holmes YC, Bridgeman-Shah S et al. A clinical pathological study of acne vulgaris in black females. *J Invest Dermatol.* 1996;106:888.
23. Taylor SC. Skin of color: Biology, structure, function, and implications for dermatologic disease. *J Am Acad Dermatol.* 2002;46(Suppl):S41–62.
24. Poli F. Acne on pigmented skin. *Int J of Dermatol.* 2007;46(Suppl 1):39–41.
25. Jacyk WK, Mpofu P. Adapalene gel 0.1% for topical treatment of acne vulgaris in African patients. *Cutis.* 2001;68(Suppl 4):48–54.
26. Bulengo-Ransby SM, Griffiths CE, Kimbrough-Green CK et al. Topical tretinoin (retinoic acid) therapy for hyperpigmented lesions caused by inflammation of the skin in black patients. *N Engl J Med.* 1993;328:1438–43.
27. Grimes P, Callender VD. Tazarotene cream for postinflammatory hyperpigmentation and acne vulgaris in darker skin: A double-blind, randomized, vehicle–controlled study. *Cutis.* 2006;77(1):45–50.
28. Halder RM, Richards GM. Topical agents used in the management of hyperpigmentation. *Skin Therapy Lett.* 2004;9(6):1–3.
29. Draelos ZD. Skin lightening preparations and the hydroquinone controversy. *Dermatol Ther.* 2007;20(5):308–13.
30. Handog EB, Datuin MS, Singzon IA. Chemical peels for acne and acne scars in asians: Evidence based review. *J Cutan Aesthet Surg.* 2012;5(4):239–46.
31. Garg VK, Sinha S, Sarkar R. Glycolic acid peels versus salicylic-mandelic acid peels in active acne vulgaris and post-acne scarring and hyperpigmentation: A comparative study. *Dermatol Surg.* 2009;35(1):59–65.
32. Roberts WE. Chemical peeling in ethnic/dark skin. *Dermatol Ther.* 2004;17(2):196–205.
33. Sobanko JF, Alster TS. Management of acne scarring, part I: A comparative review of laser surgical approaches. *Am J Clin Dermatol.* 2012;13(5):319–30.
34. Fabbrocini G, Annunziata MC, D'Arco V et al. Acne scars: Pathogenesis, classification and treatment. *Dermatol Res Pract.* 2010;2010:893080.
35. Ud-Din S, Bayat A. New insights on keloids, hypertrophic scars, and striae. *Dermatol Clin.* 2014;32(2):193–209.
36. Tuan TL, Nichter LS. The molecular basis of keloid and hypertrophic scar formation. *Mol Med Today.* 1998;4:19–24.
37. Jacob CI, Dover JS, Kaminer MS. Acne scarring: A classification system and review of treatment options. *J Am Acad Dermatol.* 2001;45(1):109–17.
38. Fulton JE. Dermabrasion, chemabrasion and laser abrasion. *Dermatol Surg.* 1996;22:619–28.
39. Kadunc BV, Trindale de Albeida AR. Surgical treatment of facial acne scars based on the morphologic classification: A Brazilian experience. *Dermatol Surg.* 2003;29:1200–9.
40. Gold MH, Berman B, Clementoni MT et al. Updated international clinical recommendations on scar management: Part 1 – Evaluating the evidence. *Dermatol Surg.* 2014;40(8):817–24.
41. Jalali M, Bayat A. Current use of steroids in management of abnormal raised skin scars. *Surgeon.* 2007;5:175–80.

42. Asilian A, Darougheh A, Shariati F. New combination of triamcinolone, 5-fluorouracil, and pulsed-dye laser for treatment of keloid and hypertrophic scars. *Dermatol Surg.* 2006;32:907–15.
43. Davison SP, Dayan JH, Clemens MW et al. Efficacy of intralesional 5-fluorouracil and triamcinolone in the treatment of keloids. *Aesthet Surg J.* 2009;29:40–6.
44. Darougheh A, Asilian A, Shariati F. Intralesional triamcinolone alone or in combination with 5-fluorouracil for the treatment of keloid and hypertrophic scars. *Clin Exp Dermatol.* 2009;34:219–23.
45. Phillips TJ, Gerstein AD, Lordan V. A randomized controlled trial of hydrocolloid dressing in the treatment of hypertrophic scars and keloids. *Dermatol Surg.* 1996;22:775–8.
46. Shah S, Alster TS. Laser treatment of dark skin: An updated review. *Am J Clin Dermatol.* 2010;11(6):389–97.
47. Alster TS, Zaulyanov-Scanlon L. Laser scar revision: A review. *Dermatol Surg.* 2007;33:131–40.
48. Lee JB, Chung WG, Kwahck H et al. Focal treatment of acne scars with trichloroacetic acid: Chemical reconstruction of skin scars method. *Dermatol Surg.* 2002;28(11):1017–21.
49. Khunger N, Bhardwaj D, Khunger M. Evaluation of CROSS technique with 100% TCA in the management of ice pick acne scars in darker skin types. *J Cosmet Dermatol.* 2011;10(1):51–7.
50. Levy LL, Zeichner JA. Management of acne scarring, part II: A comparative review of non-laser-based, minimally invasive approaches. *Am J Clin Dermatol.* 2012;13(5):331–40.
51. Cohen BE, Elbuluk N. Microneedling in skin of color: A review of uses and efficacy. *J Am Acad Dermatol.* 2016;74(2):348–55.
52. Fabbrocini G, De Vita V, Monfrecola A et al. Percutaneous collagen induction: An effective and safe treatment for post-acne scarring in different skin phototypes. *J Dermatolog Treat.* 2014;25(2):147–52.
53. Sharad J. Combination of microneedling and glycolic acid peels for the treatment of acne scars in dark skin. *J Cosmet Dermatol.* 2011;10(4):317–23.
54. Klein AW. Skin filling: Collagen and other injectables of the skin. *Dermatol Clin.* 2001;19:491–508.
55. Odunze M, Cohn A, Few JW. Restylane in people of color. *Plast Reconstr Surg.* 2007;120(7):2011–6.
56. Alster TS, Tanzi EL. Laser surgery in dark skin. *Skin Med.* 2003;2:80–5.
57. Tanzi EL, Alster TS. Cutaneous laser surgery in darker skin phototypes. *Cutis.* 2004;73:21–30.
58. Ho C, Nguyen Q, Lowe NJ et al. Laser resurfacing in pigmented skin. *Dermatol Surg.* 1995;21:1035–7.
59. Tanzi EL, Lupton JR, Alster TS. Review of lasers in dermatology: Four decades of progress. *J Am Acad Dermatol.* 2003;49:1–31.
60. Alster TS, Lupton JR. Prevention and treatment of side effects and complications of cutaneous laser resurfacing. *Plast Reconstr Surg.* 2002;109:308–16.
61. Walia S, Alster TS. Prolonged clinical and histological effects from CO_2 laser resurfacing of atrophic acne scars. *Dermatol Surg.* 1999;25:926–30.
62. Tanzi EL, Alster TS. Side effects and complications of variable pulsed erbium:YAG laser skin resurfacing: Extended experience with 50 patients. *Plast Reconstr Surg.* 2003;111:1524–9.
63. Tanzi EL, Alster TS. Single-pass carbon dioxide versus multiple pass Er:YAG laser skin resurfacing: A comparison of postoperative wound healing and side effect rates. *Dermatol Surg.* 2003;29:80–4.
64. Bhatt N, Alster TS. Laser surgery in dark skin. *Dermatol Surg.* 2008;34:184–95.
65. Jeong JT, Kye YC. Resurfacing of pitted facial acne scars with a long-pulsed Er:YAG laser. *Dermatol Surg.* 2001;27(2):107–10.
66. Alster TS. Preoperative patient considerations. In: *Manual of Cutaneous Laser Techniques.* 2nd ed. Alster TS. eds. Philadelphia: Lippincott Williams & Wilkins, 2000, 13–32.
67. West TB, Alster TS. Effect of pretreatment on the incidence of hyperpigmentation following cutaneous CO_2 laser resurfacing. *Dermatol Surg.* 1999;25:15–7.
68. McDonald WS, Beasly D, Jones C. Retinoic acid and CO_2 laser resurfacing. *Plast Reconstr Surg.* 1999;7:2229–35.
69. Manstein D, Herron GS, Sink RK, Tanner H, Anderson RR. Fractional photothermolysis: A new concept for cutaneous remodeling using microscopic patterns of thermal injury. *Lasers Surg Med.* 2004;34:426–38.
70. Hasegawa T, Matsukura T, Mizuno Y et al. Clinical trial of a laser device called fractional thermolysis system for acne scars. *J Dermatol.* 2006;33:623–7.
71. Alster TS, Tanzi EL, Lazarus M. The use of fractional laser phothermolysis for the treatment of atrophic scars. *Dermatol Surg.* 2007;33:295–9.
72. Alajlan AM, Alsuwaidan SN. Acne scars in ethnic skin treated with both non-ablative fractional 1,550 nm and ablative fractional CO_2 lasers: Comparative retrospective analysis with recommended guidelines. *Lasers Surg Med.* 2011;43(8):787–91.

73. Wilkins JW, Voorhees JJ. Prevalence of nodulocystic acne in white and Negro males. *Arch Dermatol.* 1970;102:631–4.
74. Kelly AP, Sampson DD. Recalcitrant nodulocystic acne in black Americans: Treatment with isotretinoin. *J Nat Med Assoc.* 1987;79:1266–70.
75. Fleischer AB Jr, Simpson JK, McMichael A, Feldman SR. Are there racial and sex differences in the use of oral isotretinoin for acne management in the United States? *J Am Acad Dermatol.* 2003;49(4):662–6.
76. Perez A, Sanchez JL. Treatment of acne vulgaris in skin of color. *Cosmetic Derm.* 2003;16:23–8.

16

Treatment Algorithm for Acne Scars

Daniele Innocenzi*, Ilaria Proietti, Concetta Potenza, Patrick M. Zito, and Kenneth R. Beer

KEY FEATURES

- Scarring that results from acne is a very distressing and difficult problem for physician and patient alike. The type of scarring following acne eruptions is also variable and each type requires a different treatment strategy. The most common permanent findings are diffuse, depressed scars. Other forms of irregularities include hypo- or hyper-pigmentation, hypertrophy, keloids, and cutaneous fistula. In order to treat the patient with scarring, a true knowledge of the pathophysiology and anatomy of the different types of scars should be sought. Although this classic pathophysiology is shared, the subsequent evolution of the acne lesion and the degree of inflammation at clinical presentation may vary among individuals according to all skin phototypes. The morphology of each scar must be assessed and treatment designed accordingly.
- Therapy needs to reflect patient characteristics such as age, gender, pubertal status, lifestyle, motivation, and coexisting conditions. Acne scars may have a negative psychological impact on social life and relationship.
- Recently, newer techniques and modifications to older ones may make this refractory problem more manageable. Options and treatment algorithms for dealing with post-scar scarring are explored and a systematic review of literature is performed. The advent of fractionated lasers is one of the most important tools for treating acne. Depending on whether or not the scars cover a large percentage of the face or just a few areas, treatments can be calibrated to fit each scenario.
- The wide variety of new treatment methods for post-acne scarring includes the advent of tissue undermining, newer resurfacing tools, and possibly some future surgical and laser techniques. There are multiple medical and surgical devices useful in acne scar treatments. Many of these techniques may be performed in a single treatment session, but multiple treatments are often necessary.

Introduction

Scarring occurs in all types of acne, not linked tonodulocystic disease, but does vary with the severity and delay until effective treatment is organized. Some degree of post-acne scarring is an outcome in 95% of patients with acne [1,2].

Acne scars can be particularly devastating and may even trigger suicidal ideation [3]. Interventions are needed to limit the course of disease, and thereby, its long-lasting fallout of both physical and emotional scars. Aggressive treatment of acne that is prone to scarring occasionally prevents this outcome [3–5]. Once scarring has occurred, patients and physicians are left to struggle with the options available for improving the appearance of the skin.

* Deceased

Treating acne scars, according to Fulton, "is perhaps the most difficult cosmetic surgery procedure that exists" [6]. It is really challenging to achieve total correction of tissue destruction caused by severe inflammatory acne, which can destroy the epidermis, dermis and the underlying fat. The main treatment goal is to obtain as much improvement as possible rather than perfection.

Diffusion Treatments

Acne vulgaris is a common disorder in people of all ethnic skin types. This ubiquitous disease of early and midlife occurs across the range of skin phototypes, from pale-white to dark-brown or black (in 95%–100% of 16- to 17-year-old boys and 83%–85% of 16- to 17-year-old girls) [7].

Acne has been shown to persist into adult life and a recent study of adults over 25 years of age revealed at least mild disease in 3% of men and 12% of women [8]. In recent years, the literature has begun to acknowledge that race and ethnicity are also parameters that need to be considered in acne management. The current (very limited) evidence base indicates that there are probably no fundamental differences in acne epidemiology, pathophysiology (except for so called pomade acne in African-American patients) [9], or basic treatment options across the spectrum of skin types. However, given the prevailing racial and ethnic disparities in access to healthcare [10], such survey results must be interpreted cautiously. Several key differences related to acne sequelae do stand out—especially the elevated risk of hyperpigmentation and keloids formation in those with darker skin [11,12]. Clinicians need to be aware of these differences because they may require additions to the "standard" treatment algorithms to accommodate patients with darker skin. As the US population of individuals with dark skin continues to increase (e.g., the proportion of the US population that is White, non-Hispanic, is projected to decline steadily from 70% in 2003 to 50% in 2060) [13], these issues will soon spread beyond the domain of dermatologists specializing in ethnic skin to all dermatologists and primary care practitioners.

For most patients, acne remains a nuisance with occasional flares of unsightly comedones, pustules and nodules. For other less fortunate persons, the severe inflammatory response to *Propionibacterium acnes* results in permanent disfiguring scars. Acne scarring was recorded in 14% of women and 11% of men [14].

History

As far back as 1905, surgical methods have been used to improve the skin that has been scarred by facial acne [15]. The work of the dermatologist Kromayer at the beginning of the twentieth century [16,17] was instrumental in the development of dermabrasion, once the main treatment modality for skin resurfacing [18]. Advances in equipment, techniques, and anesthesia have steadily occurred over the last three decades with wire brushes, diamond-embedded fraises, and serrated wheels being utilized [19,20]. In 1941, Eller and Wolff [21] first performed phenol peelings. Mechanisms used to resurface the epidermis and tighten the dermal collagen have included laser skin resurfacing carbon dioxide (CO_2) [22,23] and erbium:yttrium–aluminum garnet (Er:YAG) [24] lasers or their combination [25]. Removal or leveling (or both) of individual scars has been achieved via excision, punch excision, punch elevation, dermal grafting, punch grafting, and subcision [26,27].

Multiple other methods have been added to ablative techniques, including injections of collagen [28], silicone [29] or fat, facelifts [30], and needling [31,32].

Newer permanent injections such as methylmethacrylate are also helpful in correcting acne scars. Collagen stimulators such as poly-L-lactic acid have been used on a limited basis to treat acne scars [33].

Different authors have also tried to facilitate acne scar treatment by suggesting schematic diagrams that correlate scars morphology and treatment [34,35], whereas others have used sequential therapeutic plans in treating theses scars.

Several excellent reviews of these scar revision modalities have been published [36–40]. However, according to the literature, the results of isolated ablative techniques are extremely variable, presenting effectiveness of outcomes that ranges from 25 to 81.4% [41].

Structure and Function and Developments in Pathophysiology

The first element in the evolution of an acne scar is evolution of acne itself. Acne vulgaris most commonly begins with a non-inflammatory comedone of the pilosebaceous unit. In the lower part of the follicular wall, the horny cells become stickier, causing impaction of these horny cells and dilatation of the sebaceous follicle [42].

Furthermore, in comedonic skin condition *Propionibacterium acnes* flourishes and triggers production of the inflammatory stage of acne.

In uncomplicated cases, the comedone spontaneously uncaps to release the contained sebum and keratinous debris and may go on to develop into an inflamed acne lesion such as a papule, pustule, nodule or cyst from, which likely leads to scarring (Figure 16.1). A perifollicular abscess is due to ruptures through the weakened infrainfundibular section of the follicle. If the abscess rapidly encapsulates and communicates with the cornified layer, full release is still possible in 7–10 days with no sequelae [43,44].

Scarring results when this process is incomplete or delayed. Failure to encapsulate results in further inflammatory progression and rupture. With this follicular explosion, hairs, lipids, keratin, free fatty acids and released *Propionibacterium acnes* activate both classic and alternative complement pathways, amplifying the inflammation [45] in the dermis and leading to irritation in their new environment [46]. Thus, grouped open comedones or multichanneled fistulous tracts with interconnected keratinized tunnels may appear [46]. Prolonged inflammation of the follicular unit also promotes hyperplastic epithelialization, which is reflected clinically as ice pick scars [47].

Other scars owe their appearance to the extent and the depth of the inflammation or perifollicular abscess formation that may directionally extend away from the cutaneous surface. If the dermal inflammation is severe and left untreated, sloughing is significant with total necrosis of the follicle, leading to severe dermal scarring as its sequela. Additional involvement of adjacent structures in the subcutis shows inflammatory migration along sweat glands and destruction of subcutaneous fat. When such deep inflammation occurs and transdermal abscess expulsion is not accomplished, nodules and cysts occur [47].

Ongoing deep infection and inflammatory modulation of the pilosebaceous units often result in scarring that is either atrophic (Figure 16.2) or hyperplastic (hypertrophic or keloidal) [48] (Figures 16.3 and 16.4). As the scars mature, along with myoepithelial contraction caused by wound healing, they draw in the

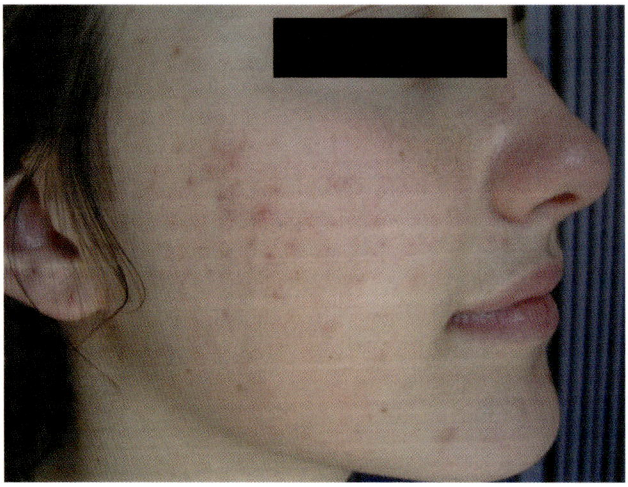

FIGURE 16.1 Grade I post-acne scarring. A patient whose acne is coming under control with erythematous lesions treatment.

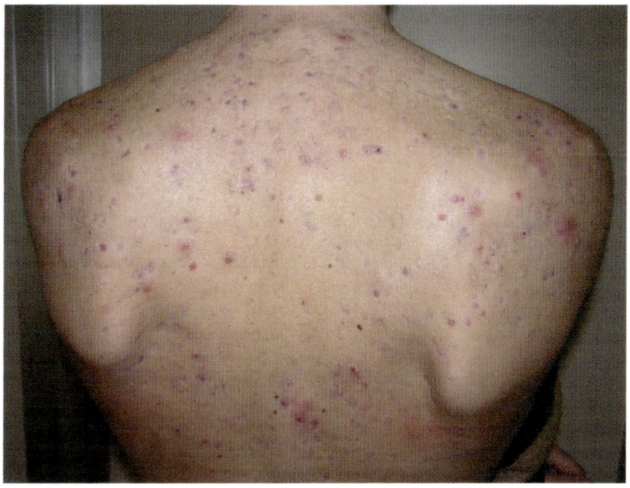

FIGURE 16.2 Inflammatory lesions and atrophic scars co-exist in the same patient.

surface layers and cause atrophy, depressed craters or indention. Much less commonly, acne scarring may become thickened (hypertrophic or keloidal) rather than atrophic. Certain individual characteristics seem to predispose patients to this type of acne scarring. These include family history, being between the ages of 10 and 30 years, and severity and site of the inflammation. Keloid formation is also more common following acne in African-American, Hispanic and Asian patients compared with White patients. These keloidal overgrowths of scar tissue are seen five to 16 times more frequently in patients with skin of color [2].

If the acneiform activity is limited to the epidermis and superficial dermis, the disconcerting appearance may be only dyschromatic. It is common to observe immature processes as erythematous macules, especially within the first year of their onset. The return to normal pigmentation is often more prolonged in these lesions than other cutaneous trauma. Chronic macular inflammation may lead to permanent hypopigmentation or hyperpigmentation (especially seen in Fitzpatrick IV to VI skin types) [2].

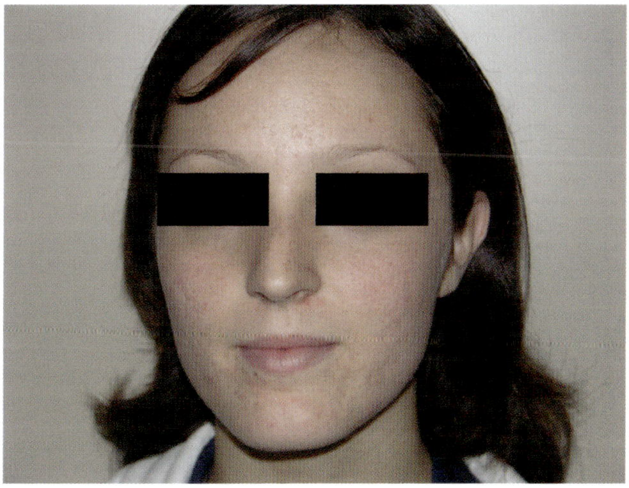

FIGURE 16.3 Grade II post-acne scarring.

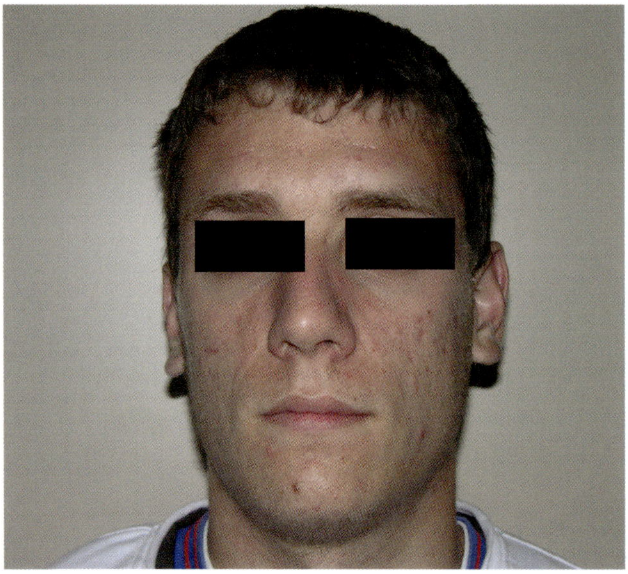

FIGURE 16.4 Grade III post-acne scarring.

Treatment

Therapeutic intervention for post-acne scarring has historically been limited by the considerable morbidity of most treatments for only marginal disease improvement [49].

Within the past decade, a requirement for developing successful treatments for post-acne scarring is a greater understanding of its pathogenesis and variability of inflammatory mediators among afflicted individuals [49].

New techniques have been added and older ones modified in attempts to improve risk–benefit profiles and less recuperation. One should assess both the overall appearance and the morphology of each scar and adjust the treatment accordingly. In literature authors have been using their own acne scar denominations. There are a lot of methods that encompass the majority of acne scar types and correlate the lesions and the specific techniques used to repair them [50,51].

To perform a treatment algorithm for dealing with post-acne scarring we use the qualitative grading system of Goodman and Baron (Tables 16.1–16.3), which, in our opinion, is used as a template for describing the most suitable techniques to improve burden of disease of patients.

TABLE 16.1

Grades of Post-Acne Scarring

Grade and Level	Characteristics
I. Macular	Erythematous, hyper- or hypo-pigmented flat marks visible to patient or observer at any distance
II. Mild	Mild atrophy or hypertrophy that may not be obvious at social distances of 50 cm or greater and may be covered adequately by makeup or the normal shadow of shaved beard hair in men or normal body hair if extrafacial
III. Moderate	Moderate atrophic or hypertrophic scarring that is obvious at social distances of 50 cm or greater and is not covered easily by makeup or the normal shadow of shaved beard hair in men or body hair if extrafacial, but is still able to be flattened by manual stretching of the skin (if atrophic)
IV. Severe	Severe atrophic or hypertrophic scarring that is obvious at social distances greater than 50 cm and is not easily covered by makeup or the normal shadow of shaved beard hair in men or body hair if extrafacial and is not able to be flattened by manual stretching of the skin

TABLE 16.2

Global Acne Scarring Classification: Types of Scars Making up the Classification Grades

Grade and Level	Examples of Scars
I. Macular	Erythematous, hyper- or hypo-pigmented flat marks
II. Mild	Mild rolling, small soft papular
III. Moderate	More significant rolling, shallow boxcar, mild-to-moderate hypertrophic or papular scars
IV. Severe	Punched-out atrophic (deep boxcar), ice pick, bridges and tunnels, marked atrophy, dystrophic significant hypertrophy or keloid

TABLE 16.3

Global Acne Scarring Classification and Likely Treatment Options

Grade and Level	Examples of Scars
I. Macular	Time, optimized home skin care, light-strength peels, microdermabrasion, vascular or pigmented lasers, or IPL
II. Mild	Non-ablative lasers, blood transfer, skin needling or rolling, microdermabrasion, dermal fillers
III. Moderate	Ablative lasers, dermabrasion, medical skin rolling, fractionated resurfacing, dermal fillers if focal, subcision and blood transfer. Intralesional corticosteroids steroids or fluorouracil and/or vascular laser if hypertrophic
IV. Severe	Punch techniques (float, excision grafting), focal trichloroacetic acid (CROSS technique) with or without resurfacing techniques (including fractionated resurfacing); fat transfer; occasionally rhytidectomy if grossly atrophic; intralesional corticosteroids steroids or fluorouracil and/or vascular laser if hypertrophic

Macular Acne Scarring and Marking (Grade-1 Acne Scarring)

The first grade of scarring is macular changes of color and not of contour. Scars are visible irrespective of distance and may be red, white or various shades of brown to black.

Erythematous Macules

Clinical Aspects

If the scarring process is relatively superficial, only the epidermis and superficial dermis are involved. The scars may result as macules that may be erythematous if inflamed and comparatively early or young scars (under 1 year) or with altered pigmentation [44] (Figure 16.5).

Often red macules improve over ensuing months spontaneously. Vascular laser therapy is useful for erythematous macules because red changes are quite well targeted by these light sources In theory, lasers may be useful for maturation of these scars more rapidly and useful for prevention of progression to scarring of inflamed healing acne lesions [52].

Patients affected by acne excoriée with erythematous macules can be treated with psychotherapy associated with lasers (e.g., neodymium-doped:YAG [Nd:YAG], Er:YAG, diode and intense pulsed light [IPL]) with success [66].

Hyperpigmented Macules

Clinical Aspects

Pigmentation of scars may be increased in more olive-skinned patients and represents mostly a post-inflammatory response that will fade in 3–18 months [53].

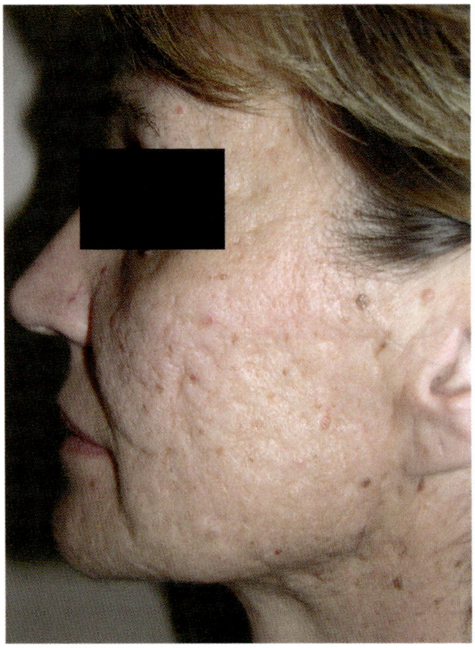

FIGURE 16.5 Grade IV post-acne scarring.

Treatment

These scars need strict sun protection to guard against aggravation of the hyperpigmentation, further reparative treatment is not usually required. If patients seek treatment, medical therapy with topical reparative creams such retinol (vitamin A), tretinoin (retinoic acid) or hydroxyl acids in conjunction with topical corticosteroids, hydroquinone, topical synthetic epidermal growth factor serum, kojic acid, and azelaic acid used in other examples of post-inflammatory pigmentation may be useful [53–55]. Alternatively, or additionally, low-strength skin peels with glycolic and retinoic acids and Jessner's solution or its variants may also be utilized effectively [56,57], although their efficacy in the treatment of post-inflammatory acne marking is not established.

Even if there is a risk of inducing post-inflammatory hyperpigmentation (PIH) with pigmented lesion lasers or light sources such as Nd:YAG, Q-switching or IPL, these devices occasionally may be useful for resistant cases [58].

Hyperpigmented Macules in Ethnic Skin

Clinical Aspects

PIH presents clinically as hyperpigmented macules that correspond to the area of inflammation [2]. These lesions can be diffuse or localized and they can occur with or without secondary excoriation. The discoloration persists for months to years—much longer than the acne lesions themselves. For many patients, the lingering PIH is more psychologically disturbing than the original or residual acne itself [2].

Treatment

In patients with darker skin, early aggressive therapy for inflammatory acne combined with careful consideration of the patient's risk of irritation will help clinicians to eliminate PIH. Clinicians can achieve this balance in patients with ethnic skin with judicious use and prescription of widely available products. In addition, use of prevention strategies (e.g., sunscreen), special depigmenting agents (e.g., hydroquinone)

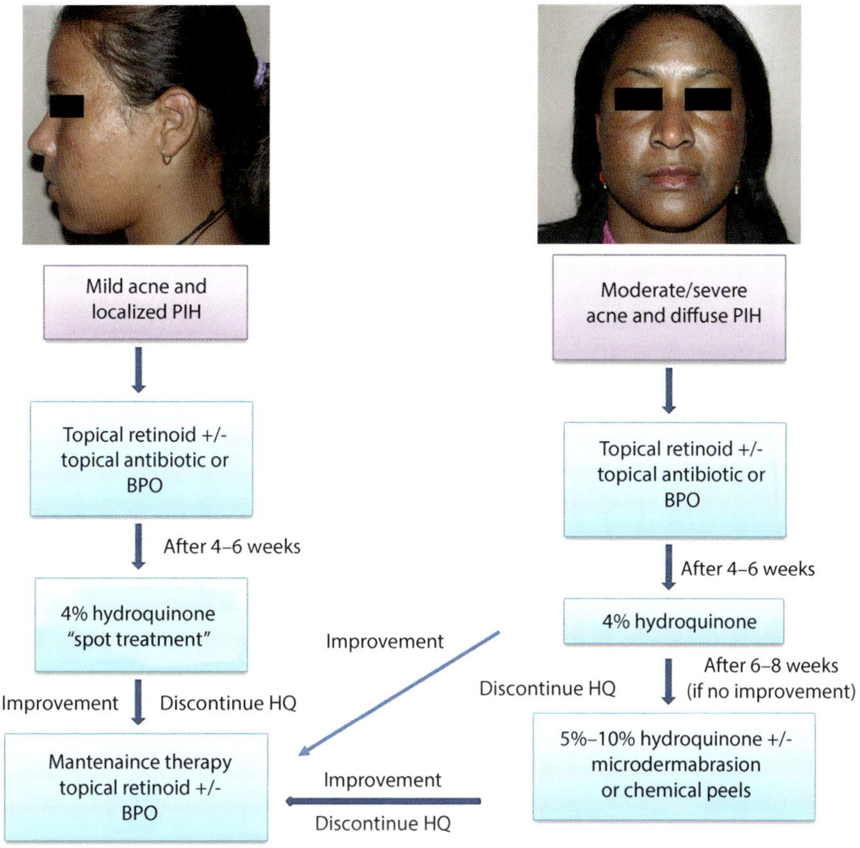

FIGURE 16.6 Treatment algorithm for acne and post-inflammatory hyperpigmentation. BPO, benzoyl peroxide; HQ, hydroquinone. (Adapted from Callender VD. Cutis. 2005;76(2 Suppl):19–23.)

and even adjunctive therapies (e.g., chemical peels or microdermabrasion) can be essential [59]. Following Callender we purpose the simplified algorithm in Figure 16.6 [60].

Hypopigmented Macules

Clinical Aspects

The white macules visible in the post-acne scarring may be true scars or post-inflammatory leukoderma.

Treatment

Treatment of these lesions are very difficult and it is often without significant outcomes. In literature there is the description of an 11-year-old White female patient who was successfully treated with manual dermabrasion for a hypochromic scar on the left forearm [61]. Reports of improvement of these lesions by needle dermabrasion utilizing a tattoo gun without pigment [62] and pigment transfer procedures have been attempted.

Hypopigmented macular scarring also called perifollicular scarring has been reasonably refractory to treatment.

Perifollicular acne inflammation may result in small hypopigmented macular scars from destruction of dermal components around the hair follicles and they are largely untreatable at the present time [63].

Minigrafting also utilized for treatment of vitiligo, holds some promise in the treatment of post-acne scarring [64]. The most known epidermal suspensions are cultured for 24 hours, but an automated commercial kit for trypsin dermal epidermal separation may improve the ease of the technique of minigrafting and allow immediately available, autologous, non-cultured epidermal suspension (Re-Cell, Clinical Cell Culture Americas, Coral Springs, FL, USA). This is now the most effective method [65].

Mild Atrophy (Grade 2 Acne Scarring)

Clinical Aspects

This grade of scarring includes those scars that may not be obvious at social distances of 50 cm or greater and may be covered adequately by makeup or the normal shadow of shaved beard hair in men or normal body hair if extrafacial (Figure 16.7).

This equates to a superficial type of atrophic scar or mild rolling scar. Mild rolling scars are usually wider than 4–5 mm and have abnormal fibrous anchoring of the dermis to the subcutis. Correction of the subdermal component is essential for treatment success [33].

Treatment of Patients with Few Scars

Tissue Augmentation

The group with few scars benefits from fairly simple treatments. The past decade has seen the advent of many non-autologous biologic and non-biologic tissue augmentation agents that may be used for atrophic scar contour correction. Achievement of safe, long-term or permanent correction using a tissue augmentation agent is a burgeoning area of interest [66].

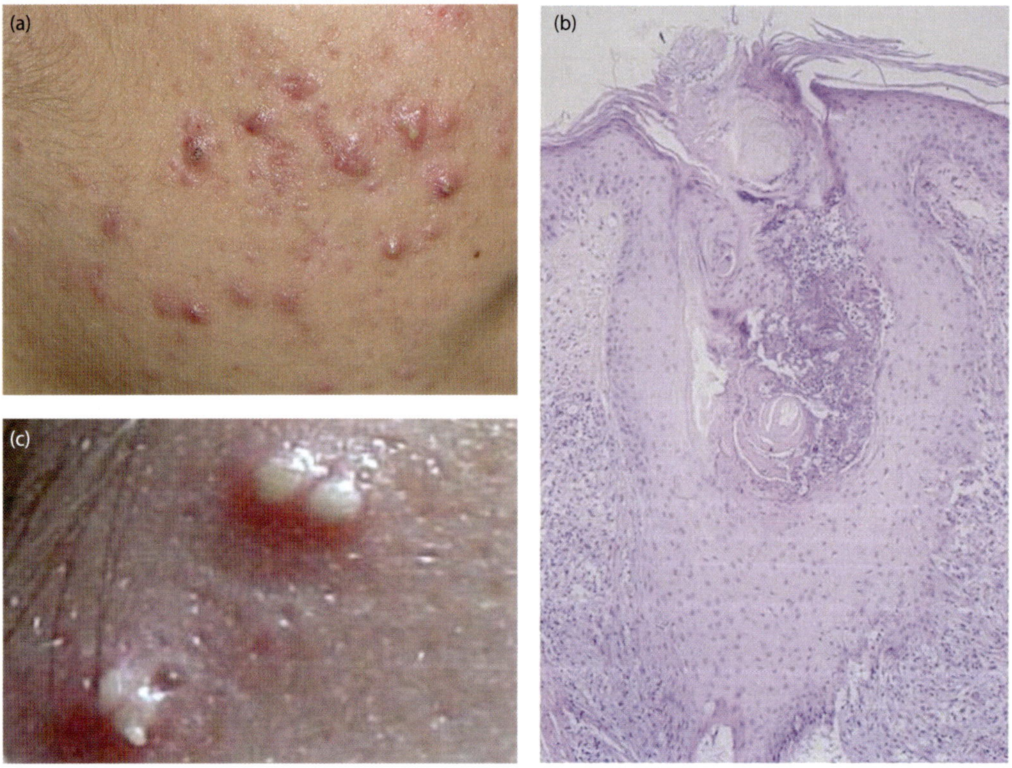

FIGURE 16.7 (a) Clinical and (b) histological features of inflamed acne lesions. I phase (6–24 hours) increase of neutrophilic cells into follicle (suppurative folliculitis) and of lymphocytes around pilosebaceus unit (perifolliculitis). (c) Grade 3 acne scarring.

The short-term correction agents that are in use include injectable fillers, including bovine collagen mixed with methylmethacrylate beads, polylactic acid and hyaluronic or agarose acid. Usually two or three treatment sessions are required for the best possible skin correction, which may need time in the range of 6 months to 1 or 2 years for correction to be attained.

Silicon variations of polyacrylamides and expanded polytetrafluoroethylene are agents used for longer correction [33]. They are not sufficiently accurate for improvement of mild scarring due to important local immunologic events.

However, all dermal augmentation agents may cause immunomediated adverse events or simply not be perfectly placed [33].

Goodman [67] described hematogenous transfer for tissue augmentation by the use of the patient's whole blood. This agent was investigated for its ability to present an exogenous chromophore that can be used by monochromatic laser or polychromatic light as a suitable target.

Blood is injected immediately after drawing by simple injection with a 1-mL syringe with attached 30-gauge needle high up in the dermis distending the scar giving a bleb with a bruised appearance. This treatment may be repeated at monthly intervals until adequate improvement is attained. Excessive fluence may be counterproductive because further collagen deposition may be induced by a low-level heat injury.

Treatment of Patients with Many Scars

Microdermabrasion

Dermabrasion was the first resurfacing technique that aided patients with this disorder. Over the last three decades we have observed advances in techniques, equipment and anesthesia and the exceeding of the manual dermabrasion.

New handpieces with 20,000–30,000 rpm have helped to control the depth of injury and reproducibility of treatment. Performed on frozen or tumesced facial skin, dermabrasion removes tissue to the level of the papillary dermis, or in significant scarring, the upper reticular dermis [68].

Microdermabrasion using aluminum oxide crystals has attracted some considerable attention for acne scarring [68]. Small crystals of aluminum oxide are fired against the skin from a nozzle housing a compression and aspiration system; this causes multiple small lacerations, and used crystals are aspirated back from the skin surface and discarded. Multiple treatments are required.

Before starting any resurfacing procedure, it is exceptionally important to discuss with the patient the possible outcomes, including nature of healing, postsurgical care, and potential complications. Specific inquiries about infectious conditions, prior herpetic outbreaks, keloid formation, bleeding diathesis and prior isotretinoin treatment are required [68].

Even if dermabrasion as a procedure is risk prone and may lead to scarring and dyschromia and results point to substantial variation in clinical outcomes, it is indeed a low-cost alternative to laser therapy and forms an integral part of the armamentarium of the practitioner involved in the treatment of acne scarring.

Skin Needling

Skin needling is an effective method for treating acne scars because it involves puncturing the skin multiple times with a small needle to induce collagen growth. Since 1995, Orentreich and Orentreich [26] have used this technique to achieve percutaneous collagen induction. Desmond Fernandes [31], simultaneously and independently, used skin needling to treat the upper lip by inserting a 15-gauge needle into the skin and then tunneling under the wrinkles in various directions. Scars were treated with a tattoo gun to "needle abrade" them. Although this technique could be used on many areas, it was laboriously slow and the holes in the epidermis were too close and too shallow. All these techniques worked because the needles break old collagen strands in the most superficial layer of the dermis that tether scars or wrinkles. It is presumed that this process promotes removal of damaged collagen growth and induces more collagen immediately under the epidermis.

A special new device covered with 30-gauge needles (Dermaroller) is now available. It may be rolled horizontally, vertically and diagonally, right and left, over the areas affected by acne scars. The microneedles penetrate through the epidermis and for about 1.5–2 mm into the dermis. The epidermis is only punctured and rapidly heals. After the treatment, the skin bleeds for a short time. When bleeding stops, the serous ooze formed may be removed from the surface of the skin using sterile saline solution. After each session of treatment, patients' facial skin appear reddened and swollen but redness and swelling disappear in 2–3 days. No side effect was described or found and every area of the face and the body may be treated [32,69].

With this technique the rolling is continued and done once a month until some bruising is noted.

The mechanism of action of the collagen induction therapy (CIT) is based on scientific facts that skin cells communicate by electrical signals. When the skin is microneedled, cells react to this intrusion by changing their internal electrical potential. This electrical charge in return stimulates skin cells to release chemical compositions, protein and growth factors. Proliferated skin cells, such as fibroblasts, migrate to the point of injury and transform into collagen fibers [69].

CIT is a simple technique and can have an "immediate effect" on the improvement of rolling acne scars. In accordance with the literature, a complete result after CIT may be observed after 8–12 months of treatment as the deposition of new collagen takes place slowly. Compared with other ablative methods, CIT has advantages. The most important one is that the epidermis remains intact because it is not damaged, eliminating most of the risks and negative side effects of chemical peeling, laser resurfacing or dermabrasion.

This treatment appears to be synergistic with other methods such as non-ablative lasers, blood transfer and vascular lasers. Goodman and Barron [49] suggest to always supplement the procedure of skin rolling with other procedures, both simultaneously (blood transfer, vascular laser and subcision for bigger scars) and sequentially starting 1 month after the procedure and continuing monthly for three treatments (non-ablative 1450-nm diode laser).

A recently introduced laser employing the concept of "fractionated photothermolysis" produces small, vertical zones of full-thickness thermal damage by a midinfrared laser [70,71]. This is a method of ablative resurfacing without a pronounced and long healing phase and conceptually it may be the laser equivalent of skin needling.

Non-ablative Lasers

Laser skin resurfacing has become a popular therapeutic modality for the correction of acne scars, but it is not always effective in all types of acne scars. Non-ablative dermal remodeling has gained acceptance in the treatment of atrophic scars and has a role especially in rolling and shallow boxcar scars. With respect to ice pick and deep boxcar scars, ablative lasers are the better treatment choice [72].

Although improvement is seen with non-ablative lasers, most investigators conclude that the results do not approach those of ablative lasers requiring subsequent re-epithelialization. For the patient, the trade-off is between reduced improvement and more recovery time, as a longer recovery time is necessary to ensure proper healing.

The major lasers used for this purpose are the mid-infrared lasers such as diode, short-pulsed, variable-pulsed, and dual-mode Er:YAG, Nd:YAG lasers, and fractionated photothermolysis [73,74].

As opposed to CO_2 laser resurfacing, these lasers minimize epidermal damage by cooling the epidermis while targeting water within the dermis to produce a diffuse dermal injury by heating above 501°C. As a result, re-epithelialization is avoided during the recovery period. In addition, new models in this area have further reduced epidermal injury by cooling the skin with a cryogen spray (CoolTouch, Laser Aesthetics) to maintain an epidermal temperature between 42 and 481°C [75,76].

Repeated treatments are required with a suitably higher benefit–risk ratio, but longevity of result is still largely unknown.

Much speculation surrounds the mechanisms by which non-ablative dermal remodeling occurs, despite its documented clinical and histologic efficacy in the treatment of rhytides [77]. The concept of a beneficial subclinical epidermal injury has been raised with non-ablative laser resurfacing [78]. Such superficial dermal blood vessel injury and cytokine release, with potentially enhanced dermal remodeling, could explain the results.

Subcision techniques or skin needling in conjunction with non-ablative lasers may be used in patients presenting milder to slightly more severe scarring.

Moderate Atrophy (Grade 3 Disease)

Clinical Aspects

This level of scarring is obvious at social distances of 50 cm or greater and is not covered easily by makeup or the normal shadow of shaved beard hair in men or body hair if extrafacial, but is still able to be flattened by manual stretching of the skin (Table 16.1; Figure 16.8).

It equates to the deep rolling and shallow boxcar atrophic-type scars.

Shallow (0.1–0.5 mm) boxcar atrophic-type scars are round-to-oval depressions with sharply demarcated vertical edges, similar to varicella scars. They are clinically wider at the surface than ice pick scars and do not taper to a point at the base.

Treatment of Patients with Few Scars

If there are few scars then their augmentation by temporary or longer-term autologous or external agents may be appropriate. Combinations of techniques such as subcision, blood transfer, non-ablative or vascular laser, and skin needling may be useful for more significant scarring.

Subcision

The technique of subcutaneous incision, or subcision, is used to free the tethering fibrous bands that cause deep rolling and shallow boxcar atrophic-type scars.

For this procedure, the entire area to be subcised is marked and subcutaneous anesthetic is administered. A hypodermic needle may be used (18–26 gauge, depending on scar size and depth) to cut the adherent bands beneath the skin. Excellent results can be achieved by using an 18-gauge, 11/2-inch NoKor Admix needle (Becton Dickinson and Co, Franklin Lakes, NJ, USA). The triangular tip (similar to a No. 11 blade) allows smooth and thorough separation of the fibrous cords. The actions consist in tunneling parallel to the skin surface using a gentle piston-like motion to advance the needle through the fibrous bands in order to release epidermis from upper dermis [26].

This process leads to a pooling of blood under the defect, keeping the scar base from immediately reattaching to the surface layers. Blood accumulates under the defect, and its subsequent organization

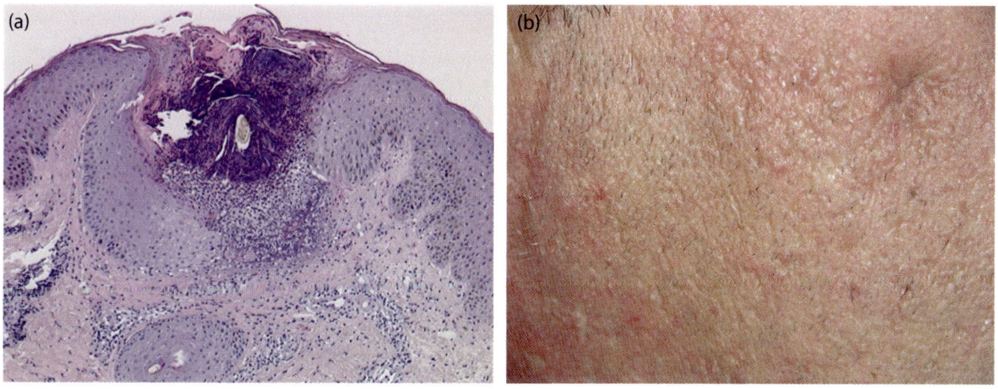

FIGURE 16.8 (a) II phase (48 hours). Ruptures through the weakened infrainfundibular section of the follicle cause perifollicular abscess (suppurative perifolliculitis). (b) Clinical aspect of atrophic scars.

is thought to result in connective tissue formation. Most atrophic acne scars improve well with one to three treatments. This technique may be readily combined with resurfacing and this leads to long-term correction of the defect.

The technique of undermining scars has been practiced as an adjunct to fibrin foam or collagen implantation, dermal grafting, and microlipoinjection [79].

Risks of subcision include bleeding (which is uncommon with proper anesthesia and pressure bandages) and excessive fibroplasia leading to nodule formation. This rare outcome can be improved with low-dose intralesional steroid injections, but often resolves without treatment in 2–3 months. Bruising from the procedure fades within 1–2 weeks.

As a simple technique that appears to produce long-term correction of contour defects, it deserves to be a first-line treatment for many isolated moderate atrophic scars [79].

Treatment of Patients with Many Scars

Technique-Sensitive Resurfacing (Lasers, Radiofrequency, Medium-Strength Peels, Plasma, and Abrasion)

The atrophic forms in this group are improved by ablative laser resurfacing if widespread atrophy is seen. CO_2 laser was the laser system first utilized for post-acne scarring, commonly replacing dermabrasion (drywall/plaster-sanding screen [80] or moistened silicon carbide sandpaper and strong chemical peeling). These newer adaptations of older techniques still suffer from a prolonged healing phase and morbidity. Although other lasers have been added to the armamentarium, it is uncertain whether they add much to the efficacy [80,81]. Modulating the erbium laser has meant that it behaves more like a CO_2 laser with arguably a better safety profile. Another popular method has been to combine erbium and CO_2 lasers either simultaneously or sequentially [81].

The statements made above regarding the excessive morbidity of resurfacing techniques, however, are almost as true for these newer lasers [82].

The greatest fear for those performing laser resurfacing is the incidence of hypopigmentation. The use of trypsin-digested donor epidermal cells after the resurfacing may allow a protection from this complication and a more rapid epithelialization. In an effort to increase penetration depth and strive toward collagen shrinkage and skin tightening, radiofrequency (RF) wavelengths have been extensively employed [105]. RF and fractionated microneedle RF devices produce electrical energy that heats the dermis without plume and at relatively low temperatures [83].

The first energy source in this arena was the monopolar RF device, ThermaCool (Thermage, Inc, Hayward, CA, USA), which demonstrated improvement in skin laxity and acne scars. The most recent development is the Accent device (Alma Lasers, Ltd, Caesarea, Israel), which offers alternatively bipolar and a novel unipolar RF modes [84]. The treatment of photoaging through non-ablative photorejuvenation encompasses the use of photodynamic therapy [85,86]. The application of topical photosensitizers, namely 5-5-aminolevulinic acid (ALA), for short incubation times combined with newer laser and light sources has been shown to be safe and effective. It may have a role in the collagen growth and thus in improvement of atrophic scars.

This may also benefit from the treatments described in the milder group, especially medical skin rolling combined simultaneously with subcision and later by non-ablative laser [87].

Severe Atrophy (Grade 4 Acne Scarring)

Clinical Aspects

This is represented by severe atrophic scarring that is obvious at social distances of 50 cm or greater and is not covered easily by makeup or the normal shadow of a shaved beard hair in men or body hair if extrafacial and is not able to be flattened by manual stretching of the skin (Table 16.1; Figures 16.9 and 16.10).

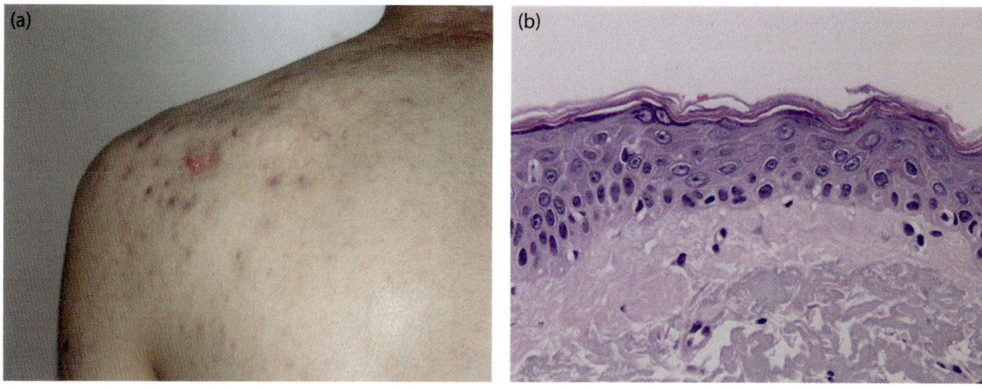

FIGURE 16.9 (a) Clinical and (b) histological features of hypertrophic scars.

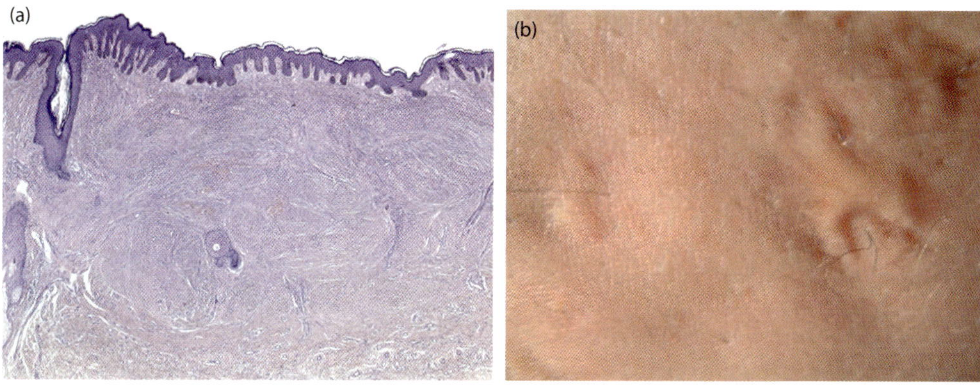

FIGURE 16.10 (a) Clinical and (b) histological features of keloid scars.

Ice Pick Scars

Deep ice pick scars are narrow (<2 mm) and fibrotic scars, with sharp shoulders perpendicular to the skin. They are epithelial invaginations that can reach the subcutaneous layer. The surface opening is usually, but not always, wider than the deeper infundibulum as the scar tapers from the surface to its deepest apex.

Punched-Out Atrophic

Punched-out atrophic or deep boxcar scars are depressions (=0.5 mm) with sharply demarcated, vertical edges (1.5–4.0 mm).

Tunnels are constituted of two or more ice picks connected by an epithelized tract. They have to be excised but can also be repaired by punch grafting [88].

Dystrophic Scars

These types of scars may have irregular or star-like shapes with a white and atrophic floor. They can also be represented by fibrotic masses with multichanneled tracts that retain sebaceous or pustular material.

Marked Atrophy

Marked atrophy is a deficit seen in patients with acne where disrupted acne follicles and cysts release inflammatory mediators that destroy facial fat. Cysts are also space-occupying lesions that leave a void after their resolution that the atrophied subcutaneous tissues cannot fill.

Aging exaggerates this lipoatrophy and the concavities of the preauricular, temples, inframalar, and perioral tissues become exaggerated and scarring in these regions appears worse.

Treatment

Larger punched-out scars (deep boxcar and larger ice pick scars) have to be excised by cylindrical punches [88], which have to be large enough to involve the entire lesion and by elevation or float techniques. They can be left to second intention healing or be replaced by full-thickness grafts from the postauricular area, which are 25%–50% larger than the defect (punch-graft technique). Direct closure of these small holes very frequently leads to enlarged and unpleasant scars, unless they are submitted to deep intradermal. The use of focal trichloroacetic acid at high concentrations (60%–100%, chemical reconstruction of skin scars technique) [89], especially in the treatment of smaller ice pick and poral-type scars, has always been difficult. This technique requires multiple sessions until the center of the scar is seen to flatten, basically scarring the inside of the cylindrical scar, making it cosmetically more appealing.

Dystrophic scars are treated by direct excision under primary elliptical or broken lines, and sometimes even "M," "Z" or "W" plasties are required for their treatment [90].

In the treatment of marked atrophy, fat is an excellent deeper augmentation material because it is cheap and readily available. This technique is also termed lipofilling, which does not result in rejection or allergic reactions. Fat is probably a permanent augmentation technique (more than 50% of transplanted fat survives), and correctly implanted, it produces accurate, longstanding and autologous correction [91]. It is useful to combine this augmentation with most other surface techniques such as resurfacing or subcision. Fat is injected through a small nick made with a vented needle (Nokor, Becton Dickinson), 11-gauge blade, or similar instrument. To achieve precision of correction, undermining or subcision [92] is used to release the scar tissue from its attachments to deeper tissues. The residual fat may always be frozen and may be used for at least 12 months after the procedure.

Most acne-scarred patients benefit from further top-up procedures 3 months after the procedure. Overcorrection should be kept to no more than 10%. Aging adds to the problems of the acne-scarred face and influences patients to seek corrective surgery. Polylactic acid and hyaluronic acid may be used to augment substantially depressed acne scarring if fat is not available.

Mild, Moderate, and Severe Hypertrophic Disease

Clinical Aspects

Much less commonly, although, acne scarring may become thickened (papular, bridges, hypertrophic or keloid scars) rather than becoming atrophic. Certain individual characteristics seem to predispose patients to this type of acne scarring.

Papular Scars

Papular scars may be small, soft, popular scars (grade 2 mild) or more significant papular scars (grade 3 moderate). Papules are soft elevations, like anetodermas, which are frequently observed on the trunk and chin area.

Treatment

They are largely untreatable at the present time, but if scars are facial, they can be treated by controlled CO_2 laser vaporization or light electrodesiccation of each papule [93].

Bridges

Bridge, another kind of elevated scar, is a fibrous string over healthy skin (grade 4 severe). This type of scar is common on the face.

Treatment

They are treated by tangential excision.

Hypertrophic and Keloid Scars

Hypertrophic scars are also thickened elevations, but remain within the confines of the original acne lesion with the scar progressing for a few months and then slowing before regressing after some years. Histologically, hypertrophic scars show numerous fibroblasts but relatively few collagen bundles, but with some myofibroblasts, and this may explain the scar contracture that is seen (grade 4 severe).

Keloid scars spread outside the confines of the original wound. They have differences in fibroblast size and activity, immune cell actions, and an imbalance between production and degradation of excess collagen. They are common in the mandibular arch, shoulders and sternal region and are prone to recur (grade 4 severe) [93].

Treatment

Topical Silicone-Gel Sheeting Topical silicone-gel sheeting alone or with intralesional steroids are the only evidence-based, recommendable forms of treatment to control the quality of a scar. The advantages and disadvantages of both are well known. Signorini and Clementoni [94] first verified the efficacy of a new topical self-drying spreadable silicone gel (Dermatix®, Valeant Pharmaceuticals, Milan, Italy) in a prospective trial involving a group of 160 patients. Considering the effective results obtained and the good patient compliance, the authors rated this concept of treatment as the first choice for preventing hypertrophy of recent scars (such as hypertrophic and keloidal post-acne scarring).

Intralesional Cytotoxic Therapy The use of corticosteroid injections to date is the core treatment available for the management of excessive tissue production in scars. Currently, the most effective and safe regimen for hypertrophic and keloidal acne management appears to be the use of corticotherapy injection of intradermal steroids (triamcinolone acetonide 10 or 40 mg/mL or betamethasone sodium phosphate and betamethasone acetate 5.7 mg/mL). Usually it is best to start with triamcinolone acetonide (10 mg/mL) or betamethasone sodium phosphate and betamethasone acetate (5.7 mg/mL), reserving triamcinolone acetonide (40 mg/mL) for resistant cases [95].

There has also been recent interest in the intralesional use of the cytotoxics fluorouracil and bleomycin sulfate, however, as treatments of these lesions. Fluorouracil is usually utilized at a concentration of 50 mg/mL and has been mixed 80:20 with low-strength intralesional steroid. It may be used alone, however. Usually approximately 1 mL is utilized in each session and often 0.1–0.3 mL is all that is required for an individual scar. Recently the molecular basis of the action of fluorouracil has been elucidated. Fluorouracil appears to be a potent inhibitor of transforming growth factor-β/SMAD protein signaling [96,97].

Vascular Lasers Alster and Williams first reported treatment of keloid sternotomy scars with 585 nm flash lamp-pumped pulsed-dye laser with improvement in scar height, skin texture, erythema and pruritus in the laser-treated scars [98].

Other Therapies Rusciani et al. treated 135 patients to assess the efficacy of cryotherapy in the treatment of keloids with good results. The main adverse effects reported were atrophic depressed scars and residual hypopigmentation but no recurrences arose during the follow-up period [99]. It is useful to combine cryotherapy with other modalities such as surgery or corticosteroids.

Other authors described surgical excision and immediate postoperative adjuvant use of ionizing radiation with X-rays or 1200 Gy in three or four fractions. However, recurrence rates were high and suggested use was as a last resort option [100,101]. Intralesional verapamil at a concentration of 2.5 mg/mL (0.5–2 mL injected volume depending on the size of the scar) or topical imiquimod have been suggested as post-operative adjunctive treatment to surgical excision of keloidal scars [102,103].

Outlook: Future Developments

In clinical practice, it is common to observe some patients with inflammatory acne suffer from significant scarring, while others with apparently similar severity are able to heal without scarring. It is known that there are both humoral and cellular-immune components that correlate with the severity of acne and that antigens of *Propionibacterium acnes* play a central role and the extent of this response has been found to differ among patients.

Holland et al. [104] examined this by assessing whether there were differences in the cell-mediated immune responses at different time points in inflamed lesion development between resolution in patients who were prone and those with the same degree of inflamed acne but who were not prone to develop scarring.

In lesions of non-scarring patients, the time course was typical of a type-IV, delayed-hypersensitivity response, a significant angiogenesis with preferential recruitment of macrophages and Langerhans cells with high cellular Human Leukocyte Antigen-DR isotype (HLA-DR) expression that indicates the clearance of causal antigen(s). In addition, these patients are not highly sensitized to the antigen(s) responsible for acne because they have CD4+ T cells, with an even smaller number being specifically skin homing. Thus, there is the effective removal of the causal antigen(s) and the satisfactory resolution of the inflammation.

In lesions from patients who scar, the scenario was different. In early lesions, they have a low cellular HLA-DR expression and an ineffectual early inflammatory response. In resolving lesions, the number of CD4+ T cells in the infiltrate and angiogenesis remained high and these would lead to abnormal healing and pathological scarring in these patients. Thus, based on the poorly resolving inflammation, scarring would be a more likely outcome, suggesting the requirement of anti-inflammatory medications.

In addition, prolonged angiogenesis may play an important role in the developing of post-acne atrophic scars. For blood vessels to cut a path and invade into the subcutaneous layer requires an increase in metalloproteinases (MMPs). The matrix MMPs are a family of zinc metallo endopeptidases (MMP 1F Type 1 collagenase, MMP 2F Type 4 collagenase and MMP 3F stromelysin-1) that can collectively cleave all components of the extracellular matrix and allow vascular proliferation [105]. Healing induces many changes to the collagen content of the wound; both the collagen type and positioning of the fibers are altered as the scar tissue develops. Tissue inhibitors of MMPs (TIMPs) control their activity because if MMPs are overactive or active for a longer time than required to support prolonged angiogenesis, the dissolution of dermal support or a breakdown of the normal balance of collagen production may occur.

So if we are to intervene with physical therapies, it may seem reasonable to target poorly resolving angiogenesis also, and keeping this in mind, vascular lasers and light sources could be examined for possible treatment options. Common agents such as retinoic acid, imiquimod, calcipotriol, corticosteroids, low-dose fluorouracil, diclofenac, tetracyclines, hyaluronic acid, estrogen, metabolites, genestein, heparin, cyclosporine A, steroids and COX2 inhibitors have all been suggested to be anti-angiogenesis substances. Many of these agents have both anti-inflammatory and anti-angiogenesis characteristics and may deserve investigation to help avert early acne scarring [106].

Summary for the Clinician

Acne often results in secondary damage in the form of scarring. Even with prevention and good efforts, scars may occur. The aim of this work is to give a broad overview of multiple management options, whether medically, surgically or procedurally based. It is also important to ensure that the patient is able to comply with therapy, and clear guidelines regarding treatment, possible adverse effects and realistic expectations are to be provided before commencing therapy.

REFERENCES

1. Kromayer E. Kosmetische resultate bei anwedung des stanverfahrens. *Dermatol Wochenschr.* 1935;101:1306.
2. Pereira Duquia R, da Silva Dos Santos I, de Almeida H Jr, Martins Souza PR, de Avelar Breunig J, Zouboulis CC. Epidemiology of acne vulgaris in 18-year-old male army conscripts in a South Brazilian City. *Dermatology.* 2017;233(2–3):145–54.
3. Chernyshov PV, Zouboulis CC, Tomas-Aragones L et al. Quality of life measurement in acne. Position Paper of the European Academy of Dermatology and Venereology Task Forces on Quality of Life and Patient Oriented Outcomes and Acne, Rosacea and Hidradenitis Suppurativa. *J Eur Acad Dermatol Venereol.* 2018;32(2):194–208.
4. França K, Keri J. Psychosocial impact of acne and postinflammatory hyperpigmentation. *An Bras Dermatol.* 2017;92(4):505–9.
5. Liu CW, Reed A, Sisic M, Tan J. Reconsidering accuracy of acne self-reports. *J Cutan Med Surg.* 2017;21(4):359.
6. Fulton JE. Dermabrasion, chemabrasion and laser abrasion. *Dermatol Surg.* 1996;22:619–28.
7. Lauermann FT, Almeida HL Jr, Duquia RP, Souza PR, Breunig Jde A. Acne scars in18-year-old male adolescents: A population-based study of prevalence and associated factors. *An Bras Dermatol.* 2016;91(3):291–5.
8. Skroza N, Tolino E, Proietti I et al. Women and acne: Any difference from males? A review of the literature. *G Ital Dermatol Venereol.* 2016;151(1):87–92.
9. Plewig G, Fulton JE, Kligman AM. Pomade acne. *Arch Derm.* 1970;101(5):580–4.
10. Institute of Medicine. *Unequal Treatment: Confronting Racial and Ethnic Disparities in Healthcare. Summary.* Washington, DC: National Academies of Sciences, 2003.
11. Grimes PR, Stockton T. Pigmentary disorders in blacks. *Dermatol Clin.* 1988;6:271–81.
12. Kelly AP. Keloids: Pathogenesis and treatment. *Cosmetic Derm.* 2003;16:29–32.
13. US Census Bureau. Population Projections Program, Washington D.C. Table NP-T5-B (middle series projections). January 13, 2000.
14. Tan J, Kang S, Leyden J. Prevalence and risk factors of acne scarring among patients consulting dermatologists in the Unites States. *J Drugs Dermatol.* 2017;16(2):97–102.
15. Kromayer E. Die Heilung der Akne durch ein neues narbenloses Operationverfahren. *Munchen Med Wochenschr.* 1905;52:943.
16. Kromayer E. Rotationsinstrurnente. Ein neues technisches. Veffahren in der dermatologischen Kieinchirurgie. *Dermatol Z.* 1995;12:26.
17. Kromayer E. Die Heilung der Akne durch ein neues narbenloses. Operationsverfahren: Das Stanzen. *Illustr Monatsschr Aerztl Polytech.* 1905;27:101.
18. Aronsson A, Erifsson T, Jacobsson S et al. Effects of dermabrasion on acne scarring: A review and a study of 25 cases. *Acta Derm Venereol.* 1997;77:39–42.
19. LeVan P. Mechanical method of freezing the skin for surgical planing. *Arch Dermatol Syph.* 1954;69:739–41.
20. Goodman GJ, Richards S. The treatment of facial wrinkles and scars. *Mod Med.* 1994;37:50–63.
21. Eller JJ, Wolff S. Skin peeling and scarification. *JAMA.* 1941;116:934–8.
22. Alster TS, West TB. Resurfacing of atrophic facial acne scars with a high-energy, pulsed carbon dioxide laser. *Dermatol Surg.* 1996;22:151–5.
23. Walia S, Alster TS. Prolonged clinical and histological effects from laser resurfacing of atrophic acne scars. *Dermatol Surg.* 1999;25:926–30.
24. Jeong TJ, Kye YC. Resurfacing of pitted facial acne scars with a long-pulsed Er:YAG laser. *Dermatol Surg.* 2001;27:107–10.
25. Cho SI, Kim YC. Treatment of atrophic facial scars with combined use of high-energy pulsed CO_2 laser and Er:YAG laser. *Dermatol Surg.* 1999,25.959–64.
26. Orentreich DS, Orentreich N. Subcutaneous incision less (subcision) surgery for the correction of depressed scars and wrinkles. *Dermatol Surg.* 1995;21:543–9.
27. Arouete J. Correction of depressed scars on the face by a method of elevation. *J Dermatol Surg Oncol.* 1976;2:337–9.
28. Klein AW. Implantation techniques for injectable collagen. *J Am Acad Dermatol.* 1983;9:224–8.

29. Selmanowitz VJ, Orentreich N. Medical grade fluid silicone: A monographic review. *J Dermatol Surg Oncol.* 1977;3:597–611.
30. Moritz DL. Surgical corrections of acne scars. *Dermatol Nurs.* 1992;4:291–9.
31. Fernandes D. Minimally invasive percutaneous collagen induction, oral and maxillofacial. *Surg Clin N Am.* 2005;17:51–63.
32. Fabbrocini G, Fardella N, Monfrecola A, Proietti I, Innocenzi D. Acne scarring treatment using skin needling. *Clin Exp Dermatol.* 2009;34(8):874–9.
33. Forbat E, Ali FR, Al-Niaimi F. The role of fillers in the management of acne scars. *Clin Exp Dermatol.* April 10, 2017. doi: 10.1111/ced.13058.
34. Jacob CI, Dover JS, Kaminer MS. Acne scarring: A classification system and review of treatment options. *J Am Acad Dermatol.* 2001;45(1):109–17.
35. Whang KK, Lee M. The principle of a three-staged operation in the surgery of acne-scars. *J Am Acad Dermatol.* 1999;40:95–7.
36. Cooper AJ, Harris VR. Modern management of acne. *Med J Aust.* 2017;206(1):41–5.
37. Stal S, Hamilton S, Spira M. Surgical treatment of acne scars. *Clin Plast Surg.* 1987;14:261–76.
38. Orentreich D, Orentreich N. Acne scar revision update. *Dermatol Clin.* 1987;5:359–68.
39. Alster TS, West TB. Treatment of scars: A review. *Ann Plast Surg.* 1997;39:418–32.
40. Solish N, Raman M, Pollack SV. Approaches to acne scarring: A review. *J Cutan Med Surg.* 1998;2:24–32.
41. Cohen BE, Brauer JA, Geronemus RG. Acne scarring: A review of available therapeutic lasers. *Lasers Surg Med.* 2016;48(2):95–115.
42. Kadunc BV, Trindade de Almeida AR. Surgical treatment of facial acne scars based on morphologic classification: A Brazilian experience. *Dermatol Surg.* 2003;29(12):1200–9.
43. Strauss JS. Sebaceous glands. In: *Dermatology in General Medicine.* 4th ed. Fitzpatrick TB, Eisen AZ, Wolff K, Freedburg IM, Austen KF, eds. New York: McGraw-Hill, 1993, 709–26.
44. Goodman GJ. Postacne scarring: A review of its pathophysiology and treatment. *Dermatol Surg.* 2000;26:857–71.
45. Webster GF, Leyden JJ, Nilsson UR. Complement activation in acne vulgaris: Consumption of complement by comedones. *Infect Immun.* 1979;26:183–6.
46. Tucker SB, Rogers RS, Winkelmann RK et al. Inflammation in acne vulgaris: Leukocyte attraction and cytotoxicity by comedonal material. *J Invest Dermatol.* 1980;74:21–5.
47. Tan J, Bourdès V, Bissonnette R, Petit B Eng L, Reynier P, Khammari A, Dreno B. Prospective study of pathogenesis of atrophic acne scars and role of macular erythema. *J Drugs Dermatol.* 2017;16(6):566–72.
48. Knutson D. Ultrastructural observations in acne vulgaris: The normal sebaceous follicle and acne lesions. *J Invest Dermatol.* 1974;62:288–307.
49. Goodman GJ, Baron JA. The management of post-acne scarring. *Dermatol Surg.* 2007;33:1175–88.
50. Lupton JR, Alster TS. Laser scar revision. *Dermatol Clin.* 2002;20:55–65.
51. Chen KH, Tam KW, Chen IF, Huang SK, Tzeng PC, Wang HJ, Chen CC. A systematic review of comparative studies of CO(2) and erbium:YAG lasers in resurfacing facial rhytides (wrinkles). *J Cosmet Laser Ther.* 2017;19(4):199–204.
52. Sebaratnam DF, Lim AC, Lowe PM, Goodman GJ, Bekhor P, Richards S. Lasers and laser-like devices: Part two. *Australas J Dermatol.* 2014;55(1):1–14.
53. Stratigos AJ, Katsambas AD. Optimal management of recalcitrant disorders of hyperpigmentation in dark-skinned patients. *Am J Clin Dermatol.* 2004;5:161–8.
54. Goldman MP. The use of hydroquinone with facial laser resurfacing. *J Cutan Laser Ther.* 2000;2:73–7.
55. Stoddard MA, Herrmann J, Moy L, Moy R. Improvement of atrophic acne scars in skin of color using topical synthetic epidermal growth factor (EGF) serum: A pilot study. *J Drugs Dermatol.* 2017;16(4):322–6.
56. Cuce LC, Bertino MC, Scattone L, Birkenhauer MC. Tretinoin peeling. *Dermatol Surg.* 2001;27:12–4.
57. Wang CM, Huang CL, Hu CT, Chan HL. The effect of glycolic acid on the treatment of acne in Asian skin. *Dermatol Surg.* 1997;23(1):23–9.
58. Stewart N, Lim AC, Lowe PM, Goodman G. Lasers and laser-like devices: Part one. *Australas J Dermatol.* 2013;54(3):173–83.
59. O'Connor AA, Lowe PM, Shumack S, Lim AC. Chemical peels: A review of current practice. *Australas J Dermatol.* October 24, 2017. doi: 10.1111/ajd.12715.
60. Callender VD. Considerations for treating acne in ethnic skin. *Cutis.* 2005;76(2 Suppl):19–23.

61. Bekhor PS. The role of pulsed laser in the management of cosmetically significant pigmented lesions. *Australas J Dermatol* 1995;36:221–3.
62. Chan H. The use of lasers and intense pulsed light sources for the treatment of acquired pigmentary lesions in Asians. *J Cosmet Laser Ther.* 2003;5:198–200.
63. Roxo RF, Sarmento DF, Kawalek AZ, Spencer JM. Successful treatment of a hypochromic scar with manual dermabrasion: Case report. *Dermatol Surg.* 2003;29:189–91.
64. Mulekar SV. Long-term follow-up study of segmental and focal vitiligo treated by autologous, noncultured melanocyte-keratinocyte cell transplantation. *Arch Dermatol.* 2004;140:1211–15.
65. Stoner ML, Wood FM. The treatment of hypopigmented lesions with cultured epithelial autograft. *J Burn Care Rehabil.* 2000;21:50–4.
66. Swinehart JM. Pocket grafting with dermal grafts: Autologous collagen implants for permanent correction of cutaneous depressions. *Am J Cosmet Surg.* 1995;12:321–31.
67. Goodman GJ. Blood Transfer: The use of autologous blood as a chromophore and tissue augmentation agent. *Dermatol Surg.* 2001;27:857–62.
68. El-Domyati M, Hosam W, Abdel-Azim E, Abdel-Wahab H, Mohamed E. Microdermabrasion: A clinical, histometric, and histopathologic study. *J Cosmet Dermatol.* 2016;15(4):503–13.
69. Bonati LM, Epstein GK, Strugar TL. Microneedling in all skin types: A review. *J Drugs Dermatol.* 2017;16(4):308–13.
70. Bernstein EF, Schomacker KT, Basilavecchio LD, Plugis JM, Bhawalkar JD. Treatment of acne scarring with a novel fractionated, dual-wavelength, picosecond-domain laser incorporating a novel holographic beam-splitter. *Lasers Surg Med.* 2017;49(9):796–802.
71. Manstein D, Herron GS, Sink RK et al. Fractional photothermolysis: A new concept for cutaneous remodeling using microscopic patterns of thermal injury. *Lasers Surg Med.* 2004;34:426–38.
72. Kim KH, Geronemus RG. Nonablative laser and light therapies for skin rejuvenation. *Arch Facial Plast Surg.* 2004;6:398–409.
73. Elcin G, Yalici-Armagan B. Fractional carbon dioxide laser for the treatment of facial atrophic acne scars: Prospective clinical trial with short and long-term evaluation. *Lasers Med Sci.* 2017;32(9):2047–54.
74. Crispin MK, Hruza GJ, Kilmer SL. Lasers and energy-based devices in men. *Dermatol Surg.* 2017;43 Suppl 2:S176–S184.
75. Chua SH, Ang P, Khoo LS, Goh CL. Nonablative 1450 nm diode laser in the treatment of facial atrophic acne scars in type IV to V Asian skin: A prospective clinical study. *Dermatol Surg.* 2004;30:1287–91.
76. Goldberg DJ. Nonablative dermal remodeling (does it really work?). *Arch Dermatol.* 2002;138:1366–7.
77. Trelles MA, Allones I, Luna R. Facial rejuvenation with a nonablative 1320 nm Nd:YAG laser: A preliminary clinical and histologic evaluation. *Dermatol Surg.* 2001;27:111–6.
78. Fatemi A, Weiss MA, Weiss RA. Short-term histologic effects of nonablative resurfacing: Results with a dynamically cooled millisecond-domain 1320 nm Nd:YAG laser. *Dermatol Surg.* 2002;28:172–6.
79. Tenna S, Cogliandro A, Barone M, Panasiti V, Tirindelli M, Nobile C, Persichetti P. Comparative study using autologous fat grafts plus platelet-rich plasma with or without fractional CO(2) laser resurfacing in treatment of acne scars: Analysis of outcomes and satisfaction with FACE-Q. *Aesthetic Plast Surg.* 2017;41(3):661–6.
80. Yu PX, Diao WQ, Qi ZL, Cai JL. Effect of Dermabrasion and ReCell(®) on large superficial facial scars caused by burn, trauma and acnes. *Chin Med Sci J.* 2016,31(3):173–9.
81. Chen KH, Tam KW, Chen IF, Huang SK, Tzeng PC, Wang HJ, Chen CC. A systematic review of comparative studies of CO(2) and erbium:YAG lasers in resurfacing facial rhytides (wrinkles). *J Cosmet Laser Ther.* 2017;19(4):199–204.
82. Juhász ML, Levin MK, Marmur ES. A review of available laser and intense light source home devices: A dermatologist's perspective. *J Cosmet Dermatol.* 2017;16(4):438–43.
83. Faghihi G, Poostiyan N, Asilian A, Abtahi-Naeini B, Shahbazi M, Iraji F, Fatemi Naeini F, Nilforoushzadeh MA. Efficacy of fractionated microneedle radiofrequency with and without adding subcision for the treatment of atrophic facial acne scars: A randomized split-face clinical study. *J Cosmet Dermatol.* 2017;16(2):223–9.
84. Sadick N, Alexiades-Armenakas M, Bitter P, Hruza G, Mulholland S. Enhanced full-face skin rejuvenation using synchronous intense pulsed optical and conducted, bipolar radiofrequency energy (ELOS): Introducing selective radiophotothermolysis. *J Drugs Dermatol.* 2005;4:181–6.

85. Barbaric J, Abbott R, Posadzki P, Car M, Gunn LH, Layton AM, Majeed A, Car J. Light therapies for acne: Abridged Cochrane systematic review including GRADE assessments. *Br J Dermatol.* 2018;178(1):61–75.
86. Stevenson ML, Karen JK, Hale EK. Laser-assisted photodynamic therapy: Two novel protocols for enhanced treatment results. *J Drugs Dermatol.* 2017;16(4):329–31.
87. Orentreich DS. Punch graft. In: *Principles and Techniques of Cutaneous Surgery.* Lask GP, Moy RL, eds. New York: McGraw-Hill, 1996, 283–95.
88. Johnson WC. Treatment of pitted scars: Punch transplant technique. *J Dermatol Surg Oncol.* 1986;12:260–5.
89. Lee JB, Chung WG, Kwahck H, Lee KH. Focal treatment of acne scars with trichloroacetic acid: Chemical reconstruction of skin scars method. *Dermatol Surg.* 2002;28:1017–21.
90. Kroepfl L, Emer JJ. Combination therapy for acne scarring: Personal experience and clinical suggestions. *J Drugs Dermatol.* 2016;15(11):1413–19.
91. Ellenbogen R. Invited comment on autologous fat injection. *Ann Plast Surg.* 1990;24:297.
92. Ersek RA. Transplantation of purified autologous fat: A 3-year follow up is disappointing. *Plast Reconstr Surg.* 1991;87:219–27.
93. Ogawa R. Keloid and hypertrophic scars are the result of chronic inflammation in the reticular dermis. *Int J Mol Sci.* 2017;18(3).
94. Signorini M, Clementoni MT. Clinical evaluation of a new self-drying silicone gel in the treatment of scars: A preliminary report. *Aesthetic Plast Surg.* 2007;31(2):183–7.
95. Roques C, Téot L. The use of corticosteroids to treat keloids: A review. *Int J Low Extrem Wounds.* 2008;7(3):137–45.
96. Uppal RS, Khan U, Kakar S et al. The effects of a single dose of 5-fluorouracil on keloid scars: A clinical trial of timed wound irrigation after extralesional excision. *Plast Reconstr Surg.* 2001;108:1218–24.
97. Wendling J, Marchand A, Mauviel A, Verrecchia F. 5-Fluorouracil blocks transforming growth factor-beta-induced alpha 2 type I collagen gene (COL1A2) expression in human fibroblasts viac-Jun NH2-terminal kinase/activator protein-1 activation. *Mol Pharmacol.* 2003;64:707–13.
98. Alster TS, Williams CM. Treatment of keloid sternotomy scars with 585 nm flashlamp-pumped pulsed-dye laser. *Lancet.* 1995;345:1198–2000.
99. Rusciani L, Paradisi A, Alfano C et al. Cryotherapy in the treatment of keloids. *J Drugs Dermatol.* 2006;5(7):591–5.
100. Annacontini L, Parisi D, Maiorella A et al. Long-term follow-up in the treatment of keloids by combined surgical excision and immediate postoperative adjuvant irradiation. *Plast Reconstr Surg.* 2008;121(2):700–1.
101. Arons JA. The results of surgical excision and adjuvant irradiation for therapy-resistant keloids: A prospective clinical outcome study. *Plast Reconstr Surg.* 2008;121(2):685–6.
102. Copcu E, Sivrioglu N, Oztan Y. Combination of surgery and intralesional verapamil injection in the treatment of the keloid. *J Burn Care Rehabil.* 2004;25:1–7.
103. Berman B, Villa A. Imiquimod 5% cream for keloid management. *Dermatol Surg.* 2003;29:1050–1.
104. Holland DB, Jeremy AH, Roberts SG et al. Inflammation in acne scarring: A comparison of the responses in lesions from patients prone and not prone to scar. *Br J Dermatol.* 2004;150:72–81.
105. Gillard JA, Reed MW, Buttle D et al. Matrix metalloproteinase activity and immunohistochemical profile of matrix metalloproteinase-2 and -9 and tissue inhibitor of metalloproteinase-1 during human dermal wound healing. *Wound Repair Regen.* 2004;12:295–304.
106. Ogawa R, Akaishi S. Endothelial dysfunction may play a key role in keloid and hypertrophic scar pathogenesis—Keloids and hypertrophic scars may be vascular disorders. *Med Hypotheses.* 2016;96:51–60.

Index